AF682599

Low-Molecular-Weight Heparins in Prophylaxis and Therapy of Thromboembolic Diseases

FUNDAMENTAL AND CLINICAL CARDIOLOGY

Editor-in-Chief

Samuel Z. Goldhaber, M.D.

Harvard Medical School
and Brigham and Women's Hospital
Boston, Massachusetts

Associate Editor, Europe

Henri Bounameaux, M.D.

University Hospital of Geneva
Geneva, Switzerland

1. *Drug Treatment of Hyperlipidemia*, edited by Basil M. Rifkind
2. *Cardiotonic Drugs: A Clinical Review. Second Edition, Revised and Expanded*, edited by Carl V. Leier
3. *Complications of Coronary Angioplasty*, edited by Alexander J. R. Black, H. Vernon Anderson, and Stephen G. Ellis
4. *Unstable Angina*, edited by John D. Rutherford
5. *Beta-Blockers and Cardiac Arrhythmias*, edited by Prakash C. Deedwania
6. *Exercise and the Heart in Health and Disease*, edited by Roy J. Shephard and Henry S. Miller, Jr.
7. *Cardiopulmonary Physiology in Critical Care*, edited by Steven M. Scharf
8. *Atherosclerotic Cardiovascular Disease, Hemostasis, and Endothelial Function*, edited by Robert Boyer Francis, Jr.
9. *Coronary Heart Disease Prevention*, edited by Frank G. Yanowitz
10. *Thrombolysis and Adjunctive Therapy for Acute Myocardial Infarction*, edited by Eric R. Bates
11. *Stunned Myocardium: Properties, Mechanisms, and Clinical Manifestations*, edited by Robert A. Kloner and Karin Przyklenk
12. *Prevention of Venous Thromboembolism*, edited by Samuel Z. Goldhaber
13. *Silent Myocardial Ischemia and Infarction: Third Edition*, Peter F. Cohn
14. *Congestive Cardiac Failure: Pathophysiology and Treatment*, edited by David B. Barnett, Hubert Pouleur, and Gary S. Francis
15. *Heart Failure: Basic Science and Clinical Aspects*, edited by Judith K. Gwathmey, G. Maurice Briggs, and Paul D. Allen

16. *Coronary Thrombolysis in Perspective: Principles Underlying Conjunctive and Adjunctive Therapy*, edited by Burton E. Sobel and Désiré Collen
17. *Cardiovascular Disease in the Elderly Patient*, edited by Donald D. Tresch and Wilbert S. Aronow
18. *Systemic Cardiac Embolism*, edited by Michael D. Ezekowitz
19. *Low-Molecular-Weight Heparins in Prophylaxis and Therapy of Thromboembolic Diseases*, edited by Henri Bounameaux

Additional Volumes in Preparation

Valvular Heart Disease, edited by Muayed Al Zaibag and Carlos G. Duran

Automatic Implantable Cardioverter-Defibrillators: A Comprehensive Text, edited by Paul J. Wang, N. A. Mark Estes III, and Antonis Manolis

Low-Molecular-Weight Heparins in Prophylaxis and Therapy of Thromboembolic Diseases

edited by
Henri Bounameaux
Geneva University School of Medicine
University Hospital of Geneva
Geneva, Switzerland

Marcel Dekker, Inc. New York • Basel • Hong Kong

Library of Congress Cataloging-in-Publication Data

Low-molecular-weight heparins in prophylaxis and therapy of thromboembolic diseases / edited by Henri Bounameaux.
p. cm. — (Fundamental and clinical cardiology ; 19)
Includes bibliographical references and index.
ISBN 0-8247-9174-6 (alk. paper)
1. Heparin—Therapeutic use. 2. Thromboembolism—Chemotherapy. I. Bounameaux, H. II. Series: Fundamental and clinical cardiology ; v. 19.
[DNLM: 1. Heparin—pharmacology. 2. Heparin—therapeutic use. 3. Thromboembolism—therapy. W1 FU538TD v. 19 1994 / QV 193 L9122 1994]
RC694.3.L68 1994
616.1'45061—dc20
DNLM/DLC
for Library of Congress 93-38785
CIP

The publisher offers discounts on this book when ordered in bulk quantities. For more information, write to Special Sales/Professional Marketing at the address below.

This book is printed on acid-free paper.

Copyright © 1994 by MARCEL DEKKER, INC. All Rights Reserved.

Neither this book nor any part may be reproduced or transmitted in any form or by any means, electronic or mechanical, including photocopying, microfilming, and recording, or by any information storage and retrieval system, without permission in writing from the publisher.

MARCEL DEKKER, INC.
270 Madison Avenue, New York, New York 10016

Current printing (last digit):
10 9 8 7 6 5 4 3 2 1

PRINTED IN THE UNITED STATES OF AMERICA

To those remarkable persons
who initiated and sustained my passion for
medicine, blood vessels and thrombosis,
and clinical research,

my father, the late Yves Bounameaux,
Alex-F. Müller, François Duckert, and Marc Verstraete.

To Anne, Claire, and Dominique

Series Introduction

Marcel Dekker, Inc., has focused on the development of various series of beautifully produced books in different branches of medicine. These series have facilitated the integration of rapidly advancing information for both the clinical specialist and the researcher.

My goal as editor-in-chief of the Fundamental and Clinical Cardiology series is to assemble the talents of world-renowned authorities to discuss virtually every area of cardiovascular medicine. In the current monograph, my associate editor, Dr. Henri Bounameaux, has edited a much-needed and timely book. Future contributions to this series will include books on molecular biology, interventional cardiology, and clinical management of such problems as coronary artery disease and ventricular arrhythmias.

Samuel Z. Goldhaber

Foreword

It is becoming recognized that there is far more at stake in the endeavor to understand the mechanism of blood coagulation than the mere satisfaction of academic curiosity or the settling of differences of opinion. Thrombosis and embolism have become one of the main causes of death in developed countries, and their causation and treatment cannot be determined without reference to the coagulation process and its interconnection with the vascular wall and dynamics of the circulation. The time has come that an academic exercise has full bearing on the practice of medicine. Although novel therapeutic agents are sometimes discovered by chance, as was the case for heparin, their refinement and clinical application are possible only on the background of clinical science.

The aim of a book is to inform the reader and to present in a well-structured fashion the prevailing opinion on issues centered around a central theme. Thus in a book on heparin the reader expects to find solid information and the experts' opinion in areas of doubt. I myself have a series of propositions and questions that are challenged and addressed in this book. I am therefore unbiased, but not completely free of prejudice, in listing in a candid manner my own spectrum of uncertainties.

1. Clinical-grade, unfractionated heparin is a mixture of over a hundred closely related substances, differing in molecular weight, chain length, uronic acid, amino sugar, electrostatic charge, and negative charge distribution along the chain. Fractionation or fragmentation of the present molecule by any procedure, e.g., on the basis of molecular weight, will give heparins differing in any other parameters (sugars, negative charge, density, affinities). Although the molecular-weight distributions of different brands of low-molecular-weight heparins are rather close, each of them should be tested for efficacy and safety in patients and used at an individual dose regimen.

2. In unfractionated heparin those molecules with low affinity for antithrombin III have only a limited anticoagulant effect but can still potentiate the antithrombotic activity of high-affinity, low-molecular-weight heparin fractions, inhibit hyperplasia of vascular smooth muscle, activate lipoprotein lipase, suppress aldosterone secretion, and induce platelet aggregation.

3. The interindividual variability of anticoagulant response of unfractionated heparin is related to its binding to platelet factor 4 and a variety of plasma proteins (among others, histidine-rich glycoprotein, vitronectin, fibronectin, von Willebrand factors) whose concentration may vary considerably in normal persons and even more in a patient population. However, there is still a considerable interindividual variation of the anticoagulant effect of a given low-molecular-weight heparin, although binding to platelet factor 4 and the above-mentioned plasma factors is remarkably and uniformly less than for unfractionated heparin.

4. At high doses of unfractionated heparin-binding sites on plasma proteins, endothelial cells and macrophages are saturated and the bioavailability becomes essentially the same as for low-molecular-weight heparin. Why in this setting is the half-life of low-molecular-weight heparins two- to fourfold longer than that of unfractionated heparin?

5. The commercially developed low-molecular-weight heparins have anti-factor Xa to anti-II ratios varying between 4 : 1 and 2 : 1 based on in vitro assays in platelet-poor plasma. The high specific activity of fragments is due to the large number of molecules per milligram as the molecular weight decreases. The relationship between these two anticoagulant activities and their relative contribution to the antithrombotic effect is still a matter of debate. There are arguments that a delayed and/or decreased thrombin generation is primarily a function of the thrombin inhibitory capacity of low-molecular-weight heparins, affecting the thrombin feedback loops and decay of formed thrombin. If the antithrombotic activity of low-molecular-weight heparins were due only or mainly to the inhibition of thrombin, why is there no correlation between the antithrombotic effect and ex vivo measurement of anti-IIa? Does one have to (re)consider the impact of anti-Xa activity on the prevention of thrombin generation? If so, this effect becomes more important than anticipated, because after subcutaneous injection, the absorption process favors the passage of the lowest-molecular-weight molecules. Moreover, owing to the preferential binding of platelet factor 4, more high-molecular-weight molecules will be neutralized. Both phenomena shift the balance toward a higher concentration of anti-factor X molecules in circulating blood.

6. It has been shown that heparin injection is associated with a release of the extrinsic pathway inhibitor. The antithrombotic role played by this inhibitor of the activated factor VIIa–tissue factor complex, which also has anti-Xa properites, is still to be defined.

7. In some studies on the prevention of postoperative deep venous throm-

bosis, the low-molecular-weight heparin used was more effective than low-dose unfractionated heparin, both being administered subcutaneously. With other brands of low-molecular-weight heparin no difference in antithrombotic effectiveness was found in a similar comparison. Whether one brand of low-molecular-weight heparin is superior in terms of antithrombotic efficacy to another low-molecular-weight heparin is still to be tested in a direct comparative trial. A similar and also unanswered—but most difficult to answer—question is whether two different brands of low-molecular-weight heparins with the same antithrombotic efficacy differ in their minor or (and) major bleeding complications when used in postoperative patients.

8. It was shown in one trial in patients with deep venous thrombosis that fixed doses of low-molecular-weight heparin, or doses adjusted to obtain ex vivo anti-Xa activities in the range of 0.5–1.0 IU/ml, result in equivalent antithrombotic effect and similar bleeding incidence. This important conclusion should be confirmed in other trials.

9. In some experimental animal models, low-molecular-weight heparins were shown to induce less bleeding for an equivalent antithrombotic effect than unfractionated heparin. Except for one of six major trials in orthopedic surgery and one of eight large trials in general surgery, no difference in major or minor bleeding incidence was noted between patients randomized to low-molecular-weight heparin, used at the presently recommended dose regimen, and those receiving subcutaneously unfractionated heparin. Also, one of six published trials on the treatment of established deep venous thrombosis with low-molecular-weight heparin administered subcutaneously (weight adjusted but not monitored) versus intravenous unfractionated heparin (monitored and adjusted) showed a significantly reduced bleeding incidence in the low-molecular-weight group.

10. One of the principles of meta-analysis is that the trials considered for inclusion have to comply with rigid selection criteria and, of course, must all be conducted with the same drug. As low-molecular-weight heparins are distinct compounds differing among each other in their molecular weight distribution, specific activities (anti-Xa to anti-IIa ratio), and plasma clearance, a meta-analysis of clinical results conducted with different low-molecular-weight heparins might not be appropriate.

11. One should realize that although the activated partial thromboplastin time and prothrombin time are used to monitor heparin and anticoagulant treatment for excessive anticoagulation and possible bleeding, they are not suited to measure the antithrombotic potential.

12. The question whether unfractionated heparin and low-molecular-weight heparin are as safe when administered before or after spinal anesthesia is unsettled. The same holds for the pre- or postoperative administration of these drugs in patients with major trauma.

13. The research group at the University of Saskatchewan has shown that

unfractionated heparin and hydrogenated or nonhydrogenated dextran sulfate (mean molecular weight 8000) are recovered from the endothelium less than 10 min after intragastric administration in rats. A substantial proportion is retained in the large endothelial surface of the splanchnic area, but enough reaches the vascular endothelium to prevent formation of experimental venous thrombi. Similar experiments were apparently not reported with low-molecular-weight heparins.

14. Unfractionated heparin binds to endothelium and leads by inhalation to measurable amounts of heparin in the plasma. Similar experiments with low-molecular-weight heparins were not reported, possibly because of their decreased affinity to endothelium or simply because nobody has tried.

15. Low-molecular-weight heparins interact less with platelets than does unfractionated heparin. It is logical that larger heparins would have greater affinity than smaller ones of equivalent sulfation, as the larger species would represent more negatively charged areas for binding to positively charged regions of the platelet surface; a secondary factor may be the balance of sugar moieties. Although the expectation is that low-molecular-weight heparins induce less thrombocytopenia than unfractionated heparin, such cases have already been described for all brands of low-molecular-weight heparins.

16. Unfractionated heparin does not cross the human placenta, but low-molecular-weight heparin appears to release dermatan sulfate–like molecules in the fetal circulation of sheep. It is unknown whether the same phenomenon occurs in humans.

17. Whether the long-term use of low-molecular-weight heparin would induce osteoporosis, particularly in elderly patients, in a similar manner as unfractionated heparin, is unknown. Both drugs inhibit type 1 collagen and DNA synthesis in fetal rat calvaria.

18. Protamine sulfate used at an equimolar concentration neutralizes the effects on hemostasis of unfractionated heparin but neutralizes only the anti-factor IIa activity of low-molecular-weight heparins. The search continues for a more effective antidote that would bind to the very-low-molecular-weight fragments of heparin.

In wishing the book all success it deserves, I ask consideration for a foreword which does not follow a classical path and for which I have no apologies.

Marc Verstraete, M.D.
Professor of Medicine
Center for Molecular and Vascular Biology
Catholic University of Leuven
Leuven, Belgium

Sometimes in science we read of an apparently simple experiment that results in an observation so fundamental in its implications that we can never again think about an entire field of inquiry the way we thought about it before. An example of such an exciting turn of events occurred in 1976, when three laboratories (those of Lam and Rosenberg, Höök, and Andersson) independently but almost simultaneously announced their discovery that the familiar anticoagulant drug heparin was not the homogeneous solution of identical molecules it was previously assumed to be, but instead was a heterogeneous mixture of linear polysaccharide chains that varied in molecular weight and in biological activity so that over 80% of its anticoagulant effect could be account for by the activity of only 30% of its molecules. The remainder were found to be essentially inert as cofactors for antithrombin III, the chief inhibitor of thrombin-induced conversion of fibrinogen to fibrin, which at that time was regarded as the predominant action of heparin in blood.

The subsequent elucidation of heparin's structure and the identification of the pentasaccharide that was its minimal active fragment, the recognition that heparin-like glycosaminoglycans were incorporated in the endothelial surface of blood vessels and the revelation of their role in maintenance of the normal fluidity of the blood, the demonstration of the nonhematological actions of heparin and the appreciation of its function as a regulator of cell growth and differentiation, the description of heparin-platelet interaction and the awareness of heparin-induced thrombocytopenia as a clinical entity, and, most important in terms of its immediate relevance to this volume, the story of low-molecular-weight heparin (LMWH)—can be traced back to the discovery, either by design or by serendipity, of the heterogeneity of heparin.

Among the therapeutic advances that contributed to the current excitement over the new look in heparin, the so-called LMWHs lead the way. Usually between 5000 and 8000 Da, these are either natural constituents of pharmaceutical-grade heparin or products of its chemical or enzymatic hydrolysis. Generally the latter are preferred, as the fraction of natural heparin whose M_r is under 8000 comprises only a few percent of the total, making it a less economical source material than are the large heparin species that can be converted to small molecules by chemical hydrolysis.

The pharmacology of the low-molecular-weight preparations has been extensively studied. They are readily absorbed from extravascular sites and survive in the circulation longer than conventional heparin, so long in fact that they need only be administered subcutaneously once daily and can conveniently be prescribed for outpatients. They are largely free of side reactions with platelets and have even been given to patients with heparin-induced thrombocytopenia with satisfactory maintenance of anticoagulation, return of the platelet count to normal, and restoration of hemostasis.

Quick off the mark, clinical investigators have applied themselves to evaluation of the efficacy and safety of LMWHs, following encouraging preliminary assessments in animals that suggested an unprecedented degree of freedom from hemorrhagic side effects compared with their antithrombotic effectiveness. Time will tell whether these early impressions will be confirmed by more extensive trials.

This timely volume faces these issues squarely. Only a few minutes spent thumbing through it are needed to satisfy one that here is a comprehensive overlook at what is known and what is not known about LMWHs. The careful reader is rewarded by a critical but balanced treatment of the details. This is the work of experts.

Mostly European or Canadian in origin, this book is a reminder that the United States lags behind in availability of the LMWHs. At the time of this writing, no LMWH preparation has yet been licensed here. We look foward to an early correction of this therapeutic deficiency and to any expansion of our understanding of other innovative applications of the discovery of the heterogeneity of heparin.

Edwin W. Salzman, M.D.
Professor of Surgery
Beth Israel Hospital
Boston, Massachusetts

Preface

In the 1980s, a new class of antithrombotics was developed in Europe, the low-molecular-weight heparin (LMWH) fractions. These compounds offer certain advantages in comparison with unfractionated heparin (UFH). Their longer half-life permits once-daily subcutaneous injections under certain circumstances instead of two or three injections per day. Moreover, the increased bioavailability of LMWHs might also simplify further heparin dosing adjustments in the treatment of established venous thromboembolism by allowing weight-adjusted dosing rather than dosing based on expensive and cumbersome in vitro clotting tests, such as the activated partial thromboplastin time (APTT) or the thrombin clotting time. In 1993, enoxaparin was the first LMWH to receive approval by the Food and Drug Administration (for the sole indication of prophylaxis in elective hip replacement).

This timely book on LMWHs provides fundamental basic science as well as clinical information about this new class of antithrombotic agents which is progressively replacing the "old" heparin. Researchers in the fields of thrombosis and antithrombotics should find this book most useful. Insights are also given into the interactions of LMWHs with the endothelium, platelets, the fibrinolytic system, and even the proliferation of smooth muscle cells. The clinician (surgeon, internist, gynecologist, cardiologist, vascular medicine specialist, or hematologist) confronted with prevention or treatment of deep venous thrombosis and pulmonary embolism should also find this book to be informative. Last but not least, it is also our hope that this book will contribute to the widespread spirit of prevention in medicine today.

We appreciate the enthusiasm and efficiency of all the contributors. Graham Garratt, Executive Vice President, and Henry Boehm, Production Supervisor, at Marcel Dekker, Inc., were most helpful and supportive.

Henri Bounameaux

Contents

Series Introduction v
Foreword Marc Verstraete vii
Edwin W. Salzman
Preface xiii
Contributors xvii

1. Pharmacology of Unfractionated and Low-Molecular-Weight Heparins 1
Frederick A. Ofosu

2. Mode of Action of Low-Molecular-Weight Heparins in Plasma and Its Consequences for the Clinical Laboratory 21
H. Coenraad Hemker and Suzette Béguin

3. Laboratory Control of Low-Molecular-Weight Heparins: Needs and Possibilities 43
Martine Alhenc-Gelas and Martine Aiach

4. Deep Venous Thrombosis: An Overview of Diagnosis, Treatment, and Prevention 55
Samuel Z. Goldhaber

5. Interaction of Heparins with Platelets, Including Heparin-Induced Thrombocytopenia 75
Theodore Earl Warkentin and John G. Kelton

6. Interactions Between Glycosaminoglycans and Endothelial Cells 129
Gérard Tobelem

7. Interactions Between Heparin and Fibrinolysis 143
Henri Roger Lijnen and Désiré Collen

8. Low-Molecular-Weight Heparins for Prevention of Venous Thromboembolism Following General Surgery 169
David Bergqvist

9. Low-Molecular-Weight Heparins for Prevention of Venous Thromboembolism Following Orthopedic Surgery 187
Fedor Bachmann and Pierre-François Leyvraz

10. Low-Molecular-Weight Heparins and Heparinoids for Prevention of Venous Thromboembolism in Stroke and Neurosurgical Patients 213
Alexander G. G. Turpie

11. Low-Molecular-Weight Heparins for Prevention of Venous Thromboembolism in Medical Patients 225
Meyer M. Samama and Gregory T. Gerotziafas

12. Low-Molecular-Weight Heparins for Prevention of Venous Thromboembolism Following Lumbar Regional Anesthesia 241
Thomas Mätzsch and David Bergqvist

13. Low-Molecular-Weight Heparins in Extracorporeal Circuits 247
M. T. Nurmohamed, H. R. Büller, and J. W. ten Cate

14. Low-Molecular-Weight Heparins for Prevention of Restenosis Following Coronary Angioplasty 273
F. W. Amann, B. J. Meyer, C. Neuenschwander, and H. Drexel

15. Low-Molecular-Weight Heparins for Treatment of Established Venous Thromboembolism 283
Dieter Lockner

16. Conclusion: Current Controversies About Low-Molecular-Weight Heparins in Prevention and Therapy of Venous Thromboembolism 307
Henri Bounameaux

Index *319*

Contributors

Martine Aiach, Ph.D. Laboratoire d'Hémostase, Hôpital Broussais, Paris, France

Martine Alhenc-Gelas, Ph.D. Laboratoire d'Hémostase, Hôpital Broussais, Paris, France

F. W. Amann, M.D. Associate Professor, Leitender Arzt, Kardiologie DIM, University Hospital, Zurich, Switzerland

Fedor Bachmann, M.D., F.A.C.P. Professor Emeritus, University of Lausanne Medical School, Lausanne, Switzerland

Suzette Béguin, Ph.D. Department of Biochemistry, Cardiovascular Research Institute and University of Limburg, Maastricht, The Netherlands

David Bergqvist, M.D., Ph.D. Professor of Vascular Surgery, Department of Surgery, University Hospital, Uppsala, Sweden

Henri Bounameaux, M.D. Chief, Division of Angiology and Hemostasis, Department of Medicine, Geneva University School of Medicine and University Hospital of Geneva, Geneva, Switzerland

H. R. Büller Centre for Haemostasis, Thrombosis, Atherosclerosis and Inflammation Research, Academic Medical Centre, Amsterdam, The Netherlands

Désiré Collen, M.D., Ph.D. Professor of Medicine, Department of Pathophysiology, Center for Molecular and Vascular Biology, University of Leuven, Leuven, Belgium

H. Drexel, M.D. Associate Professor, Department of Medicine, University Hospital, Zurich, Switzerland

Gregory T. Gerotziafas, M.D. Resident, Central Laboratory of Hematology, Hôtel Dieu Hospital, Paris, France

Samuel Z. Goldhaber, M.D. Associate Professor, Department of Medicine, Harvard Medical School, and Staff Cardiologist, Brigham and Women's Hospital, Boston, Massachusetts

H. Coenraad Hemker, M.D., Ph.D. Department of Biochemistry, Cardiovascular Research Institute and University of Limburg, Maastricht, The Netherlands

John G. Kelton, M.D. Professor, Departments of Medicine and Pathology, McMaster University, Hamilton, Ontario, Canada

Pierre-François Leyvraz, M.D. Privatdocent, Service Universitaire d'Orthopédie, Hôpital Orthopédique de la Suisse Romande, Lausanne, Switzerland

Henri Roger Lijnen, Ph.D. Associate Professor, Department of Pathophysiology, Center for Molecular and Vascular Biology, University of Leuven, Leuven, Belgium

Dieter Lockner, M.D., Ph.D. Associate Professor, Thrombosis Unit, Department of Medicine, University Hospital, Huddinge, Sweden

Thomas Mätzsch, M.D., Ph.D. Assistant Professor, Department of Surgery, Lund University and Malmö General Hospital, Malmö, Sweden

B. J. Meyer, M.D. University Hospital, Zurich, Switzerland

C. Neuenschwander, M. D. University Hospital, Zurich, Switzerland

M. T. Nurmohamed, M.D. Centre for Haemostasis, Thrombosis, Atherosclerosis and Inflammation Research, Academic Medical Centre, Amsterdam, The Netherlands

Frederick A. Ofosu, Ph.D. Professor, Department of Pathology, McMaster University, and Canadian Red Cross Society, Hamilton, Ontario, Canada

Meyer M. Samama, M.D. Professor, Department of Hematology, and Director, Central Laboratory of Hematology, Hôtel Dieu Hospital, Paris, France

J. W. ten Cate Centre for Haemostasis, Thrombosis, Atherosclerosis and Inflammation Research, Academic Medical Centre, Amsterdam, The Netherlands

Gérard Tobelem, M.D., Ph.D. Professor, Department of Hematology, INSERM 348, Hôpital Lariboisière, Paris, France

Alexander G. G. Turpie, M.D., F.R.C.P. (Lond. Glasg.), F.A.C.P., F.A.C.C., F.R.C.P.C. Professor, Department of Medicine, McMaster University and Hamilton General Hospital, Hamilton, Onario, Canada

Theodore Earl Warkentin, M.D. Assistant Professor, Departments of Pathology and Medicine, McMaster University and Hamilton Civic Hospitals, Hamilton, Ontario, Canada

1

Pharmacology of Unfractionated and Low-Molecular-Weight Heparins

Frederick A. Ofosu
McMaster University and Canadian Red Cross Society, Hamilton, Ontario, Canada

I. INTRODUCTION

The pharmacology of drugs deals with their chemistry, uses, and effects on living organisms. This chapter will discuss in brief the clinical uses of unfractionated heparins (UFH) and low-molecular-weight heparins (LMWH), focusing on their inhibitory effects and catalytic actions on prothrombin activation and thrombin inhibition, respectively. While it probably has other effects in vivo, UFH is used in clinical situations requiring increased inhibition of blood coagulation. UFH is used: to prevent the development of deep vein thrombosis (DVT) (1–10); to initiate the treatment of DVT (11–14); to permit cardiopulmonary bypass surgery (15, 16); during percutaneous transluminal coronary angioplasty (PTCA) (17); and in hemodialysis (18). The above uses constitute the major antithrombotic (in vivo) uses of UFH. The laboratory use of heparin as an anticoagulant constitutes its major in vitro use. LMWH are also used to prevent thrombosis (1, 5, 6, 8–10), to inhibit thrombus growth and prevent its recurrence (19–21), and in hemodialysis (22, 23) but thus far not during cardiopulmonary bypass surgery or PTCA, or as in vitro anticoagulants.

UFH and LMWH probably achieve their antithrombotic actions by catalyzing antithrombin III–mediated inhibition of several serine proteases of blood coagulation. As should become evident during this review and elsewhere in this volume, the common link between the in vivo antithrombotic and in vitro anticoagulant effects of UFH and LMWH is their ability to inhibit prothrombin activation. Whether UFH and LMWH heparins influence the same coagulation reactions in vivo and in vitro to suppress prothrombin activation remains to be established. The net effects of UFH and LMWH on in vivo coagulation, when given to prevent thrombosis or to initiate the treatment of existing DVT, will be first reviewed. This will be followed by a discussion on how UFH and LMWH influence in vitro coagulation. The next section will briefly discuss the survival of the drugs in the intravascular space after they are given parenterally. The final section will speculate on the additional knowledge that might be necessary to establish how UFH and LMWH achieve their prophylactic and therapeutic antithrombotic actions in humans.

II. EFFECTS OF UFH AND LMWH ON IN VIVO COAGULATION

Since the primary goal of antithrombotic prophylaxis and therapy is to moderate in vivo coagulation to the levels normally required for hemostasis, it is not surprising that plasmas of patients at high risk for developing DVT, and of patients with thrombosis, have higher concentrations of the markers thought to reflect in vivo coagulation than are normally found in the plasmas of healthy volunteers (24–30). During coagulation, the enzyme complex prothrombinase, consisting of factor Xa (enzyme), its cofactor factor Va, and ionic calcium bound to an appropriate coagulant surface, converts prothrombin into equimolar concentrations of prothrombin fragment 1 + 2 and thrombin (31, 32). The concentration of prothrombin fragment 1 + 2 endogenous to carefully prepared plasma, therefore, represents one index of in vivo coagulation (Fig. 1). Two routinely available markers of in vivo coagulation indirectly estimate the concentrations of thrombin produced in vivo. The first measures the concentrations of fibrinopeptide A, a product released when thrombin interacts with fibrinogen, one of its major plasma substrates. The second marker thought to reflect thrombin generation is thrombin-antithrombin III, the inactivate product formed when thrombin reacts with antithrombin III, one of its major inhibitors in plasma. In addition to converting fibrinogen into fibrin and fibrinopeptides A and B by limited proteolysis (33), thrombin accelerates fibrin stabilization by activating factor XIII in a reaction accelerated by fibrin (34). Thrombin also accelerates its own generation by activating platelets, factor V, factor VIII, and factor XI during coagulation (35–38). Factor Va is the cofactor in prothrombinase, and factor VIIIa is the cofactor for factor X activation by the enzyme factor IXa (31, 32). Therefore, the availability of factor Va and factor VIIIa accelerates the generation of prothrombinase. For these reasons, effective inhibition of thrombin in vivo is crucial if the direct actions of thrombin on fibrinogen and platelets (which directly facilitate thrombus formation and growth) are to be minimized. Effective in vivo inhibition of thrombin also has the potential to suppress further prothrombin activation since this would decrease the availability of factor Va, factor VIIIa, and coagulantly active platelets. A key action of UFH and LMWH is to catalyze the inhibition of thrombin by antithrombin III (39–42 and Fig. 2), thereby

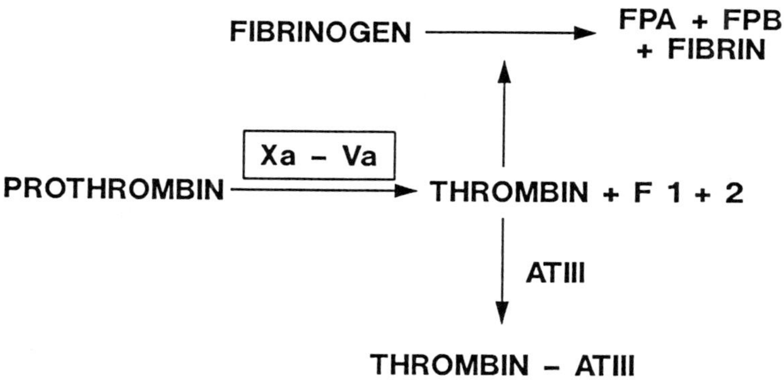

Figure 1 Markers of *in vivo* coagulation. The concentration of prothrombin fragment 1 + 2 (F1 + 2) in carefully collected plasma directly reflects that of prothrombin activated *in vivo* since equimolar concentrations of thrombin and F1 + 2 are generated when prothrombinase, Xa-Va, activates prothrombin. The concentration of thrombin–antithrombin III (thrombin-ATIII) is another marker of *in vivo* coagulation since this parameter estimates the concentration of the endogenously generated thrombin inactivated by its major plasma serpin. The concentration of fibrinopeptide A (FPA) estimates the degree to which the thrombin generated *in vivo* had interacted with fibrinogen, one of its major plasma substrates.

limiting the participation of thrombin in its usual coagulant and procoagulant functions.

A. Prophylactic Use of UFH and LMWH

Available information on the actions of UFH and LMWH on in vivo coagulation, used to prevent DVT or to inhibit prothrombin activation after blood comes in contact with artificial surfaces during cardiopulmonary bypass surgery or hemodialysis, is reviewed next.

1. Orthopedic and Abdominal Surgery

The concentrations of prothrombin fragment 1 + 2 and thrombin–antithrombin III in the plasmas of patients at high risk for developing postoperative thrombosis, including patients over 40 who have undergone elective gynecological, knee, or hip surgery, increase markedly after the surgery and remain elevated for several days (43–46). Without prophylaxis with UFH or LMWH, or with oral anticoagulants, up to 70% of patients over 40 years of age who have undergone any of the above surgical procedures develop postoperative DVT (1, 3, 7, 9). The endogenous concentrations of prothrombin fragment 1 + 2 in carefully prepared plasmas represent the steady-state concentrations of prothrombin previously activated in vivo, whereas those of thrombin-antithrombin III represent the steady-state

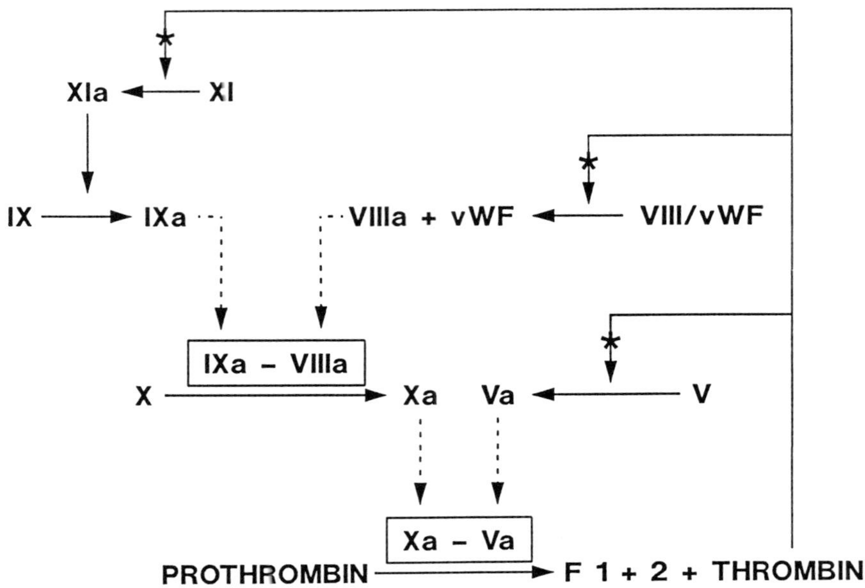

Figure 2 Steps in plasma coagulation sensitive to inhibition by UF and LMW heparins. UF and LMW heparins inhibit the formation of prothrombinase, Xa-Va, at two sites, namely thrombin-catalyzed activation of factor VIII and factor V. These sites are indicated by asterisks. By catalyzing thrombin inhibition by ATIII, UFH and LMWH prolong the times required to effect factor V and factor VIII activation. During coagulation, activation of factor V and factor VIII is usually catalyzed by the endogenously generated thrombin (9, 41, 75, 85, 87). Inhibition of factor VIII activation suppresses factor X activation by factor IXa (intrinsic tenase represented as IXa-VIIIa). Inhibition of factor V activation decreases the availability of factor Va, a critical component for the assembly of prothrombinase. Because thrombin is also able to activate factor XI (37, 38), catalysis of thrombin inhibition by ATIII has the potential to inhibit factor XI activation (indicated by asterisk) and, thus, the potential to inhibit factor IX activation by factor XIa. Whether these sites of *in vitro* coagulation inhibited by UFH LMWH are similarly subject to inhibition by these glycosaminoglycans *in vivo* remains to be established.

concentrations of the proportions of thrombin that had been inactivated by antithrombin III at the time of blood collection (47–50).

Depending on the kits used to measure it, the concentrations of prothrombin fragment 1 + 2 in the plasmas of healthy individuals vary between 0.3 and 2.5 nM (47–51). It appears that the plasma concentrations of prothrombin fragment 1 + 2 increase with age (51). Commercial kits for quantifying this parameter in plasma have been available for only a relatively short time. Therefore, there is limited information on the utility of this parameter for estimating the risk for developing DVT, the presence of thrombin, and for monitoring the effectiveness of antithrombotic prophylaxis or therapy. The mean (± 1 SD) concentration of prothrombin fragment 1 + 2 we measured in the plasmas of 53 routine blood donors (aged 16–65 years) was 1.07 ± 0.10 nM. The comparable value found in preoperative plasmas of 15 patients over 40 who underwent elective hip replacement was not significantly different from the above value. However, 12–24 hr following hip surgery, and prior to the first prophylactic injection of UFH or LMWH, this preoperative value had increased to 1.51 ± 0.20 nM ($p < 0.01$). Within 3 hr of the first prophylactic injection of UFH or the LMWH Enoxaparin, the mean concentration of prothrombin fragment 1 + 2 had decreased to the preoperative value and remained at this lower level for at least 12 hr (in preparation). These results provide direct evidence that at least the first injection of a prophylactically effective dose of UFH or a LMWH moderates prothrombin activation in vivo. As noted above, the plasma concentrations of prothrombin fragment 1 + 2 and thrombin-antithrombin III increase invariably following elective hip surgery.

Commercial kits for measuring the concentrations of thrombin–antithrombin III endogenous to plasma have been available longer than kits for estimating plasma concentrations of prothrombin fragment 1 + 2. Therefore, several studies evaluating longer-term changes in the concentrations of thrombin–antithrombin III in the plasmas of patients who have undergone high-risk orthopedic surgery, and the effects of UFH and LMWH prophylaxis on the production of thrombin–antithrombin III in vivo, have been published (43–46–56). The results demonstrate that surgery markedly increases the plasma concentrations of thrombin–antithrombin III, reflecting the increased postoperative prothrombin activation noted above. Second, following prophylaxis with UFH or LMWH or the heparinoid ORG 10172 (Orgaran), the concentrations of thrombin–antithrombin III in these plasmas then decrease significantly. Thus, the daily plasma samples obtained from patients receiving antithrombotic prophylaxis have lower concentrations of thrombin-antithrombin III than comparable plasmas of patients who received placebo (43–46, 52–55). There is also evidence that the prophylactic drugs do not suppress in vivo prothrombin activation in patients who develop postoperative DVT as effectively as they do in patients in whom antithrombotic prophylaxis is successful. In particular, the concentrations of thrombin–antithrombin III in the postheparin or post-Enoxaparin plasmas of patients who developed DVT after major orthopedic surgery remained significantly higher than the values found in plasmas of patients in whom prophylaxis was successful (46).

In summary, there is evidence for increased prothrombin activation, and consequently increased thrombin inhibition by antithrombin III in vivo, following major orthopedic or abdominal surgery in patients over 40, accounting for the high risk for developing DVT after these procedures. Prophylactic injections of

UFH, LMWH, or a heparinoid suppress prothrombin activation in these patients (43–46, 52–55). A more effective suppression of prothrombin activation is seen in plasmas of patients in whom prophylaxis is successful than is found in the plasmas of patients in whom prophylaxis fails. The reasons for the less effective inhibition of in vivo prothrombin activation and inhibition in plasmas of patients who develop postoperative DVT, in spite of prophylaxis, are not known. However, the difference probably cannot be attributed to differences in the concentrations of UFH or LMWH in the plasmas of DVT-positive and DVT-negative patients (46).

2. *Cardiopulmonary Bypass Surgery, PTC, and Hemodialysis*

Heparin is also the prophylactic antithrombotic drug used during cardiac bypass surgery. The dose used in the 90 to 180-min procedure is equivalent to the usual daily dose of heparin used to initiate therapy of DVT (15, 16). Consequently, up to 5 times higher blood levels of UFH are obtained during this procedure than during heparin therapy for proximal vein thrombosis. Although there is no doubt that heparin in the circulation inhibits prothrombin activation during cardiac bypass surgery, heparin does not suppress prothrombin activation and the associated generation of thrombin–antithrombin III as effectively as it does during the prophylaxis of postoperative DVT or treatment of DVT (54, 55). Heparin is also used during PTCA, and the levels of prothrombin fragment 1 + 2 thrombin–antithrombin III generated during this procedure are significantly lower than the levels generated during cardiopulmonary bypass surgery (56). LMWH are not routinely used in cardiac surgery or in PTCA, and therefore, their effects on in vivo coagulation during these procedures are not known.

UFH and LMWH are equally effective in preventing clots from forming during routine hemodialysis (18, 22, 23). The effective doses of UFH and LMWH markedly suppress production of fibrinopeptide A during hemodialysis (22, 23). It is likely, therefore, that the doses used in hemodialysis also inhibit in vivo prothrombin activation and the formation of thrombin–antithrombin III. Note, however, that the levels of UFH or LMWH that permit successful hemodialysis do not reduce the concentrations of fibrinopeptide A or thrombin–antithrombin III to the predialysis levels. The concentrations of the two parameters indeed increase during the course of successful dialysis (22, 23), as they do during cardiac bypass surgery or PTCA (54, 56, 57).

3. *Other Prophylactic Uses of Heparin*

Heparin has also proved to be effective for preventing DVT after acute stroke (58–60), after myocardial infarction (61, 62), for preventing thromboembolism in high-risk pregnancy (63), and for preventing thrombosis in patients undergoing elective intracranial neurosurgery (64, 65). The direct effects of heparin on in vivo coagulation when used for these indications have not been reported.

B. Therapeutic Use of UFH and LMWH

Plasmas of patients with DVT or pulmonary embolism have significantly elevated concentrations of prothrombin fragment 1 + 2, thrombin–antithrombin III, and fibrinopeptide A than are normally found in the plasmas of healthy individuals (30, 66–69). The elevated levels of the three markers indicate that higher-than-normal concentrations of circulating thrombin are available in the patients to convert fibrinogen into fibrin and fibrinopeptide A. Therapeutic doses of heparin decrease the levels of fibrinopeptide A (FPA) found in these patients' plasmas. When heparin infusion is discontinued, the levels of FPA increase subsequently to the preheparin levels (26, 69), suggesting that heparin does not eliminate the thrombogenic stimulus. Only one study has reported the effects of continuous heparin infusion over 10 days on the concentrations of prothrombin fragment 1 + 2 and thrombin–antithrombin III in the plasmas of patients with DVT (70). Heparin suppressed production of both markers of in vivo coagulation. However, even 10 days of continuous heparin infusion failed to suppress production of the two markers of prothrombin consumption to the levels usually found in the plasmas without thrombosis (70). These results are consistent with prior observations that production of FPA in patients with DVT or pulmonary embolism increases after the heparin infusion is stopped (28, 69). The failure of therapeutic heparin to reduce prothrombin activation in the levels appropriate for hemostasis also explains for the need for oral anticoagulant therapy to minimize the occurrence of DVT after the course of heparin therapy (71).

Several recent studies have demonstrated that UFH and LMWH are equally effective for initiating the treatment of DVT (19–21). However, none of these studies reported the direct effects of UFH or LMWH on in vivo coagulation. Given how important the suppression of in vivo prothrombin activation by UFH and LMWH appears to be for efficacy during prophylaxis of venous thrombosis with UFH and LMWH (44–46, 52), it is highly likely that the effective therapeutic doses of the LMWH also inhibit prothrombin activation in vivo.

III. MECHANISMS FOR THE ANTICOAGULANT ACTIONS OF UFH AND LMW

The saturating concentration of prothrombinase generated in situ to essentially convert all plasma prothrombin to thrombin within 60 sec has been estimated by Hemker and associates to be $\geqslant$0.3 nM (72). Prothrombinase consists of the enzyme factor Xa and an equimolar concentration of the cofactor factor Va bound to an appropriate coagulant surface in a Ca^{2+}-dependent reaction (31, 32). There are two distinct but linked pathways for generating factor Xa in vitro. In the first, factor X is activated by the enzyme factor IXa in a reaction critically dependent on factor VIIIa, the cofactor for factor IXa (31, 32). Thrombin is the only enzyme likely to activate factor VIII in plasma, where factor VIII is complexed to von Willebrand factor and thus cannot be activated by factor Xa (73). The second enzyme complex for activating plasma factor X consists of the enzyme factor VIIa and its cofactor tissue factor (31, 32). The factor VIIa–tissue factor enzyme complex can also activate factor IX (31, 32). Both factor Xa and thrombin activate factor V (74,75), and thus their actions on factor V make the cofactor factor Va available in situ for the generation of prothrombinase. The key anticoagulant action of UFH and LMWH on prothrombin activation is the ability to delay the onset of the generation of prothrombinase in situ (39–42).

With respect to antithrombin III, UF heparin can be considered to consist of two components, namely catalytic and inert fractions. The catalytic fraction of UFH binds to antithrombin III with high affinity and accelerates the antithrombin III–dependent inactivation of thrombin, factor Xa, and factor IXa (75). The minimum M_r of high-affinity heparin fragments able to catalyze the antithrombin III–mediated inhibition of all three coagulant enzymes is $\geqslant$5000 (76). Since all the constituent chains of UFH have M_r $\geqslant$5000, high affinity of fractions of UFH can functionally be considered to be a single entity with respect to their ability to catalyze the inhibition of the three enzymes by antithrombin III. In contrast, two distinct catalytic components, namely the subfraction able to catalyze the inhibition of all three enzymes by antithrombin III (M_r $\geqslant$5000), and the fraction only able to catalyze factor Xa inhibition by antithrombin III (M_r $\geqslant$5000), are found in LMWH preparations (42, 77, 78). An additional catalytic difference between UFH and LMWH is that on average, the catalytic moieties in UFH also have higher molar specific activity than LMWH fraction (79–81). This is one reason why the specific activities of UFH (usually reported in international units/milligram) exceed those of LMWH. A second reason for the higher specific activity of UFH is that there may be up to three of the pentasaccharide sequence that bind antithrombin III with high affinity in a single UFH oligosaccharide chain (82) compared to only one in LMWH. A third reason for the lower specific activity of LMWH is that some of the processes used to depolymerize heparins lead to loss of sulfate residues (83). In general, the catalytic effectiveness of heparin fragments increases with both their degree of sulfation and M_r (83, 84).

To inhibit prothrombin activation in plasma, UFH and LMWH must delay the onset of the generation of prothrombinase in situ and/or inactivate prothrombinase. The latter action would only be accomplished if the UFH and LMWH can effectively catalyze the inactivation of factor Xa within prothrombinase. The minimum antithrombin concentration of UFH and LMWH used clinically able to delay the onset of prothrombin activation in contact-activated plasma (evaluated using the APTT test) is ~0.2 antithrombin units/ml of plasma (40). At this concentration, each drug can simultaneously delay the onset of intrinsic factor X and factor V activation (see Fig. 2). Factor Xa and factor Va are critical constituents of prothrombinase. By delaying their generation *in situ*, UFH and

LMWH thereby prolong the onset of prothrombin activation (75, 85). Available experimental evidence, which is summarized in Figure 2, is consistent with the idea that UFH and LMWH delay the onset of both factor X and factor V activation in contact-activated plasma by catalyzing the inhibition of endogenous thrombin (39–42, 75, 85–87). This action probably increases the time required for the concentration of endogenously generated thrombin to reach the threshold level required to activate factor VIII (a prior step required for intrinsic factor X activation). In support of this idea, the availability of $\leq$1.0 n factor Xa in plasma abrogates the ability of 0.2 antithrombin units of UFH or LMWH to delay the onset of prothrombin activation (41). While $\leq$1.0 nM factor Xa abrogates the ability of heparin to delay prothrombin activation, factor Va is unable to reverse the anticoagulant action of heparin (41). These results are consistent with both factor Xa and thrombin being able to activate plasma factor V, while only thrombin is able to activate factor VIII in plasma (73–75).

Whether UFH or LMWH can also can effectively catalyze factor Xa inhibition when the enzyme is prothrombinase-bound and thereby inhibit prothrombin activation remains unresolved. Using purified prothrombinase and antithrombin III, it is clear that UFH and most LMWH can catalyze the inactivation of prothrombinase-bound factor Xa by antithrombin III, but at rates significantly slower than those seen when antithrombin III–UFH or antithrombin III–LMWH complex inactivates factor Xa in solution (79, 80). Whether the catalytic actions of UFH and LMWH, at concentrations that can delay the onset of prothrombin activation in contact-activated plasma, can effectively inhibit prothrombinase generated in plasma has not yet been determined directly. Published results that evaluated the inhibition of plasma prothrombinase by UFH and LMWH employed plasmas that also had the potential to generate additional prothrombinase. In addition, the studies did not directly measure time-dependent changes in prothrombin or prothrombin fragment 1 + 2 concentrations. Rather, the concentrations of enzymatically active thrombin were used to estimate prothrombinase activity (86, 87). It should be recalled that UFH and LMWH also catalyze thrombin inhibition. Therefore, the direct effects of UFH and LMWH on prothrombinase remain equivocal.

UFH and LMWH do not effectively inhibit plasma prothrombin activation initiated by adding concentrations of tissue factor usually employed for prothrombin time tests to plasma (75). This is because the concentration of factor Xa needed to activate factor V to the level required to generate saturating concentrations of prothrombinase is readily attained in the presence of the heparins. Using highly diluted tissue factor as the coagulant stimulus, however, it is clear that UFH and LMWH can inhibit extrinsic prothrombin activation (86, 87). Initiated with highly dilute tissue factor, thrombin-mediated activation of factor VIII probably becomes essential to ensure production of saturating concentrations of factor Xa. Effective factor X activation in these circumstances is likely attributable to the enzymatic action of the factor IXa–factor VIIIa complex (intrinsic tenase) on factor X. Consistent with these ideas, UFH and LMWH prolong the times required to generate plasma prothrombinase initiated by adding dilutions of tissue factor that clot normal plasmas in approximately 30 sec, i.e., a time comparable to the clotting time of contact-activated plasmas (unpublished).

IV. PHARMACODYNAMICS OF UFH AND LMWH

UFH and LMWH are highly heterogenous for two reasons: (1) the M_r of constituent chains in UFH preparations can vary from ~7000 to 30,000, while those of LMWH vary between <2000 and ~10,000 (78); (2) less than 40% of the constituent chains of UFH and LMWH have the pentasaccharide sequence required for high-affinity interactions with antithrombin III (78). Both the antithrombotic (in vivo) and anticoagulant (in vitro) actions of UFH and LMWH largely result from their catalyzing thrombin and factor Xa inhibition by antithrombin III. This high-affinity pentasaccharide must be present before any given oligosaccharide chain can catalyze factor Xa inhibition by antithrombin III (88, 89). Additional structural elements are no doubt important for optimizing the catalytic actions of UFH and LMWH, for beginning with high-affinity hexasaccharides, the anti-factor Xa activities of heparin oligosaccharides increase with M_r (79–81). The minimum M_r of high-affinity oligosaccharides able to catalyze thrombin inhibition by antithrombin III is ⩾5000, i.e., ⩾18 monosaccharide residues long (79–81). The antithrombin activity of heparin oligosaccharides also increases with both M_r and degree of sulfation (79–81). These additional features, which partly define the catalytic effectiveness of UFH and LMWH, clearly influence their measurable pharmacodynamic parameters. It is worth noting that the principal sites for clearance of UFH and LMWH differ. UFH is taken up by the liver, spleen, and lungs to undergo desulfation and depolymerization and subsequent elimination by the kidneys. Thus, reticuloendothelial cell blockade prolongs the clearance of the UFH from the circulation. Because of their reduced affinity for the reticuloendothelial system, the kidneys are the principal organs that account for the elimination of LMWH (90–94). Whether impaired renal function has the potential to lead to the accumulation of LMWH given therapeutically remains to be established.

UFH and LMWH are given by subcutaneous injection to prevent deep vein thrombosis (1–10). Used in higher doses therapeutically, the drugs can be given either by continuous intravenous infusion or by once- to twice-daily subcutaneous injections (11–14, 19–21). The measured pharmacodynamic parameters of UFH and LMWH in man humans will next be considered only briefly as the topic has been recently reviewed extensively by others (90–94).

A. Intravenous Injection

Three activities of UFH and LMWH, readily measured in plasma after the drugs are injected intravenously, are used to derive their pharmacodynamic parameters: (1) prolongation of global coagulation tests; (2) anti-factor Xa; and (3) antithrombin catalytic activities. Manufacturers of UFH routinely assign potency to each preparation by reference to the international standard for UF heparins. Manufacturers of LMWH now assign potency to their products using the international standard for LMWH as the reference preparation (95). Therefore, the concentrations of UFH and LMWH in plasma are usually reported in international units. The potency of UFH is also stated in pharmacopoeial units. For most practical purposes, the international and pharmacopoeial units of UFH can be considered to be equivalent. It is worth noting that collaborative studies have demonstrated the inappropriateness of the UFH standard for assigning potency to LMWH preparations (95). Assayed in vitro by the APTT, anti-factor Xa, and antithrombin activity assays, $\geqslant$0.05 units of UFH can readily be detected in plasma. By convention, the in vitro APTT, antithrombin, and anti-factor Xa activities of UFH are usually equal. However, the ratios of the three activities change markedly after UFH is injected into humans or experimental animals (90–94).

The clearance curves of intravenous UFH are dose-dependently concave-convex, with three distinct components: a rapid initial clearance phase (reflecting the high-affinity binding of UFH to the endothelium and other saturable reticulo-endothelial sites); a saturable clearance phase at low doses; and an exponential first-order kinetics at high (therapeutic) doses (90–94). Of the three biological activities, the half-life of intravenous heparin is significantly shorter when measured by its APTT or antithrombin activity than by its anti-factor Xa activity. One consequence of these differences is that following subcutaneous injections, the ratios of the anti-factor Xa to the other two activities become significantly greater than 1 and also continue to increase with time. Like the antithrombin activity, the APTT activity depends predominantly on the fractions of UFH that catalyze thrombin inhibition (75, 90–94). Since these larger and more sulfated fractions (i.e., fractions that contribute to the APTT and antithrombin activities) of UFH have higher affinity for the endothelium than fractions with predominantly anti-factor Xa activity (96, 97), they are cleared from plasma more rapidly at low doses.

Intravenous injection of LMWH also leads to an increase in the APTT and antithrombin activities, and for the same reasons as UFH, the anti-factor Xa half-life of LMWH is significantly longer than the antithrombin or APTT half-life (90–94). In addition, when equivalent anti-factor Xa activities of UFH and LMWH are injected subcutaneously into healthy human volunteers, at least twice more anti-APTT activity is recovered after the LMWH than after the UFH injection (93). An even higher difference in recovery is observed when the recoveries of the anti-factor Xa activities of UFH and LMWH are compared (93). The higher recoveries of LMWH largely reflect their lower affinity for the endothelium relative to UFH. Plasma also contains several moieties that interact with heparin oligosaccharides to modulate the catalytic activities of the glycosaminoglycans on thrombin and factor Xa inhibition (98). To a certain extent, the neutralizability of the catalytic activities of heparin oligosaccharides increases with M_r and degree of sulfation (81). UFH have higher charge density (higher sulfation) and obviously have higher M_r than LMWH.

B. Subcutaneous Injection

Subcutaneous administration of UFH and LMWH also results in the recovery of APTT, anti-factor Xa, and antithrombin activities (90–94). The activities thus recovered from subcutaneously injections of LMWH are equal to or approach those obtained by the intravenous route of administration (90–94). This fact has led to the choice of subcutaneous injections of LMWH as the preferred route of administration for prophylaxis and therapy of DVT. In contrast to LMWH, significantly lower activities are recovered after subcutaneous injections of UFH than after intravenous injections. Thus, while the bioavailability of LMWH is or approaches 100%, that of UFH is <40% (90–94).

V. RELATIONSHIPS BETWEEN BLOOD LEVELS OF UFH AND LMWH AND ANTITHROMBOTIC EFFICACY

The establishment of clear relationships between blood levels of UFH and LMWH and efficacy, on the one hand, and the risk of bleeding, on the other hand, could simplify the clinical use of UFH and LMWH. Prolongation of the APTT to 1.5–2.5 times normal values within 24–48 hr after initiation of heparin therapy is the minimum ex vivo action of the drug that must be achieved to reduce the frequency of recurrence of DVT to ≤10% (14, 99). The relationship between the blood levels of UFH and bleeding, however, is not clearly established. Blood levels of LMWH, when given therapeutically, need not be monitored since the drugs are given in units/kilogram when they are used to initiate treatment of DVT (19, 21), and close and predictable relationships exist between the concentrations recovered ex vivo and the doses of LMWH injected (93).

Attempts to establish relationships between blood levels of UFH and efficacy, when UFH is used to prevent postoperative thrombosis, have been and may continue to be futile. The drug is usually given by twice-daily subcutaneous injections, and no ex vivo activity attributable to the injections of UFH can be readily measured for significant periods between injections. This is due in part to the short *plasma* half-life associated with prophylactic doses of UFH. The suppression of postoperative prothrombin fragment 1 + 2 production to the preoperative values by heparin can be demonstrated up to 12 hr after the first prophylactic injection of heparin. In contrast, ex vivo activities can usually be detected for no more than 6 hr after prophylactic injections of UFH. Therefore, the relationship between blood levels of UFH and its prophylactic efficacy remains in doubt. This doubt heightens somewhat when one considers that in healthy volunteers, prophylactic doses of UFH do not inhibit production of prothrombin fragment 1 + 2 or thrombin–antithrombin III (in preparation). Intravenous injections of heparin to cancer patients also fail to suppress the increased coagulation (measured as elevation of plasma fibrinopeptide A concentrations) in these patients (100).

The longer duration of the anti-factor Xa activity, compared to the antithrombin activity, and the higher recovery anti-factor Xa activity from LMWH than UFH injections, has led to the idea that the anti-factor Xa activity may be an important parameter for estimating prophylactic antithrombotic efficacy of UFH and LMWH. The relationship between the ex vivo levels of LMWH activities and prophylactic efficacy remains controversial, however, despite the longer duration of the anti-factor Xa activity after each injection of LMWH compared to UFH (93). Indeed, the consensus has emerged that it is unnecessary to monitor during levels when UFH and LMWH are used prophylactically.

The lack of clear relationships between blood levels of UFH or LMWH and prophylactic effectiveness raises fundamental questions regarding the anatomical site(s) for the excessive thrombin production that can lead to the development of DVT in high-risk situations. The specific steps of in vivo coagulation the drugs must moderate for prophylaxis to be successful are also not yet defined. The ability of UFH to inhibit prothrombin activation in postoperative patients and its failure to inhibit prothrombin activation in healthy volunteers (unpublished) and cancer patients (100) raise the possibility that the sites where excessive thrombin is generated during postoperative thrombosis differ from the site where thrombin is produced for hemostasis. The sites of thrombin generation for thrombosis and hemostasis also appear to be differentially accessible to inhibition by UFH or LMWH, raising the possibility that prothrombinase is assembled on different cell surfaces for hemostasis and thrombosis. Since UFH and LMWH heparins also inhibit factor X and factor IX activation (101) and accelerate the inhibition of factor Xa and factor IXa by antithrombin III, reliable kits for measuring the extents of factor IX and factor X activation in vivo (activation peptide assays), and for measuring complexes of factor IXa and factor Xa with their inhibitors will probably be necessary before the critical reactions that must be adequately regulated for antithrombotic efficacy can be discerned.

ACKNOWLEDGMENTS

The experimental studies carried out by the author, and which are described in this manuscript, were funded by grants-in-aid by the Heart and Stroke Foundation of Ontario and the Canadian Red Cross Society, Blood Services R&D Fund.

REFERENCES

1. Kakkar VV, Djazaeri B, Fok J, Fletcher M, Scully M, Westwick J. Low molecular weight heparin and prevention of post-operative vein thrombosis. Br Med J 1982; 284:375–397.
2. Kakkar VV, Corrigan T, Spindler J, Fossard DP, Flute PT, Crellin RQ. Efficacy of low doses of heparin in prevention of deep-vein thrombosis after major surgery. A double blind randomized trial. Lancet 1972; 2:101–106.
3. Gallus AS, Hirsh J, Tuttle RJ, Trebilcock R, O'Brien SE, Carroll JJ, Minden JH, Hudecki SM. Small subcutaneous doses of heparin in prevention of venous thrombosis. N Engl J Med 1973; 288:545–551.
4. Clarke-Pearson DL, Colman RE, Synan IS, Hinshaw W, Creasman WT. Venous thromboembolism prophylaxis in gynecologic oncology: a prospective, controlled trial of low-dose heparin. Am J Obstet Gynecol 1983; 145:606–613.
5. European Fraxiparin Study (EFS) Group. Comparison of a low molecular weight heparin and unfractionated heparin for the prevention of deep vein thrombosis in patients undergoing abdominal surgery. Br J Surg 1988; 75:1058–1063.
6. Bergqvist D, Burmark US, Frisell J, Hallbrook T, Lindblad B, Risberg B, Torngren S, Wallin G. Low molecular weight heparin once daily compared with conventional low dose heparin twice daily: a prospective double-blind multicentre trial on prevention of postoperative thrombosis. Br J Surg 1986; 73:204–208.
7. Turpie AGG, Levine MN, Hirsh J, Carter CJ, Jay RM, Powers PJ, Andrew M, Hull RD, Gent M. A randomized controlled trial of a low-molecular weight heparin (Enoxaparin) to prevent deep vein thrombosis in patients undergoing elective hip surgery. N Engl J Med 1986; 315:925–929.
8. Caen JP. A randomized double-blind study between a low molecular weight heparin Kabi 2165 and standard heparin in the prevention of deep vein thrombosis in general surgery: a French multicenter trial. Thromb Haemost 1988; 59:216–220.
9. Leclerc JR, Geerts W, Desjardin L, Jobin F, Laroche F, Delorme F, Haviernicks S, Atkinson S, Bourgouin J. Prevention of venous thrombosis after major knee surgery—a randomized, double-blind trial comparing a low molecular weight heparin fragment (Enoxaparin) to placebo. Thromb Haemost 1992; 67:417–423.
10. Levine MN, Hirsh J, Gent M, Turpie AGG, Leclerc J, Powers PJ, Jay RM, Neemeth J. Prevention of deep vein thrombosis after rlective hip surgery. A randomized trial comparing low molecular weight heparin with standard unfractionated heparin. Ann Intern Med 1991; 1[illegible]4:545–551.
11. Salzman EW, Deykin D, Shapiro RM, Rosenberg R. Management of heparin therapy: controlled prospective trial. N Engl J Med 1976; 292:1046–1050.

12. Glazier RL, Crowell EB. Randomized prospective trial of continuous versus intermittent heparin therapy. JAMA 1976; 236:1365–1367.
13. Hyers TM, Hull RD, Weg JG. Antithrombotic therapy for venous thrombotic disease. Chest 1989; 95(Suppl):37S–51S.
14. Hull RD, Raskob GE, Hirsh J, Jay RM, Leclerc JR, Geerts WH, Rosenblooom D, Sackett DL, Anderson C, Harrison L, Gent M. Continuous intravenous heparin compared with intermittent subcutaneous heparin in the initial treatment of proximal vein thrombosis. N Engl J Med 1986; 315:1109–1114.
15. Bull BSJ, Korpman RA, Huse M, Briggs BD. Heparin therapy during extracorporeal circulation. I. Problems inherent in existing heparin protocols. The use of a dose response curve to individualize heparin and protamine dosages. J Thorac Cardiovasc Surg 1975; 69:674–689.
16. Jobes DR, Schwartz AJ, Ellison N, Andrews R, Ruffini RA, Ruffini JJ. Monitoring heparin anticoagulation and its neutralization. Ann Thorac Surg 1981; 31:161–166.
17. Stein PD, Dalen JE, Goldman S, Schwartz L, Turpie AGG, Theroux P. Antithrombotic therapy in patients with saphaneous vein and internal mammary artery bypass grafts following percutaneous transluminal coronary angioplasty. Chest 1992; 102:(Suppl) 508S–515S.
18. Anastassiades E, Ireland H, Flynn A, Lane DA, Curtis JR. A low-molecular-weight heparin (Kabi 2165, fragmin) in repeated use for haemodialysis: prevention of clotting and prolongation of the venous compression time in comparison with commercial unfractionated heparin. Nephrol Dial Transplant 1990; 5:135–140.
19. Hull RD, Raskob GE, Pineo GF, Green D., Trowbridge AA, Elliott CG, Lerner RG, Norton J, Carter CJ, George R, Merli G, Ward J, Mayo W, Rosenbloom D, Brant R. Subcutaneous low-molecular-weight heparin compared with continuous intravenous heparin in the treatment of proximal-vein thrombosis. N Engl J Med 1992; 326:975–982.
20. Albada J, Niewenhuis HK, Sixma JJ. Treatment of acute venous thromboembolism with low molecular weight heparin (Fragmin): results of a double-blind randomized study. Circulation 1989; 80:935–940.
21. Prandoni P, Lensing AWA, Buller HR, Carta M, Cogo A, Vigo M, Casara D, Ruol A, ten Cate JW. Comparison of subcutaneous low molecular weight heparin with intravenous heparin in proximal vein thrombosis. Lancet 1992; 339:441–445.
22. Anastassiades E, Lane DA, Ireland H, Flynn A, Curtis JR. A low molecular weight heparin (''Fragmin'') for routine hemodialysis: a crossover trial comparing three dose regimens with a standard regimen of commercial unfractionated heparin. Clin Nephrol 1989; 32:290–296.
23. Ireland H, Lane DA, Flynn A, Pegrum AC, Curtis JR. Low molecular weight heparin in haemodialysis for chronic renal failure: dose finding study of CY222. Thromb Haemost 1988; 59:240–247.
24. Nossel HL. Radioimmunoassay of fibrinopeptides in relation to intravascular coagulation. N Engl J Med 1976; 242:428–432.
25. Peuscher F, van Aken W, Flier O. Effect of anticoagulant treatment measured by fibrinopeptide A (FPA) in patients with venous thromboembolism. Thromb Res 1980; 18:33–43.

26. Speiser W, Mallek R, Koppensteiner R, Stumpflen A, Kapiotis S, Minar E, Ehringer H, Lechner K. D-dimer and TAT measurement in patients with deep vein thrombosis: utility in the diagnosis and judgement of anticoagulant treatment effectiveness. Thromb Haemost 1990; 64:196–201.
27. Takano K, Yamaguchi T, Uchida K. Markers of a hypercoagulable state following acute ischemic stroke. Stroke 1992; 23:194–198.
28. Uno M, Tsuji H, Watanabe M, Takada O, Kobayashi K, Takabuchi H, Shirai K, Sawada S, Toyoda T, Yamamoto K, Katoh K, Nakagawa M. Application of thrombin-antithrombin III complex for detecting a latent hypercoagulable state in patients with coronary artery disease. Jpn Circ J 1989; 53:1185–1191.
29. Wojciechewski J, Olausson M, Bengtsen KK. Fibrinopeptide A, β-thromboglobulin and fibrin degradation products as screening tests for the diagnosis of deep vein thrombosis. Haemostasis 1983; 13:254–261.
30. Yudelman IM, Nossel HL, Kaplan K, Hirsh J. Plasma fibrinopeptide A levels in symptomatic venous thromboemolism. Blood 1978; 51:1189–1195.
31. Jackson CM, Nemerson Y. Blood coagulation. Annu Rev Biochem 1980; 49:785–811.
32. Mann KG, Jenny RJ, Krishnaswamy S. Cofactor proteins in the assembly and expression of blood clotting enzyme complexes. Annu Rev Biochem 1988; 57:915–956.
33. Blomback B, Hessel B, Hogg D, Therkildsen L. A two-step fibrinogen-fibrin transition in blood coagulation. Nature 1978; 275:501–505.
34. Janus TJ, Lewis SD, Lorand L, Shafer JA. Promotion of thrombin-catalyzed activation of factor XIII by fibrinogen. Biochemistry 1983; 22:6269–6272.
35. Vehar GA, Davie EW. Preparation and properties of bovine factor VIII. Biochemistry 1980; 19:401–410.
36. Suzuki K, Dahlback B, Stenflo J. Thrombin-catalyzed activation of human coagulation factor V. J Biol Chem 1982; 257:6656–6664.
37. Gailani D, Broze G. Factor XI activation in a revised model of blood coagulation. Science 1991; 253:909–912.
38. Naito K, Fujikawa K. Activation of human blood coagulation factor XI independent of factor XII. J Biol Chem 1991; 266:7353–7358.
39. Ofosu FA, Sie P, Modi J, Hirsh J, Fernandez F, Buchanan MR, Blajchman MA. The inhibition of thrombin catalyzed positive-feedback reactions is critical to the expression of the anticoagulant effect of heparin. Biochem J 1987; 243:579–588.
40. Ofosu FA, Smith LM, Anvari N, Blajchman M. An approach to assigning in vitro potency to unfractionated and LMWH based on the inhibition of prothrombin activation and catalysis of thrombin inhibition. Thromb Haemost 1988; 60:193–198.
41. Ofosu FA, Hirsh J, Esmon CT, Modi GJ, Smith LM, Anvari N, Buchanan MR, Fenton JW II, Blajchman MA. Unfractionated heparin inhibits thrombin-catalyzed amplification reaction of coagulation more efficiently than those catalyzed by factor Xa. Biochem J 1989; 257:143–149.
42. Ofosu FA, Barrowcliffe TW. Mechanism of action of low molecular weight heparins and heparinoids. Balliere's Clin Hematol 1990; 3:505–529.
43. Bogaty-Yver J, Samama M. Thrombin-antithrombin III complexes for detection of post-operative hypercoagulable state in surgical patients receiving prophylaxis. Thromb Haemost 1989; 61:528–539.

44. Hoek JA, Nurmohamed MT, ten Cate JW, Buller HR, Knipscheer HC, Hamelynck KJ, Marti RK, Sturk A. Thrombin–antithrombin III complexes in the prediction of deep vein thrombosis following total hip replacement. Thromb Haemost 1989; 62:1050–1052.
45. Ofosu FA, Leclerc J, Delorme F, Craven S, Shafai S, Frewin L, Blajchman MA. The low molecular weight Enoxaparin inhibits the consumption of factor VII and prothrombin activation in vivo associated with elective knee replacement surgery. Br J Haematol 1992; 82:391–399.
46. Ofosu FA, Levine M, Craven S, Dewar L, Shafai S, Blajchman MA. Prophylactically equivalent doses of Enoxaparin and unfractionated heparin inhibit in vivo coagulation to the same extent. Br J Haematol 1992; 82:400–405.
47. Teitel JM, Bauer KA, Lau H, Rosenberg RD. Studies on the prothrombin activation pathway utilizing radioimmunoassays for the F_2/F1 + 2 fragment and thrombin–antithrombin III. Blood 1982; 59:1086–1097.
48. Bauer KA, Goodman TL, Kass BL, Rosenberg RD. Elevated factor Xa activity in the blood of asymptomatic patients with congenital antithrombin III deficiency. J Clin Invest 1985; 76:826–836.
49. Bauer KA, Rosenberg RD. The pathophysiology of the pre-thrombotic state in humans. Insights gained from studies using markers of hemostatic system activation. Blood 1987; 70:343–350.
50. Pelzer H, Schwartz A, Stuber W. Determination of prothrombin activation fragment 1 + 2 in plasma with an antibody against synthetic peptides. Thromb Haemost 1991; 65:153–159.
51. Bauer KA, Weiss LM, Sparrow D, Vokonas PS, Rosenberg RD. Aging-associated changes in indices of thrombin generation and protein C activation in humans. Normative aging study. J Clin Invest 1987; 80:1527–1534.
52. Jorgensen LN, Lind B, Hauch O, Leffers A, Albrecht-Beste E, Konradsen LAG. Thrombin–antithrombin III-complex and fibrin degradation products in plasma: surgery and postoperative deep venous thrombosis. Thromb Res 1990; 59:69–76.
53. Sorensen JV, Borris LC, Lassen MR, Christiansen HM, Schott P, Olsen AD. Levels of thrombin–antithrombin III complex and factor VIII activity in relation to postoperative deep vein thrombosis and influence of prophylaxis with low molecular weight heparin. Blood Coagul Fibrinol 1990; 1:389–392.
54. Boisclair MD, Lane DA, Phillipou H, Sheikh S, Hunt B. Thrombin production, inactivation and expression during open heart surgery measured by assays for activation fragments including a new ELISA for prothrombin fragment 1 + 2. Thromb Haemost (in press).
55. Lu H, Soria C, Commin P-L, Soria J, Piwnica A, Schumann F, Regnier FO, Legrand Y, Caen JP. Hemostasis in patients underoing extracorporeal circulation. The effect of trasylol. Thromb Haemost 1991; 66:633–637.
56. Brister SJ, Ofosu FA, Buchanan MR. Thrombin generation during cardiac surgery: is heparin the ideal anticoagulant? Thromb Haemost (in press).
57. Gill JB, Fondevila CG, Brister SJ, Turpie AGG, Holder DA, Ofosu FA, Buchanan MR. Contrast media induces thrombin generation during PTCA. Proc Roy Coll Phys Surg Can 1992.

58. McCarthy ST, Robertson D, Turner JJ, Hawkey CJ, Macey DJ. Low dose heparin prophylaxis against deep vein thrombosis after acute stroke. Lancet 1977; 2:800–801.
59. Prins MH, den Ottolander GJH, Gelsema R, van Woerkom TCM, Sing AK, Heller I. Deep vein thrombosis prophylaxis with a low molecular weight heparin (Kabi 2165) in stroke patients. Thromb Haemost 1987; 58 (Suppl):117.
60. Turpie AGG, Gent M, Cole R, Levine MN, Ginsberg J, Powers PJ, Leclerc J, Geerts W, Jay R, Neemeth J, Klimek M, Hirsh J. A low molecular weight heparinoid compared with unfractionated heparin in the prevention of deep vein thrombosis in patients with acute ischemic stroke. Ann Intern Med 1992; 117:353–357.
61. Handley AJ, Emerson PA, Fleming PR. Heparin in the prevention of deep vein thrombosis after myocardial infarction. Br Med J 1972; 2:436–438.
62. Wray R, Maurer B, Shillingford J. Prophylactic anticoagulant therapy in the prevention of calf-vein thrombosis after myocardial infarction. N Engl J Med 1973; 288:815–817.
63. Ginsberg JS, Hirsh J. Use of antithrombotic agents during pregnancy. Chest 1992; 102 (Suppl):385–390.
64. Cerrato D, Adriano C, Fiacchino F. Deep vein thrombosis and low-dose heparin prophylaxis in neurosurgical patients. J Neurosurg 1978; 49:378–381.
65. Lane DA, Wolff S, Ireland H, Gawel M, Foadi M. Activation of coagulation and fibrinolyytic systems following stroke. Br J Haematol 1983; 53:655–658.
66. Boisclair MD, Ireland H, Lane DA. Assessment of hypercoagulable states by measurement of activation fragments and peptides. Blood Rev 1990; 4:25–40.
67. Bounameaux H, Slosman D, de Moerloose P, Reber G. Laboratory diagnosis of pulmonary embolism: value of increased levels of plasma D-dimer and thrombin–antithrombin III complexes. Biomed Pharmacother 1989; 43:385–388.
68. Eisenberg PR, Sherman LA, Schectman K, Perez J, Sobel BE, Jaffe AS. Fibrinopeptide A: a marker of acute coronary thrombosis. Circulation 1985; 71:912–918.
69. Nossel HL, Butler HL Jr, Canfield RE, Yudelman I, Ti M, Spanondis K, Soland T. Potential use of fibrinopeptide A measurements in the diagnosis and management of thrombosis. Thromb Diathes Haemorrh (Stuttg) 1975; 33:426–434.
70. Estivals M, Pelzer H, Sie P, Pichon J, Boccalon P. Prothrombin fragment 1 + 2, thrombin-antithrombin III complexes and D-dimers in acute deep vein thrombosis: effects of heparin treatment. Br J Haematol 1991; 78:421–424.
71. Lagerstedt CI Olsson C-G Fagher BO, Oqvist BW, Albrechtson U. Need for long-term anticoagulant treatment in symptomatic calf-vein thrombosis. Lancet 1985 1:515–518.
72. Hemker HC, Beguin S, Berdetowicz AV, Wielders S. Determination of the levels of unfractionated and low-molecular-weight heparins in plasma: their effect on thrombin-mediated feedback reactions in vivo. Haemostasis 1991; 21:258–272.
73. Koedam JA, Hamer RJ, Beeser-Visser NH, Bouma BN, Sixma JJ. The effect of von Willebrand factor on activation of factor VIII by factor Xa. Eur J Biochem 1990; 189:229–234.
74. Monkovic DD, Tracey PB. Activation of human factor V by factor Xa and thrombin. Biochemistry 1990; 29:1118–1128.
75. Yang X, Blajchman MA, Craven S, Smith LM, Anvari N, Ofosu FA. Activation of

factor V during intrinsic and extrinsic coagulation. Inhibition by heparin, hirudin and H-*D*-PHE-PRO-ARGCH$_2$Cl. Biochem J 1990; 272:399–406.
76. Jordan RE, Oosta GM, Gardner WT, Rosenberg RD. The kinetics of hemostatic enzyme-antithrombin interactions in the presence of low molecular weight heparin. J Biol Chem 1980; 255:10081–10090.
77. Holmer E, Kurachi E, Soderstrom G. The molecular-weight dependence of the rate-enhancing effect of heparin on the inhibition of thrombin, factor Xa, factor IXa, factor XIa, factor XIIa and kallikrein by antithrombin. Biochem J 1981; 193:395–400.
78. Barrowcliffe TW, Johnson EA, Thomas DP. Biochemistry of anticoagulant actions in vitro. In: Low Molecular Weight Heparin. Chichester, UK: Wiley, 1992:17–44.
79. Barrowcliffe TW, Havercroft SJ, Kemball-Cook G, Lindahl U. The effect of Ca^{+2}, phospholipid and factor V on the anti-(factor Xa) activity of heparin and its high affinity oligosaccharides. Biochem J 1987; 243:31–37.
80. Ellis V, Scully MF, Kakkar VV. The relative molecular mass dependence of the anti-factor Xa properties of heparin. Biochem J 1986; 238:329–333.
81. Lane DA, Denton J, Flynn AM, Thunberg L, Lindahl U. Anticoagulant activities of heparin oligosaccharides and their neutralization by platelet factor 4. Biochem J 1984; 218:725–732.
82. Horner AA. Heterogeneous distribution of antithrombin-binding sites in rat brain heparan sulphate proteoglycans. Biochem J 1991; 280:393–397.
83. Casu B. Structure and biological activity of heparin. Adv Carb Chem 1985; 43:51–134.
84. Ofosu FA, Modi GJ, Blajchman MA, Buchanan MR, Johnson EA. Increased sulfation improves the anticoagulant activities of heparan sulfate and dermatan sulfate. Biochem J 1987; 248:889–896.
85. Ofosu FA, Choay J, Anvari N, Smith LM, Blajchman MA. Inhibition of factor X and factor V activation by dermatan sulfate and the synthetic pentasaccharide with high affinity to antithrombin III. Eur J Biochem 1990; 193:485–493.
86. Beguin S, Lindhout T, Hemker HC. The mode of action of heparin in plasma. Thromb Haemost 1988; 60:457–462.
87. Beguin S, Mardiguian J, Lindhout T, Hemker HC. The mode of action of low molecular weight heparin preparation (PK10169) and two of its major components on thrombin generation in plasma. Thromb Haemost 1989; 61:30–34.
88. Hook M, Bjork I, Hopwood J, Lindahl U. Anticoagulant activity of heparin separation of high activity and low activity heparin species by affinity chromatography on immobilized antithrombin. FEBS Lett 1976; 66:90–93.
89. Lam LH, Silbert JE, Rosenberg RD. The separation of active and inactive forms of heparin. Biochem Biophys Res Commun 1976; 69:570–577.
90. Boneu B, Caranobe C, Sie P. Pharmacokinetics of heparin and low molecular weight heparins. Bailliere's Clin Haematol 1990; 3:531–544.
91. Albada J Nieuwenhuis HK, Sixma JJ. Pharmacokinetics of standard and low molecular weight heparin. In: Lane DA, Lindah U, eds. Heparin—Chemical and Biological Properties—Clinical Application. London: Edward Arnold, 1989:417–432.
92. Bara L, Samama M. Pharmacokinetics of low molecular weight heparins. Acta Chir Scand 1988 (Suppl. 543):65–72.

93. Barrowcliffe TW, Johnson EA, Thomas DP. Pharmacology in animals and humans. In: Low Molecular Weight Heparins. Chichester, UK: Wiley, 1992:101–123.
94. Boneu B, Dol F, Caranobe C, Sie P, Houin G. Pharmacokinetics of heparin and related polysaccharides. Ann NY Acad Sci 1989; 556:282–291.
95. Barrowcliffe TW, Curtis AD, Tomlinson TP, Hubbard AR, Johnson EA, Thomas DP. Standardization of low molecular weight heparins: a collaborative study. Thromb Haemost 1985; 54:675–679.
96. Barzu T, Lormeau JC, Petitou M, Michelson S, Choay J. Heparin derived oligosaccharides: affinity for acidic fibroblast growth factors and effect on its growth promoting activity for human endothelial cells. J Cell Physiol 1989; 140:538–548.
97. Psuja P. Effect of antithrombin III on the binding of heparin and its low molecular weight fraction CY 216 to endothelium in culture. Acta Haematol Polonica 1988; 19:143–149.
98. Barrowcliffe JW, Johnson EA, Thomas DP. Interaction with heparin-binding proteins and cells. In: Low Molecular Weight Heparins. Chichester, UK: Wiley, 1992:65–100.
99. Brandjes DPM, Buller HR, Heijboer H, Jagt J, deRijk M, ten Cate JW. Comparative trial of heparin and oral anticogulants in the initial treatment of proximal vein thrombosis. Thromb Haemost 1991; 65:703.
100. Penscher FW, Cleton FJ, Armstrong L, Stoepman EA, van Mourik JA, van Aken WG. Significance of plasma fibrinopeptide (fpA) in patients with malignancy. J Lab Clin Invest 1980; 96:5–14.
101. Ofosu FA. The anticoagulant mechanisms of Lomoparan (ORG10172) and its fraction with high affinity to antithrombin III(ORG10849). Haemostasis 1992; 22:66–72.

2

Mode of Action of Low-Molecular-Weight Heparins in Plasma and Its Consequences for the Clinical Laboratory

H. Coenraad Hemker and Suzette Béguin

Cardiovascular Research Institute and University of Limburg, Maastricht, The Netherlands

I. INTRODUCTION

The questions to be posed in heparin pharmacology are the same as those in any other field of pharmacology: what are the relevant concentrations of the acting substance at the relevant site and what are the relevant functions of the body that are influenced by these substances? Then, what is the relationship between these two; i.e., what is the dose-effect relationship? If we admit that heparin acts in the blood and on the clotting system, then physiological chemistry can help pharmacology to answer the following questions: (1) How can we determine the *concentrations* of heparin (or heparins if there appears to be more than one relevant substance)? (2) What is the relevant laboratory parameter to determine the *effect* of these concentrations in a sample of the patient's blood?

Simple and straightforward as this may seem, in the case of heparins the solutions are not immediately apparent. For more than half a century the necessity to treat patients has induced a pragmatic approach, based on the state of the art of many years ago. The introduction of low-molecular-weight heparins (LMWHs) renewed the interest in these matters and clearly showed that the traditional approach was in need of reworking. In recent years, the work of many groups slowly outlined the contours of what might be a rational approach to heparins (1). In this chapter we discuss these contours, aware that we suggest solutions for some of the problems existing in the field, but that have not as yet been extensively tested in practice.

The anticoagulant action of crude tissue extracts had already been observed in the 19th century. It is difficult to decide whether the substances under investigation have been heparins. Many inhibitory substances can be obtained from tissue apart from heparin, such as certain phospholipids (2), excess of procoagulant phospholipid (3), different types of peptides, including fibrin degradation products (4), thrombomodulin (5), Annexin V (6), and so forth. Usually McLean is cited as having discovered heparins, but chances are that he purified a phospholipid and that Howell, in modifying McLean's procedure, may at a given moment have found a polysaccharide with anticoagulant properties (7). Those interested in the early history of heparin are referred to the intriguing article of Jaques (8), who explains how the attempts of Howell to fit his observations in his theory of blood coagulation retarded progress in this field. Best ameliorated heparin production and purification to the extent of making it available as a drug (for the history of heparin discovery and the heparin units see Ref. 9).

Unfractionated heparin (UFH) thus has been available since the 1920s. There consequently is quite some established practice in dealing with these drugs. Howell, for example, defined a unit of anticoagulant material (heparin or not) as that amount of material that would retard coagulation of 1 ml of cat blood so much that it would only half-clot after one night in the refrigerator. Best adopted a similar unit for quantifying his heparin preparations and called it the "Howell unit." This is not only of historical interest because the U.S. Pharmacopoeia Unit (USP unit), which also is used as the international unit (IU) and in many national pharmacopoeias, is barely different from the Howell unit, being defined as that amount of heparin that retards coagulation of 1 ml of sheep plasma enough to make it half-clot after 1 hr at 37°C (8).

Heparin was used as an anticoagulant in the late 1930s. Thus the problems of clinical dose finding have by now been solved by trial and error. The different types of heparin used (e.g., bovine lung, pig mucosa) may indeed be different in many respects. They are, however, sufficiently similar to be compared by the global clotting test used for the determination of the USP unit. When LMWH were introduced as a drug by a trial in 1976 (10), it was natural that they were measured according to the principles established for UFH. These preparations contain material that, with regard to its action of blood coagulation, is comparable to UFH, but also other material that acts essentially different from the classical heparins. Different LMWHs contain these two materials in different proportions. It is therefore not surprising that the convenient correlation between in vitro retardation of coagulation of sheep plasma and in vivo pharmacological action in the human disappeared.

Research in the last few years has made it clear that the traditional way to approach heparin potency is not the most adequate one for this more complicated situation. Indeed, there is a considerable amount of confusion arising from attempts to define LMWHs in terms that were adequate to deal with UFH. In this chapter we propose a more logical approach to the clinical chemistry of heparins based on recent biochemical data. We will indicate what the differences are with the existing practice and we will show how existing practice can be brought in line with the new approach.

II. TYPES OF HEPARIN

We recall some of the structural data that are important for the understanding of the mode of action of heparin. Heparin is a mixture of linear polysaccharides consisting of alternating iduronic acid or glucoronate units and *N*-acetylglucosamine units joined by glycosidic 1–4 linkages. Most of the *N*-acetyls of the glucosamine are replaced by *N*-sulfo groups. Most iduronates are *O*-sulfated in their 2-position, most glucosamines in their 6-position [Fig. 1, from Barrowcliffe et al. (11)]. This results in a wide variety of different possible monosaccharides. They occur in almost random order, and the chain lengths can vary from 5 to 100 or more. This chemical diversity is reflected in a diversity of biological activities. There is one sequence known to date with a specific function: the pentasaccharide that causes the heparin to bind with high affinity to AT III (12, and references therein). This binding importantly increases the biological activity of the inhibitor. The structure of the active pentasaccharide has been confirmed by organic synthesis (13, 14). Heparins that contain this sequence we call high-affinity material (HAM).* Heparins that do not contain this sequence consequently do not bind specifically to AT III. This low-affinity material (LAM) as such is not active in AT III-dependent reactions but may influence the action of HAM by replacing it in nonspecific reactions (see below).

It appears (15–17) that 17 sugar units is a critical chain length: All the HAM heparins catalyze AT III-dependent factor Xa inactivation, but only the HAM longer than 17 units is capable of catalyzing thrombin inactivation. Heparin thus contains two subfractions: on the one hand, material with a chain length of 5–17 monosaccharide units (MW 1700–5400), which only catalyzes anti-factor Xa inactivation and which we call below critical chain length material (BCLM); on the other hand, material that is longer than 17 monosaccharide units (MW $>$ 5400), which catalyzes both thrombin and factor Xa inactivation and which we call above critical chain length material (ACLM) (Fig. 2). See also Figure 3 for a schematic representation of the MW distribution of different heparins.

As far as its anticoagulant properties are concerned, every heparin preparation, although always highly heterogeneous, can be regarded as composed of the

---

*1 USP unit of standard heparin is 6 μg of crude product, i.e., about 2 μg of HAM, or 0.15 nmol. 1 U/ml = 0.15 μmol. Due to the uncertainties about the molecular weight and the distribution of the molecular weight of HAM14, these are only approximate values.

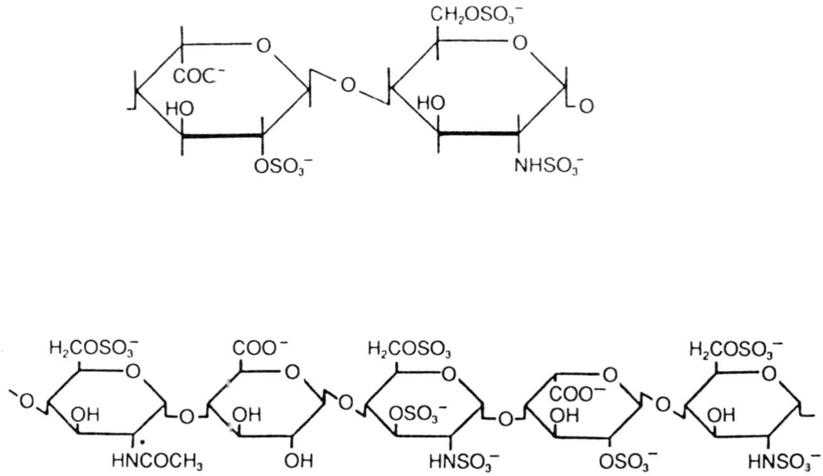

Figure 1 Structure of heparin subunits. (Top) The main repeating disaccharide subunit of heparin. (Bottom) The pentasaccharide sequence with high affinity for AT III. (From Ref. 11.)

three functionally different fractions LAM, ACLM, and BCLM (HAM is ACLM plus BCLM insofar as present). Much of the confusion existing in the field can be avoided if we realize that unfractionated heparin consists of ACLM and LAM, whereas LMWH contains a good proportion of BCLM as well (Fig. 3). It is also essential to recognize that with diminishing molecular weight, the proportion of BCLM and ACLM shifts in favor of BCLM, but also the HAM (= ACLM + BCLM) content decreases (18). As a rule, HAM represents a subpopulation of heparin molecules with a higher mean molecular weight than the total material (19).

Rendering heparin diversity by three different fractions is, of course, both a simplification of the real situation and a complication of current practice. For a logical description of the anticoagulant activity of heparin it seems to be necessary and sufficient.

Apart from anticoagulant action, two other important properties of heparin are dependent on its molecular weight: its affinity for platelet factor 4 (pf4) and its pharmacological behavior. The latter will be treated in a separate paragraph.

Platelet factor 4 is a protein contained in the α-granules of blood platelets and released when platelets are activated. Its physiological function is unknown. It binds to heparin molecules, HAM and LAM alike, with an affinity dependent on the chain length (20). From 10 to 16 saccharide units, the affinity gradually increases; above 16 units (MW ~4800) the affinity is constant and high. This

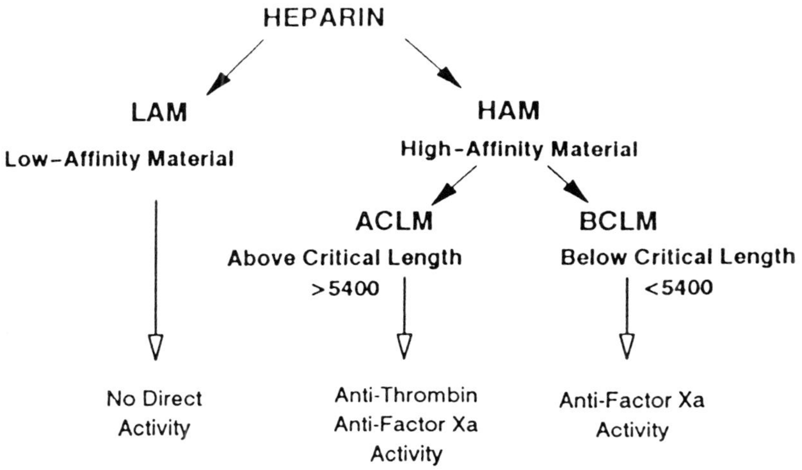

Figure 2 Subdivision of heparin species.

means that all ACLM binds maximally and is effectively neutralized. Half-neutralization requires less than 1 mol/mol, and full neutralization is observed when the ratio of pf4 to heparin molecules is 3:1 (21). For all practical purposes, the binding to ACLM may be considered irreversible; it is so strong that AT III cannot effectively compete with pf4.

BCLM escapes neutralization to a great extent because it binds to pf4 much less tightly than ACLM does. It should be stressed that pf4 binding is not dependent on the specific pentasaccharide sequence; i.e., heparin molecules of the LAM family with a sufficiently high chain length bind as tightly as ACLM (20). One of the ways in which LAM can influence heparin activity in situations where platelets are activated is precisely by their binding to pf4, which then will no longer be able to bind the catalytically active species ACLM. This may explain the potentiating effect of LAM on HAM (22).

The platelet activation that inevitably accompanies venipuncture and handling of blood samples for the clinical laboratory will always cause some pf4 to be released, which then will neutralize a certain amount of ACLM in the sample. Van Putten showed that 0.185 ± 0.072 U/ml of UFH activity on average is lost in plasma samples in the clinical laboratory (23). Apart from that, some pf4 is released from the endothelium after injection of heparin (24).

As heparin is a highly charged molecule, it will bind with a certain affinity to different positively charged plasma proteins, such as histidine-rich glycoprotein (25) and vitronectin, especially after the latter has been modified by thrombin (26–28). This binding is of comparable strength as that of AT III but yet not

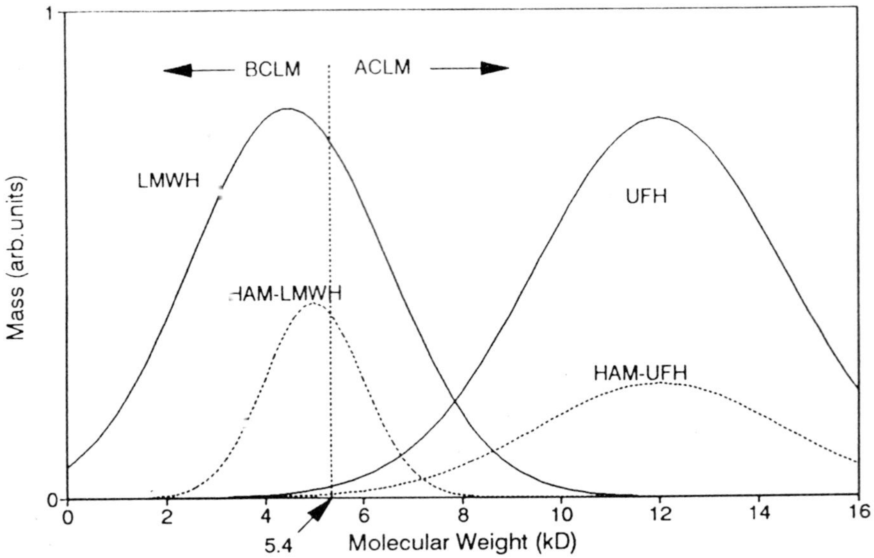

Figure 3 Schematic representation of the molecular weight distribution of different heparin species. (From Ref. 64.)

dependent on the presence of the active pentasaccharide. The HAM in a given heparin will distribute over AT III and other heparin-binding proteins in plasma. The LAM present in that heparin will bind to the other proteins. Both AT III and the other proteins occur in molar excess over heparin in therapeutic and prophylactic dosages (Table 1). The amount of HAM that binds to AT III determines the observed heparin activity. It depends on the partition of the heparin between AT III and the other proteins, which in its turn is determined by (1) the amount and the heparin affinity of AT III as compared to the amount and affinity of the other proteins, and (2) the number of heparin-binding sites on the other proteins that are occupied by LAM. This has two important consequences. First, the amount of heparin bound to AT III will be proportional to the AT III concentration, even though far from all AT III molecules will bind a heparin molecule. This is because the concentration of AT III relative to the concentration of other heparin-binding proteins will determine the probability of a free heparin molecule being bound to AT III (29). Second, LAM will occupy a certain number of binding sites for heparin on the other proteins and so make HAM material available for binding to AT III. This situation may again explain the observation that addition of LAM to HAM increases the effect of the latter (22).

Table 1 Data on Some Clotting Factors and Inhibitors

Protein	Symbol	Conc. (μM)	MW (kDa)	K_d (nM)	Peak (nM)
Prothrombin	F.II	2	66	—	200
Factor X	F.X	0.18	55	—	12
Factor IX	F.IX	0.07	70	—	2
Antithrombin III	AT III	2–3	58	5	—
Heparin cofactor II	HC II	1	65	10	—
Histidine-rich glycoprotein	HRGP	1–1.5	75	7	—
Vitronectin	Vitr.	5–5.5	75	7	—
Platelet factor 4	pf4	—	40	0.3	60

K_d is the dissociation constant for UFH in nM; kDa = kilodalton.

Peak is the approximate peak concentration of the activated factor attained in clotting plasma without heparin. For pf4 it is the amount released into platelet-rich plasma during coagulation.

III. SPECIFIC ACTIONS OF HEPARINS

It is essential to distinguish between *specific* and *composite* biological effects of heparin. The specific effects are its catalytic action on a number of well-defined biochemical reactions. The composite effects are the consequences of the specific effects in composite reaction systems. Enhancement of thrombin inactivation by AT III is one of the specific effects of heparin; prolongation of the APTT and prevention of thrombosis are two examples of composite effects.

The relative contributions of the different specific activities to the various composite effects are not exactly known as yet. There is no reason to assume that one composite action (e.g., the bleeding tendency) will depend on the specific effects (antithrombin activity, anti-thrombin Xa activity) in the same manner as another (e.g., the antithrombotic effect). This is the rationale behind the search for heparins with a more favorable distance between therapeutically active and potentially dangerous doses.

The set of specific activities of heparins is relatively large. All clotting proteases are involved (Kallikrein, Factors XIIa, XIa, Xa, IXa, and thrombin) (30–33) and two different inhibitors (AT III, HC II (34 & 35)). In practice, we do not have to deal with all of them. The contribution of HC II must be considered to be negligible (36,37) except at high concentrations of heparin, such as are seldom encountered (>5 U/ml). The effect of heparin on the inactivation of clotting factors XIa, XIIa, and kallikrein is much smaller than that on the other factors and probably without consequences for heparin action (38). Also, contact activation presumably is only of minor importance in hemostasis and thrombosis (39). These inhibitions therefore need not be considered further. We are thus left with the inactivation of thrombin, factor Xa, and factor IXa as the important specific actions of heparin.

Not all specific actions are catalyzed by the same type of heparin. There are two different families. Factors IXa and XIa follow the same pattern as thrombin inactivation (40); i.e., they are catalyzed by ACLM. Factor XIIa and kallikrein, like factor Xa, can also be catalyzed by BCLM (40). This division into two groups makes it possible to conveniently discuss the effects of ACLM and BCLM in terms of anti-factor Xa activity and antithrombin activity. A given concentration of ACLM can cause a composite effect because of its action on one or more of any of the clotting factors. It will cause an increase of the decay velocity of thrombin. Therefore, its concentration can be determined by its action on thrombin, and the magnitude of the composite effect will always correlate with the thrombin effect. In a comparable way, any global effect of BCLM will correlate with the anti-factor Xa activity.

This convenient parallelism between specific and composite actions, and therefore between composite actions among one another, has been the basis of the assessment of heparin action. It will, however, not hold as soon as mixtures of ACLM and BCLM appear. Reduction of thrombosis or induction of a bleeding tendency, for example, is an overall effect to which no doubt both ACLM and BCLM contribute, but to a different extent. Also, tests like the APTT are influenced by both ACLM and BCLM. It seems logical to assess the heparin effect in a patient by an overall test such as the APTT. This is tacitly based on the concept that the APTT would be sensitive to ACLM and to BCLM in the same way as thrombosis and bleeding are. This, however, is an unproven assumption. In fact, some substances, such as pentasaccharide and dermatan sulfate, hardly influence the APTT in doses that have a significant antithrombotic effect. Also, the prolongation of the APTT at a fixed dose of heparin is dependent on the individual plasma in which the heparin happens to be present (23).

A fixed prolongation of the APTT can be obtained by *a* ng/ml of ACLM or by *b* ng/ml of BCLM or by an infinity of mixtures of both substances (½*a* of ACLM plus ½*b* of BCLM, etc.). A given antithrombotic effect may again be obtained by *a* ng/ml of heparin in the patient's plasma, but then is not necessarily also obtained by *b* ng/ml of BCLM, but, e.g., by *c* ng/ml of BCLM. There is again an infinity of mixtures that will have the same antithrombotic effect, but this series will *not* necessarily give an identical prolongation of the APTT. This shows that the APTT can be used without problems if we deal with ACLM only (i.e., in UFH) but is no longer useful as soon as mixtures with BCLM appear, i.e., in LMWH. The only way to understand what is indicated by a given prolongation of the APTT is to determine *a* and *b* as in the example above. They will probably differ even between different types of APTT. One can imagine an ideal test that reacts to ACLM, BCLM, and all other anticoagulants in the same way as the thrombotic tendency does. For the moment we can only prove that the existing overall tests are not suitable candidates.

There is a way out of this dilemma: On basis of the specific actions on thrombin and factor Xa, we can determine the *concentrations* of ACLM and BCLM separately. This opens the possibility of studying pharmacokinetics of heparin directly, without the confusing need to compare one composite effect (e.g., APTT) to the other (e.g., bleeding).

In order to understand the quantitation of heparins on the basis of this catalytic action, we must briefly discuss the kinetics that govern this type of reactions.*

The inactivation of clotting enzymes by AT III in plasma is a bimolecular reaction ($E + A \xrightarrow{k} I$). According to standard chemical kinetics, its reaction velocity is given by $v_t = kA_tE_t$. The concentration of AT III in plasma is much higher than the highest concentration of thrombin, the most abundant enzyme in clotting plasma (AT III: 2.5 μM, thrombin about 0.2 μM at its peak). Therefore, A_t can thus be considered constant during a decay experiment, so that the decay velocity of the enzyme can be given by $v_t = kA_0E_t$, or $v = k_{dec}E_t$, where $k_{dec} = kA_0$.

The time course of E can than be given by $E_t = E_0e^{-kdec.t}$; i.e., the enzyme decays semilogarithmically. The half-life time is inversely proportional to k_{dec}; therefore, $t_{1/2} = 0.693/k_{dec}$.† The dimension of k_{dec} thus is inverse time, usually expressed in min^{-1}. Heparin catalyzes the above reaction. Although the mechanism of catalysis may be complex (41), its effect is simple: decrease of the half-life time and increase of k_{dec}. The decay constant increases proportionally to the AT III concentration and to the concentration of heparin: $k_{dec} = kAH$. This proportionality can be used to define a unit of heparin activity (see below). It should be noticed that H indicates the concentration of *active* heparin. For the decay of factor Xa, the HAM molecules count; for the decay of thrombin, only the ACLM fraction counts.

Heparins also have a number of biological activities that are not related to their anticoagulant action. They influence the growth of endothelial (42) and smooth muscle (43) cells. They also cause the release of lipoprotein lipase and tissue factor pathway inhibitor (TFPI) (44) from the vessel wall. They are neither specific nor composite effects in the sense discussed above. Here we will restrict ourselves to the effect of heparin on the blood coagulation process in plasma, because that is the basis for the assessment of the heparin effect in the clinical

---

*In the reaction equations E stands for enzyme (thrombin, factor Xa, etc.), A is AT III, I is inactive product. In the kinetic equations the same letters stand for the concentrations of these substances. The subscripts denote the time; E_0 is the enzyme concentration at zero time, and so forth.

†Because the natural logarithm of ½ equals −0.639.

laboratory. Also, the effect of nonanticoagulant actions of heparin will be difficult to establish unless the anticoagulant action can be precisely quantified. Insofar as the release effect influences overall thrombin generation, as it surely does via TFPI, it should be measured in tests that are meant to determine the overall effect and it should not influence tests that are used to measure heparin levels (see below).

IV. THE MODE OF ACTION OF HEPARINS ON THROMBIN GENERATION

Anticoagulation is the most effective way of preventing thrombosis (39). All anticoagulants have one thing in common: they diminish the amount of thrombin that is generated in clotting plasma. Occasionally an antithrombotic is announced that has no influence on blood coagulation, such as dermatan sulfate. Invariably, in our experience, such substances do not or hardly influence the APTT, but still they significantly influence the course of thrombin concentration in clotting plasma. Even aspirin need not be an exception (45). It does not seem to matter *how* the appearance of active thrombin is prevented. In principle there are two ways. Either prothrombin conversion is inhibited or thrombin inactivation is accelerated. Pentasaccharide AT III is a pure inhibitor of factor Xa, i.e., of prothrombin conversion (46). Dermatan sulfate, by enhancing the action of HC II, acts only on thrombin decay. Usually, however, the mode of action is mixed. Oral anticoagulation acts because less prothrombin is available for conversion into thrombin and conversion itself is retarded. Heparins act on all clotting enzymes, and until recently it was not clear which of its actions was the essential one. On the basis of the cascade theory of blood coagulation, it has been surmised that inhibition of factor Xa would be a more adequate way to inhibit thrombin occurrence than scavenging the thrombin by enhancing the action of AT III (47). This idea has been motivating the development of the LMWHs. Enhancing the inhibition of factor Xa relative to that of thrombin by decreasing the molecular weight of heparin was thought to be the aim. As we will see, it turned out to be false, and we will see why. Whatever the reasons for the superiority of LMWHs over UFH may be, they are not to be found in their action on the clotting mechanism per se.

The mechanism of thrombin formation is not rendered adequately by a cascade mechanism. It is a very complicated mechanism in which a number of positive and negative feedback mechanisms interact to produce a thrombin explosion that is limited both in place and in time (Fig. 4). The reader is referred to Ref. 39 for details of this mechanism. It is essential to recognize here that the product of the reaction mechanism, thrombin, both enhances and inhibits its own production. The enhancement is immediate by a direct action of thrombin on the accelerating factors V and VIII, whereas the inhibition is dependent on the

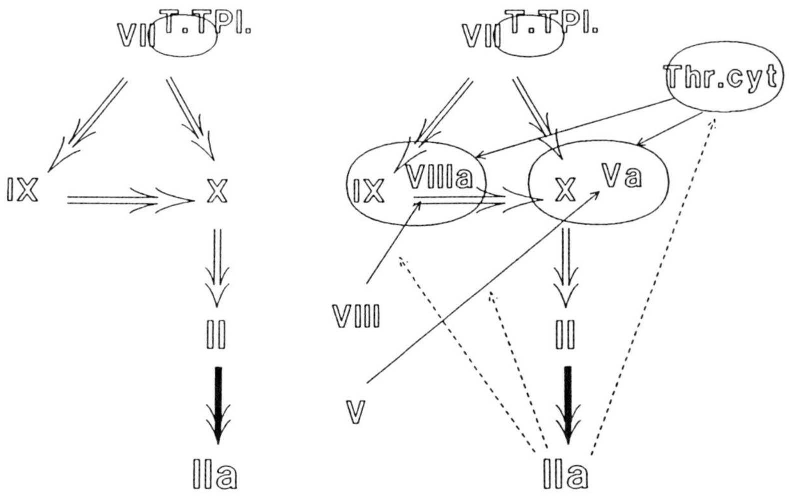

Figure 4 The clotting mechanism. (Left) The proteolytic interactions. (Right) The accelerators and feedback reactions included. Ovals indicate a phospholipid surface. (Open arrows) Proteolytic activation. (Closed arrows) Chemical conversion. (Dashed arrows) Enzymatic action. (Modified from Ref. 65.)

binding of thrombin to thrombomodulin and the activation of protein C. The important consequence for the mode of action of heparin is that accelerated thrombin disappearance in the earlier phases of the reaction will prevent the feedback activation of factors V and VIII (48–53).

We devised methods to obtain thrombin generation curves and to determine the half-life of thrombin with great precision. Via a mathematical procedure we could then, from these data, calculate the time course of prothrombin conversion (29, 54). To our surprise, it appeared that in the extrinsic system the bulk of heparin action must be attributed to its antithrombin activity (Fig. 5). This was true not only for UFH, but also for most LMWHs! It thus appeared that the enhanced inactivation of factor Xa that is undoubtedly caused by UFH and is even more important in LMWHs did not influence the coagulation mechanism very much. The reason for this unexpected finding is that factor Xa does not act as such, but as a member of the prothrombinase complex, a tripartite complex of factors Xa and Va and phospholipid. The member with the lowest concentration determines the amount of prothrombinase that can be formed. Full prothrombin conversion is observed at very low concentrations of prothrombinase: 0.3 nM. The peak concentration of factor Xa is about 12 nM, but factor Va is rate limiting in clotting plasma (51, 55). Factor Xa therefore is present in large excess,

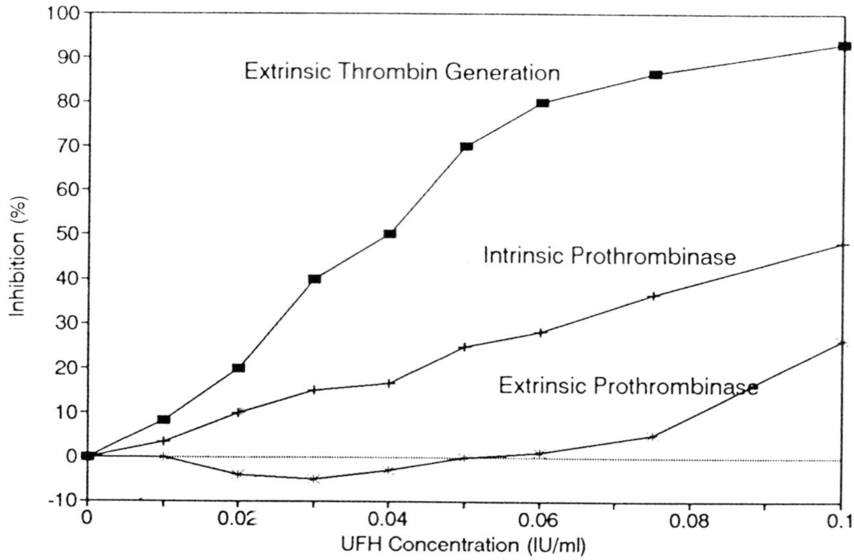

Figure 5 Inhibition of the extrinsic and the intrinsic thrombin and prothrombinase formation by heparin. (Modified from Ref. 53.)

and quite a lot of factor Xa inhibition can take place before prothrombinase is inhibited.

In the intrinsic system the inhibition of prothrombin conversion is more important than in the extrinsic system. This cannot be attributed to inhibition of factor Xa because the role of that factor is the same in the two systems. It is explained by the fact that the feedback activation of factor VIII is more sensitive to inhibition of the thrombin involved than that of factor V. The tissue factor–factor VII(a) complex of the extrinsic system is not inhibited by heparin-AT III. So in the intrinsic system the generation of factor Xa is inhibited but in the extrinsic system it is not. Further studies showed that the lag time of thrombin generation in the intrinsic system is dependent on the amount of thrombin available for the feedback activation of factor VIII and thus is prolonged in the presence of heparin (56). The amount of prothrombin eventually converted into thrombin in the intrinsic system is determined by the action of heparin on factor IXa (56). But the majority of the heparin effect also in the intrinsic system is due to direct inhibition of thrombin via AT III. From these results it is also clear why the APTT is susceptible to heparin influence: This test measures the lag time of thrombin generation in the intrinsic system. It therefore measures the time necessary for enough factor VIIIa to be formed. In other words, it is influenced by the inhibition of minute amounts of thrombin that are formed during the lag phase (Fig. 6).

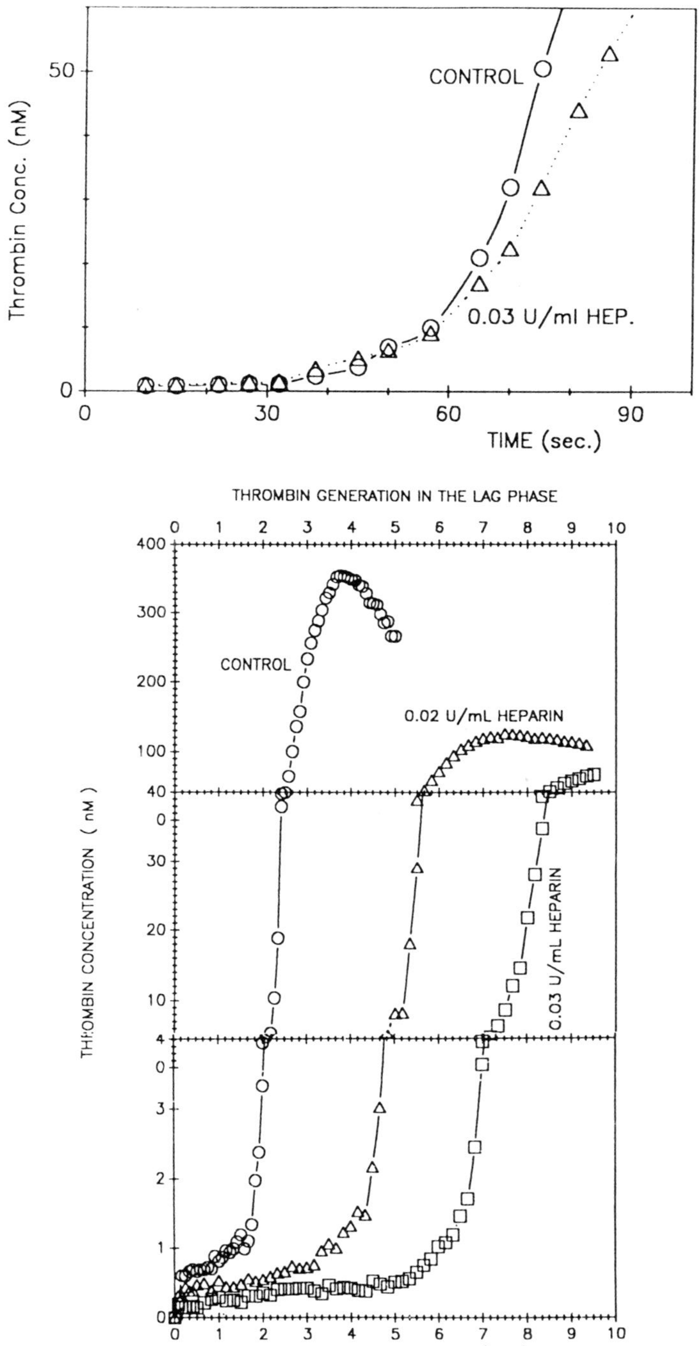

Figure 6 Early phase of thrombin formation in plasma. (Top) Extrinsic system (thromboplastin time). (Bottom) Intrinsic system (APTT). (From Ref. 66.)

In the extrinsic system no lag time of thrombin formation is seen with or without heparin. The slight prolongation of the PT that is observed is due to the fact that in the presence of heparin it takes longer to form a sufficient amount of thrombin to clot the fibrinogen present, even though thrombin formation starts directly after recalcification (53).

Compared to UFH, LMWHs are enriched in BCLM. This means that their anti-factor Xa activity will be relatively more important than their antithrombin activity. Especially when compared to a heparin standard, this effect seems impressive. By definition, 1 USP unit of standard heparin contains 1 USP unit of anti-factor Xa activity and 1 USP unit of antithrombin activity. This definition tends to obscure the fact that the anti-factor Xa activity in plasma, both in the presence and in the absence of ACLM, is always about 3 times lower than the antithrombin activity. (Table 2). The only way to enhance the anti-factor Xa activity in plasma relative to its antithrombin activity is by adding BCLM. That is what happens when LMWHs are administered. But enhancing the anti-factor Xa activity in plasma is an efficient means of inhibiting prothrombin conversion. Because factor Xa is present in excess over factor Va in clotting plasma, one can inhibit some 90% of the factor Xa activity without altering the velocity of prothrombin activation. This does not mean that it will not work. Pure BCLMs, like the synthetic pentasaccharide, can be given in such high amounts as to be efficient anticoagulants and hence efficient antithrombotics, but relatively high amounts are necessary to be effective (57). We observed that one of the LMWHs, in which the ratio BCLM/ACLM was higher than in the others, did show significant inhibition of prothrombinase (58). Indeed, there is no reason why they should not.

Other effects than the mode of action in the clotting system in platelet-poor plasma in vitro will determine whether LMWHs are useful antithrombotics. The relative enrichment of BCLM over ACLM in LMWHs may not have much influence in vitro; in vivo two circumstances favor the influence of the BCLM injected with LMWHs. First, the biological half-life time of BCLMs is signifi-

Table 2 Influence of Heparins on the Decay Constant of Thrombin and Factor Xa in Plasma

	Heparin	Factor Xa	Thrombin
No heparin	—	0.49	1.51
ACLM	UFH	4.25	13.65
BCLM	Penta	7.24	~0

The figures are in min^{-1} per μM AT III (no heparin) or in min^{-1} per μM AT III per μg heparin per ml plasma.

cantly longer than that of ACLMs (60). By this mechanism the BCLM fraction of a LMWH injected will survive longer in the circulation than the ACLM fraction, so that a "fractionation in vivo" takes place. The ratio of BCLM/ACLM in the circulation increases with time after injection. Second, activated platelets release PF4, which very efficiently neutralizes ACLM but not BCLM. Hemostasis and thrombosis inevitably entail platelet activation, hence PF4 release. In this way BCLM, but not ACLM, may escape neutralization at precisely those sites where thrombosis occurs.

V. HOW TO ASSESS THE EFFECT OF HEPARIN IN A PATIENT

As stated in the Introduction, it is of the utmost importance to dispose of a test that ex vivo, on a sample of the patient's plasma, reflects the extent of anticoagulant action in vivo. Such a test does not as yet exist, but here we would like to point to a possible candidate. Current practice provides only indirect measures that may or may not correlate with the antithrombotic effect. The prothrombin time correlates with the antithrombotic effect brought about by oral anticoagulation. The APTT indicates the effect of heparin, and so forth. The fact that different drugs, at effective concentrations, have largely different influences on these tests already indicates that neither of them can be the universal parameter that we should like to obtain. The reason for this is easy to imagine. A clotting time is essentially the time it takes before a thrombin burst takes place (60). It does not necessarily contain information about the magnitude of that burst, although it may of course do so (as in the case of the APTT at varying heparin concentrations).

It can be safely assumed that the enzymatic action of thrombin is essential in hemostasis and thrombosis and that the amount of thrombin that can act in a hemostatic or thrombotic process determines the magnitude of the hemostatic and thrombotic response (39). So what we want to know is the *amount* of thrombin formed—more precisely, the amount of thrombin formed and the time that it has the opportunity to act.

Thrombin is an enzyme, and one may expect that 1 nM of an enzyme acting for 10 sec will have the same effect as 10 nM acting for 1 sec. This means that the product of time and concentration determines the effect of thrombin. (The mathematically correct description is: the time integral of the thrombin generation curve.) A normal amount of thrombin that persists longer because of a congenital lack of antithrombin III may cause thrombosis. A tendency to thrombosis can be remedied by lowering the amount of thrombin formed via oral anticoagulation or by making a normal amount of thrombin disappear faster than normal via heparin administration.

This demonstrates that the product of concentration and time is an important variable. We called it the *thrombin potential (TP)* (61). It is not a new one; the area under the thrombin generation curve, introduced before 1950 (62), is precisely the same thing. The TP has the dimension of time multiplied by (thrombin) concentration; its value in normal plasma is around 500 nM min (61). It may depend on the experimental conditions, such as intrinsic or extrinsic clotting, but varies little if at all with thromboplastin concentration.

In our experience, all antithrombotics, including those that have little influence on the APTT (e.g., dermatan sulfate), in clinically relevant doses invariably bring about a significant decrease of the TP.

One can think of thrombin-mediated antithrombotic medication as the administration of a drug to decrease the TP value under the threshold limit of thrombogenesis but remaining above the threshold of hemostasis. It remains an open question whether the nature of the drug has an influence on the thresholds. Those who are looking for the ideal anticoagulant, one that prevents thrombosis without inhibiting hemostasis, tacitly assume that this is possible. In our opinion, this is not very likely. We think rather that the differences between drugs such as UFH and LMWH are largely due to different pharmacological properties, which means that they can be maintained more easily in the required range of plasma levels. Secondary circumstances may also intervene. Drugs that act via heparin cofactor II (dermatan sulfate, lactobionic acid) can hardly be overdosed because the plasma level of heparin cofactor II is lower than that of prothrombin, so the TP cannot be inhibited beyond a certain level.

We recently developed an easy way to determine the TP in a single spectrophotometric test (63). In this test an *inefficient* chromogenic substrate for thrombin is added to the plasma, before coagulation is triggered. The thrombin that generates and disappears will continuously convert some of the substrate, but never more than about 10% of the total amount added. In this way the final amount of chromogenic substrate converted is proportional to the concentration-time integral of thrombin.

VI. HOW TO MEASURE HEPARIN LEVELS

It is current practice to express the potency of a given heparin by comparing it to that of a standard preparation in a given clotting test. When heparin is expressed in USP units, it is assumed to be compared to the effect of a standard preparation on the clotting of sheep plasma. The outcome of any clotting test is a *composite* effect of heparin. Different combinations of ACLM and BCLM may add up to the *same final effect* on such a test. A pure BCLM, like the synthetic AT III–binding pentasaccharide, will, just like UFH, prolong the APTT or any other clotting test (except the thrombin time) to any desired length when added in high enough concentrations. Yet a given amount of pentasaccharide, which in a given clotting test is equivalent of a defined amount of standard heparin, will not automatically, in vivo, have the same antithrombotic effect as that amount of

UFH. An equivalent effect of two doses of different LMWHs in one test will not necessarily mean an equivalent effect in another test or in an in vivo situation, because LMWHs are mixtures of two fundamentally different heparins (ACLM and BCLM) that cannot be measured with the same yardstick.

Therefore, the potency of a heparin, assessed by comparison via a clotting test, is ill defined. It depends both on the nature of the standard and on the method of comparing the activities. We calculated, for example, that the activities given on the labels of LMWH vials, which are based on the current method of estimating anti-factor Xa activity (in the absence of Ca^{2+} ions), overestimate the real heparin activity in plasma 1.37–1.76 times. It is therefore necessary to define a new type of unit that allows one to express heparin activity in a standard, method-independent way.

Also, the clotting of sheep blood cannot be used to determine the heparin effect in a sample of plasma from a patient. This makes it compulsory to compare the effect in the patient's plasma to that of a standard preparation. This gives rise to the bizarre situation that LMWH in a plasma sample from a patient is compared via some type of test (e.g., an anti-factor Xa activity test) to the action of UFH in sheep blood in a quite different test. The conditions in these tests can vary so much that the behavior of heparins becomes quite different in each. The presence or absence of Ca^{2+} is often at the basis of confounding results.

The recognition of the specific actions of ACLM and BCLM on anti-factor Xa activity (both) and antithrombin activity (ACLM only) opens the possibility of a more rigorous approach. If a sample contains ACLM, then the decay of thrombin in that sample will be enhanced, or in other words, the k_{dec} of thrombin will be increased. This increase can be measured directly in min^{-1}, independent of any standard. The increase per micromole of AT III in the sample will, independent of any standard or of any method of measurement, be proportional to the amount of ACLM in the sample. The proportionality factor is the specific activity of the ACLM injected. Analogously, HAM activity can be unequivocally quantified by its anti-factor Xa activity and expressed in $min^{-1}/\mu M$ AT III, and again, via the specific anti-factor Xa activity of the HAM injected, in μg of material.

Because the decay constant, k_{dec}, is proportional to the AT III concentration and because heparin increases k_{dec} proportionally to the HAM concentration, we can define a standard, method-independent unit as: *One unit of HAM (or anti-factor Xa) activity is that amount of HAM that, in plasma with* n *μM AT III increases* k_{dec} *of factor Xa by* n *min^{-1}*.

Analogously we define: *One unit of ACLM (or antithrombin) activity is that amount of ACLM that, in plasma with* n *μM AT III increases* k_{dec} *of thrombin by* n *min^{-1}*.

It is important to note that the reaction conditions are defined to be as close as possible to the conditions in which heparin acts in vivo: normal plasma, diluted as few as the circumstances allow, and a normal concentration of free Ca^{2+} (1.15–1.32 mM).

Any LMWH preparation now can be assigned two *specific activities* (S_{ham} *and* S_{aclm}), which are simply the number of (HAM or ACLM) activity-units per unit weight (μg). The specific activity allows the determination of heparin concentrations in plasma. If we encounter a plasma sample in which we measure an anti-factor Xa activity of Z units/ml, then we can calculate the amount of HAM material as being Z/S_{ham} μg/ml. Analogously, from the antithrombin activity (say Q), we may calculate the ACLM content as Q/S_{aclm}. Finally, we can obtain BCLM from HAM minus ACLM.

For the adoption of the new unit, no important changes in everyday laboratory practice are required. Any well-designed antithrombin test is dependent on thrombin breakdown velocity only, hence will measure ACLM. Likewise, good antifactor Xa activity tests will only measure factor Xa breakdown velocity.

The results of such *monospecific* tests can be expressed directly in standard independent units. To this end one should calibrate the test against a k_{dec} ($t_{1/2}$) determination or against a heparin preparation whose potency is known in terms of SI units. This brings back the heparin standard, but this time it is no longer the standard that defines the unit. The standard is now a tool for calibration that can be abandoned by those who prefer to measure k_{dec} ($t_{1/2}$) directly. Hence the definition of the unit is no longer dependent on the standard or on the method by which the standard and the sample are compared.

A suitable ACLM preparation can be used to calibrate both anti-factor Xa tests in terms of SIU Xa and antithrombin tests in terms of SIU IIa. To determine wether the test under observation is indeed monospecific, a BCLM standard can be used. A monospecific antithrombin test will not react to BCLM at all. A monospecific anti-factor Xa test will give the same result with an ACLM and a BCLM standard.

Once the suitable calibrations are carried out, monospecific anti-factor Xa tests can then be used to determine the HAM level in samples (in μg/ml of plasma, if the specific activity of the HAM material injected is known), and monospecific anti-thrombin tests can be used to determine ACLM levels (again in μg/ml of plasma, if the specific activity of the ACLM material injected is known).

VII. CONSEQUENCES FOR HEPARIN PHARMACOKINETICS AND PHARMACODYNAMICS

The most compelling question about LMWHs was whether they were better drugs than UFHs. A number of clinical studies, referred to in other chapters, seem to point in that direction. The next question is how to explain this phenomenon. The bottom line of our biochemical studies on the mechanism of action of heparins in plasma is that LMWHs are rather more like UFHs than one would like to admit at first sight. Anyhow, as discussed above, the fact that thrombin is inhibited seems to be more important for thrombosis and hemostasis than the mechanism responsible for this inhibition.

Rather than in the biochemistry per se, we think that the difference between LMWHs and UFHs is to be found in their different pharmacological behavior. This makes it compulsory to have exact information about this behavior. A large amount of data is available in this field. Interpretation, however, sometimes poses a problem. It is not always possible to distinguish between effects on the blood levels of active materials and the consequences of these levels for functional clotting tests.

Often the effect of heparin on a blood coagulation test has been investigated rather than the amount of heparin present. The existing data on antithrombin and anti-factor Xa activity levels after heparin injection contain the relevant information. When expressed in international (= USP) (antithrombin or anti-factor Xa) units, they give levels that are proportional to, respectively, the ACLM and the HAM levels. The proportionality factor is different for the two substances, and the BCLM levels cannot immediately be calculated from the difference of the two curves. This is regrettable because the presence of BCLM constitutes the essential difference between UFH and the LMWHs, and the most important differences between the LMWHs are in the ratio ACLM/BCLM. The use of standard independent units and the determination of specific heparin activities enable us to assess separately the levels of ACLM and BCLM in the circulation. This means that we can discuss heparin pharmacokinetics in terms of concentrations of active molecules. Only then can we in a meaningful way discuss the effects of these concentrations on composite phenomena such as clotting times, thrombin formation, thrombus growth, and bleeding tendency. In this way it is possible to separate heparin pharmacokinetics from its pharmacodynamics.

It may be possible that the specific activity, when expressed per mole of active material (i.e., HAM for anti-factor Xa activity), is very similar for highly different heparin preparations. In six UFH and LMWH preparations of different origin, in which the specific activities ranged from 0.71 to 4.25 SIU Xa/μg crude material, the mean specific activity was 87 ± 13 SIU Xa per nM HAM.

In a completely analogous way, we can determine the specific antithrombin activity of a heparin. Again, from the specific activity of the crude material, one can calculate the specific activity per mole of active heparin species, i.e., of the ACLM fraction. It again seems that the specific antithrombin activity of ACLM molecules could be similar for different types of heparin (305 ± 54 SIU IIa per nM ACLM).

The constant specific activity at first sight may seem to contradict earlier findings that reported a gradual change of potency of heparin preparations with mean molecular weight (see Ref. 11 for a detailed discussion). However, in these publications the activities were expressed per unit weight of crude material, which does not take into account that the amount of active material decreases proportional to the mean molecular weight of the preparation (18). If our conjecture on the identical specific activity of all HAM is true, then the SIU Xa value would indicate the number of active HAM molecules in the sample independent of the type of heparin injected. Analogously, the ACLM level can be obtained from the SIU IIa value.

For this approach it is necessary that the heparin that is injected is well characterized as to its biochemical actions on the clotting system ex vivo.

The following data are minimally required:

1. Content of high-affinity material (% HAM).
2. Distribution of the high-affinity material around the 5400-Da limit, i.e., % ACLM and % BCLM in the HAM.
3. Specific anti-factor Xa activity of the HAM fraction.
4. Specific antithrombin activity of the ACLM fraction. Optionally the specific anti-factor Xa activity of the ACLM and the BCLM fractions may be given.

When these data are known, it is possible to express the results of common antithrombin and anti-factor Xa activity tests in terms of circulating concentrations of active (ACLM and BCLM) heparin. Also, these data will give insight in the as-yet-unsolved question of whether the different LMWH preparations have essentially different activities or differ only in their relative contents of ACLM and BCLM.

Only when a precise description is given of the pharmacology of the anticoagulant substances in UFH and the LMWHs can we start to answer the question of the importance of nonanticoagulant actions of heparin for its antithrombotic effects.

REFERENCES

1. Hemker HC, Béguin S. Nouv Rev Fr Haematol 1992; 34:5–9.
2. Kahn M, Bourgain R. Thrombine. Arch Int Pharmacodyn 1964; 149(1–2):285–289.
3. Hemker HC, Esnouf MP, Hemker PW, Swart ACW, MacFarlane RG. Nature 1967; 215:248–251.
4. Arnesen H, Godal H Chr. Scand J Haematol 1973; 10:232–240.
5. Esmon CT, Esmon NL, Harris KW J Biol Chem 1982; 257(14):7944–7947.
6. Reutelingsperger CPM, Hornstra G, Hemker HC. Cord Eur J Biochem 1985; 151:625–629.
7. Howell WH. Blood. Am J Physiol 1925; 71:553–562.
8. Jaques LB. Semin Thromb Haemost 1978; 4(4):350–353.
9. Duclos JP. L'Héparine, Fabrication, Structure, Propriétés, Analyse Paris: Masson, 1984:233–308.

10. Johnson EA, Kirkwood TBL, Stirling Y, Perez-Requejo JL, Ingram GIC, Bangham DR, Brozovic M. Thromb Haemost 1976; 35:586–591.
11. Barrowcliffe TW, Johnson EA, Thomas DP. Chichester, UK: Wiley, 1992.
12. Casu B. Adv Carboh Chem Biochem 1985; 43:51–134.
13. Choay J, Petitou M, Lormeau JC, Sinay P, Casu B, Gatti G. Biochem Biophys Res Commun 1983; 116:492–499.
14. Petitou M. Nouv Rev Franc Hematol 1984; 26:221–226.
15. Thomas DP, Merton RE, Barrowcliffe TW, Thunberg L, Lindahl U. Thromb Haemost 1982; 47:244–248.
16. Barrowcliffe TW, Merton RE, Havercroft SJ, Thunberg L, Lindahl U, Thomas DP. Thromb Res 1984; 34:125–133.
17. Lane DA, Denton J, Flynn AM, Thunberg L, Lindahl U. Biochem J 1984; 218:725–732.
18. Bendetowicz AV, Pacaud E, Béguin S, Uzan A, Hemker HC. Thromb Haemost 1992.
19. Béguin S, Wielders S, Lormeau JC, Hemker HC. Thromb Haemost 1992; 67(1):33–41.
20. Niewiarowski S, Rucinski B, James P, Lindahl U. FEBS Lett 1979; 102:75.
21. Lane DA, Denton J, Flynn AM, Thunberg L, Lindahl U. Biochem J 1984; 218:725–732.
22. Barrowcliffe TW, Merton RE, Havercroft SJ, Thunberg L, Lindahl U, Thomas DP. Thromb Res 1984; 34:125–133.
23. Putten van J, Ruit-van-de M, Beunis M, Hemker HC. Haemostasis 1984; 14:253–261.
24. Dawes J, Pumprey CW, McLaren KM, Prowse CV, Pepper DS. Thromb Res 1982; 27:65–76.
25. Lijnen HR, Hoylaerts M, Collen D. J Biol Chem 1983; 258:3803–3808.
26. Preissner KT, Wassmuth R, Muller-Berghaus G. Biochem J 1985; 213:349–355.
27. Lane DA, Flynn AM, Pejler G, Lindahl U, Choay J, Preissner K. J Biol Chem 1987; 262:16343–16348.
28. Preissner KT, Muller-Berghaus G. J Biol Chem 1987; 262:12247–12253.
29. Béguin S, Dol F, Hemker HC. Thromb Haemost 1991; 65(6):912.
30. Abilgaard U. Scand J Clin Lab Invest 1968; 21:89–91.
31. Yin ET, Wessler S, Stoll PJ. J Biol Chem 1971; 246:3703–3711.
32. Rosenberg RD, Damus PS. J Biol Chem 1973; 248:3703–3711.
33. Rosenberg RD. N Engl J Med 1975; 292:146–151.
34. Briginshaw GF, Shanberge JN. Arch Biochem Biophys 1974; 161:683–690.
35. Tollefsen DM, Blank MK. J Clin Invest 1981; 68:589–593.
36. Tollefsen DM. In: Lane DA, Lindahl U, eds. Heparin. Chemical and Biological Properties; Clinical Application. London: Edward Arnold, 1989:257–274.
37. Bray B, Lane DA, Freyssinet J-M, Pejler G, Lindahl U. Biochem J 1989; 262:225–232.
38. Colman RW, Scott CF, Pixley RA, De La Cadena RA. Acad Sci 1989; 556:95–103.
39. Hemker HC. In: Bloom AL, et al, eds. Haemostasis and Thrombosis. London: Churchill Livingstone, 1993 (in press).
40. Holmer E, Kurachi K, Soderstrom G. Biochem J 1981; 193:395–400.
41. Olson ST, Shore JD. J Biol Chem 1986; 261:13151–13159.
42. Mascellani G, Bianchini P. WO Patent no. 8606729, 1986.

43. Barrowcliffe TW, Curtis AD, Tomlinson TP, Hubbard AR, Johnson EA, Thomas DP. Thromb Haemost 1985; 54:675–679.
44. Sandset M, Abildgaard U, Larsen ML. Thromb Res 1988; 50:803–813.
45. Kessels H, Béguin S, Hemker HC. Thromb Haemost 1991; 65(6):783.
46. Béguin S, Choay J, Hemker HC. Thromb Haemost 1989; 61:397–401.
47. Yin ET, Wessler S, Stoll PJ. J Biol Chem 1971; 246(11):3712–3719.
48. Ofosu FA, Barrowcliffe TW. Bailliere's Clin Haematol 1990; 3:505–530.
49. Ofosu FA, Blajchman MA, Modi GJ, Smith LM, Buchanan MR, Hirsh J. Br J Haematol 1985; 60:695–704.
50. Ofosu FA, Hirsh J, Esmon CT, Modi GJ, Smith LM, Anvari N, Buchanan MR, Fenton JW, Blajchman MA. Biochem J 1989; 257:143–150.
51. Hemker HC, Verstraete M, Vermylen J, Arnout J, eds. Thrombosis Haemostasis. Leuven: Leuven University Press, 1987:17–36.
52. Béguin S. Thrombinoscopy—a method for the determination of prothrombinase activity in plasma, its application to the study of different types of heparin. Ph.D. thesis, Maastricht, 1987.
53. Béguin S, Lindhout T, Hemker HC. Thromb Haemost 1988; 60:457–462.
54. Hemker HC, Willems GM, Béguin S. Thromb Haemost 1986; 56:9–17.
55. Pieters J, Lindhout T. Blood 1988; 72:2048–2052.
56. Béguin S, Dol F, Hemker HC. Thromb Haemost 1991; 66(3):306–309.
57. Walenga J, Petitou M, Lormeau JC, Samama M, Fareed J, Choay J. Thromb Res 1987; 46:187–198.
58. Béguin S, Mardiguian J, Lindhout T, Hemker HC. Thromb Haemost 1989; 61:25–29.
59. Hemker HC, Béguin S, Bendetowicz AV, Wielders S. Thromb Haemost 1991; 65(6):845.
60. Béguin S, Lindhout T, Hemker HC. Thromb Haemostas 1989; 61:25–29.
61. Hemker HC, Béguin S, Wielders S, Wagenvoord R. In: Bounameaux H, Samama M, ten Cate JW, eds. Fraxiparine, Second International Symposium Recent Pharmacological and Clinical Data, Monte Carlo, October 21, 1998.
62. Biggs R, MacFarlane RG. Human Blood Coagulation and Its Disorders. Oxford: Blackwell Scientific Publications, 1953.
63. Hemker HC, Wielders S, Kessles H, Béguin S. Thromb Haemost (submitted).
64. Hemker HC, Béguin S. Thromb Haemost (submitted).
65. Hemker HC, Béguin S. Ann Pharm Fran 1992; 50:121–135.
66. Hemker HC, Béguin S. In: Lane DA, et al, eds. Heparin and Related Polysaccharides. New York: Plenum Press, 1992.

3

Laboratory Control of Low-Molecular-Weight Heparins

Needs and Possibilities

Martine Alhenc-Gelas and Martine Aiach
Hôpital Broussais, Paris, France

I. INTRODUCTION

The low-molecular-weight heparins (LMWHs) inhibit blood coagulation by potentiating the antiprotease activity of antithrombin III (AT III). Their anti-Xa activity depends only on the presence of the specific AT III-binding pentasaccharide domain. For catalysis of thrombin inactivation, simultaneous binding of thrombin on heparin chains is necessary. This binding occurs only on heparin molecules having a length of 18 monosaccharides or more (Fig. 1) (1). As LMWH preparations contain mainly short chains, they are poorly able to enhance thrombin inhibition and to prolong the clotting time of global coagulation tests like the activated partial thromboplastin time (APTT). By contrast, they are powerful enhancers of the anti-Xa activity of AT III.

LMWHs are increasingly being used in the treatment of thrombosis because they are as efficient as heparin and because they offer pharmacokinetic advantages over heparin, mainly an increased bioavailability and a longer half-life, which allows a reduction in the number of injections and in laboratory monitoring.

Plasma anti-Xa activity assay is the only method available to date to monitor the patients in clinical laboratories. At present, methods for assessment of the in vivo action of LMWHs are not available. In curative treatments, at weight-adapted dosages, no or relatively minor bleeding occurs (2). Daily monitoring is therefore generally unnecessary. However, as the risk of bleeding (which is the main side effect of LMWH administration) remains—essentially in curative treatments—laboratory control will be necessary in the following circumstances:

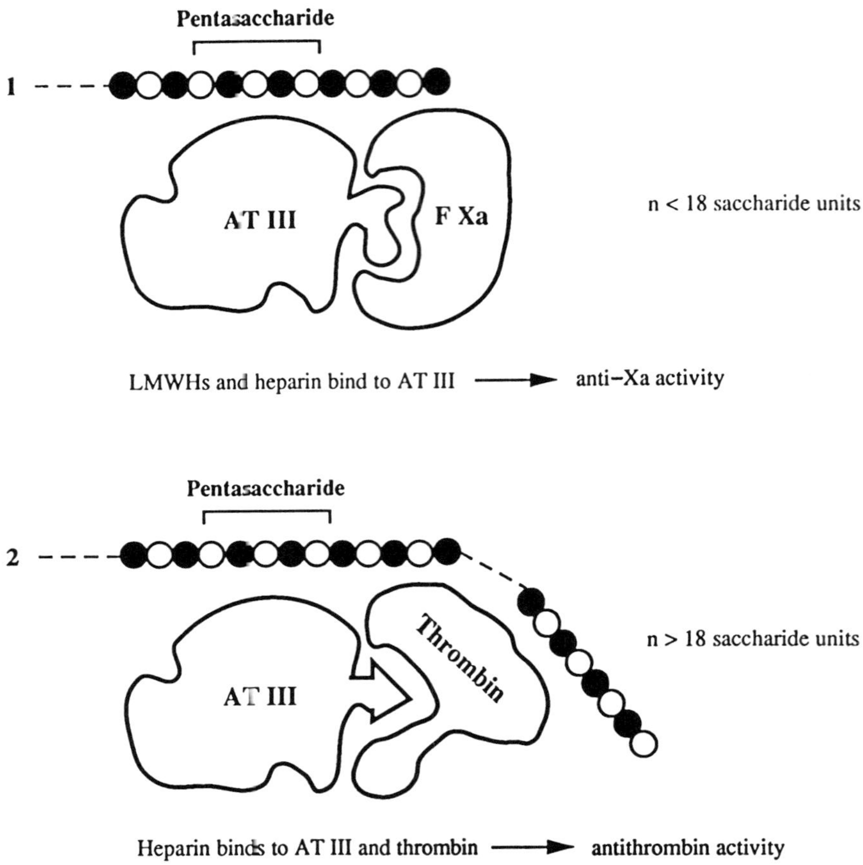

Figure 1 Specific antiprotease activities of heparins. (From Ref. 2.)

In patients in whom pharmacokinetic parameters may differ from normal, such as overweight patients or in the case of renal insufficiency

In patients at risk for hemorrhage, such as patients needing curative treatment soon after surgery

The development of tests measuring molecular markers of hemostasis activation or evaluating the ''endogeneous thrombin potential'' may provide useful information on the overall polycomponent actions of LMWHs (see also Chapters 1 and 2).

These measurements may be useful: (1) to clarify the mechanisms through which LMWHs produce their clinical effects, and (2) to define therapeutic ranges by using methods better reflecting antithrombotic activity.

We will discuss: (1) methods used to date for laboratory monitoring, and (2) new possibilities, mainly determination of the endogeneous thrombin potential determination and assays of molecular markers of thrombin generation and fibrin formation or degradation.

II. ASSAY METHODS CURRENTLY USED

The global clotting assays such as APTT have been used successfully for clinical monitoring and potency evaluation of unfractionated heparin (UFH). However, the same assays reveal little or no activity of LMWHs. Thus other, more sensitive assays are required to investigate the known measurable actions of LMWHs. Several assays have been developed to measure the anti-Xa and antithrombin actions of these agents. The anti-Xa amidolytic assays are the most commonly used in clinical practice.

A. Anti-Xa Assays

The two major types of anti-Xa assays are clotting and amidolytic assays. Their principles depend on the method used to assess residual factor Xa (Table 1).

1. Anti-Xa Clotting Assays

There are three anti-Xa clotting assays. In all these methods, a fixed quantity of bovine F Xa is added to human plasma containing LMWH. After a defined incubation time, the residual F Xa is assessed: (a) by subsampling into a clotting mixture consisting of cephalin and anticoagulant free bovine plasma (3) or of platelet substitute and bovine F X-deficient plasma (4), or (b) by addition of phospholipid and $CaCl_2$ to the mixture and measurement of the clotting time (5).

The two first assays are not easily performed. For the last one, three kits are available commercially in France (Heptest from Haemachem, Staclot heparin from Diagnostica Stago, Heparimat from Biomérieux). In these Heptest-type assays, heparin is not diluted by subsampling, so it may have an influence on prothrombin activation and thrombin inhibition as well as inhibition of F Xa (5). It has recently been demonstrated that the clotting times measured in Heptest will also reflect the plasma tissue factor pathway inhibitor (TFPI) concentration when the incubation time is prolonged to 300 sec (6). These techniques are therefore less specific than the other methods. A good correlation between the Heptest clotting time and an amidolytic anti-Xa activity has been reported in several studies for plasma samples obtained from patients treated with heparin or LMWHs (7, 8). However, the usefulness of these methods as general assay methods for LMWH has not been established.

Table 1 Principles of the Anti-Xa Assays

Anti-Xa clotting assays
With subsampling
1. Plasma + bovine F Xa
2. Incubation 2–5 min
3. Subsampling into a clotting mixture
→ coagulation time
Without subsampling
1. Plasma + bovine F Xa
2. Incubation 2 min
3. Addition of a clotting mixture
→ coagulation time
Anti-Xa amidolytic assays
Two-step assays
1. Plasma (with or without added AT III) + bovine or human F Xa
2. Incubation < 2 min
3. Addition of the chromogenic substrate
4. Optical density measurement
One-step assays
1. Plasma + chromogenic substrate + F Xa
2. Optical density measurement

2. *Anti-Xa Amidolytic Assays*

Synthetic substrates using amidolytic activity to specifically measure the enzymatic activity of the hemostatic proteases have been developed over the past few years. Numerous versions of the anti-Xa assay have been introduced for control of the LMWH therapy in clinical laboratories. Many chromogenic substrates have been designed, allowing enzymatic degradation of the substrate to be detected by simple colorimetric methods. Amidolytic assays have three major advantages:

They are specific for the activity of a given protease.
They use an enzymatic reaction whose kinetics can be defined.
They can usually be automated and adapted to instrumentation currently available in most clinical laboratories (Table 2).

Most assay procedures rely on a two-step technique:

The velocity of F Xa inhibition, which depends on the amount of LMWH present, is measured by incubating the sample with an excess of purified F Xa for a given time. Bovine F Xa is currently used. It is often preferred to human F Xa because of easier availability and increased sensitivity (9). The incubation time between the F Xa and plasma should be kept short so that the contribution of AT III in the absence of heparin is minimized. An

Table 2 Advantages and Disadvantages of Anti-Xa Activity Assays

Method	Advantages	Disadvantages
Clotting assay		
Two steps	Specificity Narrow range of linearity: 0–0.2 IU/ml	No kit available Defibrination step (Denson) Not automatized
One step	Kits available Easy to perform Range of linearity: 0–1 IU/ml	Not validated in clinical studies
Amidolytic assay	Kits available Specificity Automatization Low coefficient of variation Kinetics well defined	No correlation with antithrombotic activity Help to evaluate the hemorrhagic risk

incubation time up to 2 min is convenient and gives steep dose-response curves.

The residual F Xa activity is then evaluated after addition of a synthetic substrate. Several synthetic substrates for F Xa are commercially available. The choice of substrate has no influence on the final assay result. The velocity of chromogenic substrate hydrolysis is recorded as the increase in optical density.

As in any assay aimed at measuring an enzymatic activity, the assay conditions must be strictly defined. Some crucial steps must be emphasized:

Protease inhibition must be measured in the presence of excess amounts of AT III. To ensure pseudo first-order reaction kinetics, the AT III concentration should be at least 10 times the F Xa concentration. In several assays the plasma of the patients is supplemented with purified AT III.

The amount of substrate added must be high enough to allow measurement of the initial velocity of substrate hydrolyis.

The ionic strength, the pH, and the temperature must be rigorously defined and kept constant (10).

In some other assays (one-time assays), both protease and substrate are added simultaneously to the sample. The substrate competes with AT III for protease binding and thus the reaction is much more complex than in a two-step reaction (11).

Table 3 Comparison of Methods for Anti-Xa Amidolytic Assay

	Berichrom	Stachrom	Heparichrom	Rotachrom
Plasma	25 μl	25 μl	20 μl	25 μl
Human AT III, 1 IU/ml	25 μl			
F Xa	25 μl (human)	250 μl (bovine, 11.2 nkat/ml)		
Incubation time	60 sec	60 sec		
Chromogenic substrate	50 μl (ZD-Leu-Gly-Arg-ANBA-methylamide, 4 mM/L)	50 μl (CBS 3139: CH_3SO_2 D-Leu-Gly-Arg-pNA, ACOH, 3.2 μM/ml)	250 μl (CH3OCO D-CHG-Gly-Arg-pNA, 0.36 μM/ml)	200 μl (CBS 4803: CH30C0 D-Leu-Gly-Arg-pNA, ACOH, 0.58 mg/ml)
Incubation time			60 sec	120 sec
F Xa			75 μl (bovine, 18 nkat/ml)	200 μl (bovine, 1.68 IU/ml)
OD measurement during	60 sec	60 sec	120 sec	100 sec

Many chromogenic substrates kits are commercially available for anti-Xa activity measurements. In a recent study, we measured anti-Xa activity in plasma from 45 patients treated with LMWHs (anti-Xa activity between 0.02 and 1.2 IU/ml) using reagents from four different manufacturers (Stachrom heparin and Rotachrom heparin from Diagnostica Stago, Heparichrom from Biomérieux, Berichrom heparin from Behring). Reaction conditions are described in Table 3. Bovine F Xa was used in the first three kits. Human F Xa was used in Behring's kit. Using Rotachrom or Heparichrom, chromogenic substrate is added first to plasma before F Xa.

Calibration curves obtained using bovine F Xa were, as previously described, steeper than calibration curves obtained using human F Xa (Fig. 2).

Analysis of variance revealed a statistically significant difference between results of the four assays ($p < 0.001$).

Calibration curves have to be used in all the anti-Xa assays. In the initial studies, LMWHs were assayed against the 4th international standard (IS) for UFH. The slopes of the log-dose response lines were significantly different for the LMWHs and for this standard, and the interlaboratory variability was too high (12). It was therefore decided to proceed with the establishment of an IS

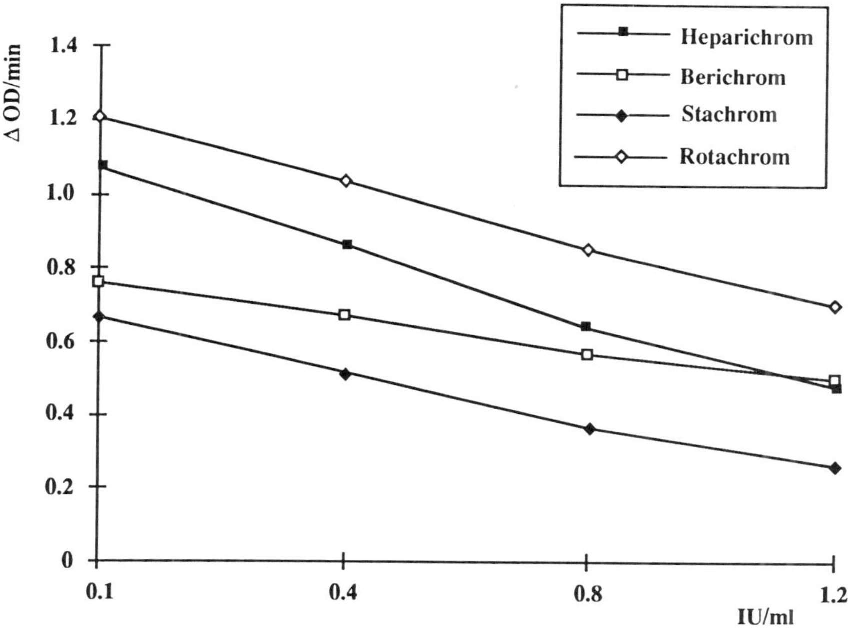

Figure 2 Calibration curves.

for LMWHs. Collaborative studies permitted the selection of a standard material with properties similar to the greatest number of LMWHs used clinically at this time. Twenty-five laboratories in 13 countries participated in the study. Potencies were determined as means of at least four independent assays with six different methods carried out in these laboratories, but against the 4th IS for UFH (13). This standard has therefore only an approximative value as it has been established by comparing materials that do not behave identically.

B. Antithrombin Assays

1. Thrombin Clotting Time

Thrombin clotting time is not often used to evaluate LMWH potency. It is not very prolonged when therapeutic levels of LMWH are achieved. Precise and reproducible measurements are, moreover, difficult to carry out in the presence of heparins.

2. Antithrombin Amidolytic Assay

The principle of this method is the same as that of the anti-Xa amidolytic assay. Thrombin is incubated for a short time with heparinized plasma, and residual thrombin activity is determined by addition of or subsampling into a chromogenic substrate for thrombin.

This test is not used to monitor treatment as antithrombin and anti-Xa activities display parallel behaviors during treatment and as low plasma antithrombin levels found are more difficult to measure accurately than anti-Xa activities.

The problems of standardization are the same as for anti-Xa assays.

III. CLINICAL USEFULNESS OF CURRENT LABORATORY MONITORING

The anti-Xa activity was first demonstrated in pharmacokinetic studies to be the best marker available of the presence of circulating LMWH. The anti-Xa amidolytic assay was then used in the first clinical studies aimed at determining efficient and safe dosages of the drugs.

A number of LMWHs have then been developed commercially and are licensed for clinical use in Europe (14). With the dosages used for the prevention of venous thrombosis, no laboratory control is necessary. In the treatment of established venous thrombosis, when higher dosages of the drug are administered, it is recommended by the manufacturer to perform a control of plasma anti-Xa activity at the beginning of the treatment to assess the individual response. For example, at the beginning of a curative treatment, injections of 120 IU anti-Xa per kg hr of Fragmin are administered twice daily to patients. It has been recommended that the dosage be adjusted to achieve an anti-Xa activity measured between 3 and 4 hr after injection in the range of 0.5–1 IU/ml. Most often, adjustment of dosage is not or is seldom required because individual responses are very similar.

The usefulness of laboratory monitoring seems highly questionable today because LMWHs were found effective and safe in the prevention and also in the treatment of deep venous thrombosis (DVT) by using fixed or weight-adapted dosages without laboratory monitoring (for review, see Ref. 2).

Moreover, the usefulness of anti-Xa activity measurements is also questionable for the following reasons:

1. For many authors, anti-Xa activity does not reflect antithrombotic activity: Holm et al. reported that improvement of the Marder score was independent of anti-Xa levels (14). Janvier et al., in an open study using Enoxaparin, did not observe any relationship between the anti-Xa activity and the changes in venograms, even among patients with less than 0.5 IU/ml (15). However, Levine et al. found a significant relationship between the anti-Xa level and the clinical outcome (16). Recently, in a multicentric study using curative dosages of Fragmin, we found a statistically significant correlation between

the anti-Xa activity and the Marder score reduction. Moreover, the efficacy of the treatment, as judged by the Marder score, seemed to be optimized by ensuring circulating activities at day 2 of treatment between 0.7 and 1 IU/ml, 3 hr after injection (17).

2. A correlation between the anti-Xa level and the hemorrhagic risk is not firmly established. However, Nieuwenhuis et al. reported an increased risk of bleeding for anti-Xa levels greater than 0.8 IU/ml. The risk of major bleeding increased from 8% for anti-Xa levels between 0.8 and 1 IU/ml to 50% for anti-Xa levels measured after the first injection greater than 1 IU/ml (18).

In a recently published study, it was appropriately pointed out that for successful and safe treatment of DVT with Fragmin, the impression is now that "the choice of an adequate Fragmin dose is more important that the adjustment of dose after anti Xa determinations" (19).

IV. NEW METHODOLOGIES

A. Endogeneous Thrombin Potential Evaluation

A computed assisted technique that permits a detailed analysis of thrombin generation curves obtained in whole plasma was recently described by Hemker et al. (20).

In this system, specific enzymatic reactions and nonspecific interactions between LMWH and plasma proteins are both evaluated. Reaction conditions are defined to be as close as possible to the in vivo conditions. Studies undertaken using this method permit the authors to postulate that to evaluate the *amount* of thrombin generated in plasma of heparinized patients during the coagulation process could give an estimation of the antithrombotic potency of the LMWHs. The *time* during which thrombin remains active during coagulation is another important factor.

Hemker et al. postulated that the area under the thrombin generation curve, named "endogeneous thrombin potential," is the parameter that must be measured (21).

It must be pointed out that correlation between determinations of the endogeneous thrombin potential and the occurrence of thrombosis has not to date been demonstrated in clinical studies. The development of a simplified spectophotometric test is absolutely necessary for routine use.

B. "Real" Specific Activities Determinations: The Choice of an Appropriate Unit System Improving Standardization

Using the same technique, Béguin et al. recently demonstrated that both in the absence and in the presence of heparin, the rate of AT III-dependent thrombin decay during the course of coagulation in plasma is proportional to the amount of AT III present. On this basis, they defined standard independent units (SIU) of heparins: 1 SIU of heparin antithrombin activity is the concentration of heparin that increases the decay constant of thrombin in plasma by one inverse minute per μM of available AT III.

The specific activity of a given heparin will therefore be expressed in SIU per unit weight of heparin. Anti-Xa activity can be treated analogously. Using this procedure to express heparin-specific activities makes it possible to be independent of an arbitrary chosen standard and of the test used to determine activity (22).

C. Assays of Molecular Markers of Coagulation Activation

A number of highly sensitive and specific tests measuring markers of the activation of the hemostatic system have recently become available. Among them, fragment 1 + 2 (F_{1+2}) measures the prothrombin molecule cleavage by F Xa, and fibrinopeptide A and thrombin–AT III complexes reflect an in vivo thrombin generation. The proteolytic action of plasmin on fibrin polymer cross-linked by F XIII generates increased levels of D-dimers in the plasma (Fig. 3).

It is thus possible to accurately define a hypercoagulable state and to detect fibrin deposition in the vascular system. The plasma levels of these markers are usually increased in the acute phase of thrombosis. Investigation of the effects of heparin treatments on the plasma levels of these markers in clinical trials could help to explain their antithrombotic effects.

Walenga et al. recently reported anti-Xa activities and F_{1+2} levels measured in two groups of postsurgical patients treated subcutaneous by with either a single daily dose of Fraxiparine (7500 ICU) or three daily dosages of Calciparin (5000 IU). Both groups of patients exhibited relatively high levels of F_{1+2} fragment on the first day of treatment. Then, F_{1+2} gradually decreased. The results were identical in both groups. In comparison, anti-Xa activity was different in the two groups. As the clinical outcome was not significantly different in both groups, it seemed clinically relevant to quantitate this marker (23). In a trial using Logiparin to prevent thrombosis in patients undergoing total hip replacement, thrombin generation evaluated with F_{1+2} measurements was also decreased by LMWH treatment. However, in this study, postoperative F_{1+2} levels in patients with thromboembolic complications were not significantly different from F_{1+2} levels in patients without complications (24). Ireland et al. studied the efficacy of four different LMWHs (Innohep, Fragmin, Org 10172, CY 222) in hemodialysis, measuring levels of FPA generated during the process and plasma anti-Xa activities. FPA and anti-Xa levels were significantly correlated. They concluded that anti-Xa activity is related to the antithrombotic effects of these compounds (25).

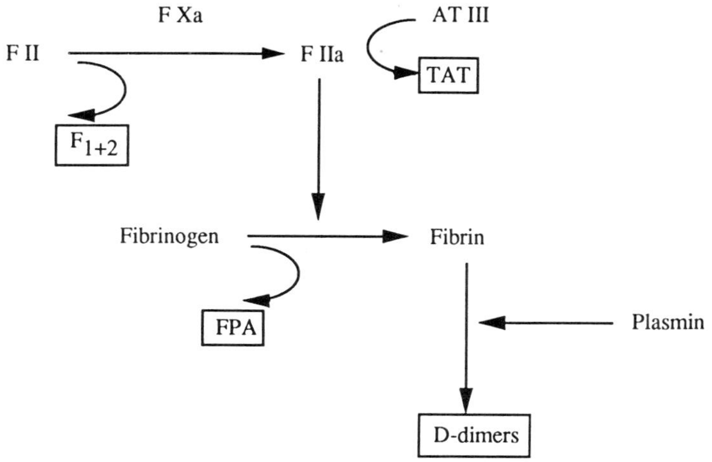

Figure 3 Simplified view of the last steps of fibrin formation and of fibrin degradation. (☐) Molecular markers of hemostatic disorders accessible to measurement.

V. POTENTIAL USEFULNESS OF THE NEW METHODOLOGIES

The LMWH treatments are to date efficient and safe even if their antithrombotic activity cannot be evaluated with the laboratory techniques currently used. The new techniques described here should therefore probably not modify routine laboratory monitoring. However, on one hand, using these techniques in large clinical studies will perhaps help to determine if lower dosages of LMWHs are as efficient as dosages administered to date. However, the results of F_{1+2} measurements reported above are rather discordant. On the other hand, using the procedure described by Béguin et al. to determine specific activities independently of an arbitrary chosen standard will help to precisely characterize these drugs.

REFERENCES

1. Choay J. Semin Thromb Haemost 1989; 15:359.
2. Hirsh J. Lewine MN. Blood 1992; 79:1.
3. Yin ET, Wessler S, Butler JV. J Lab Clin Med 1973; 81:298.
4. Denson KWE, Bonnar J. Thromb Diath Haemmorrh 1973; 30:471.
5. Yin ET. Semin Thromb Haemos 1985; 11:243.
6. Kristensen HI, Ostergaard PB, Nordfang O, Abildgaard U, Lindahl AK. Thromb Haemos 1992; 68:310.

7. Bara L, Combe-Tamzali S, Conard J, Horellou MH, Samama M. Haemostasis 1987; 17:127.
8. Harenberg J, Giese C, Knodler A, Zimmermann R. Haemostasis 1989; 1:13.
9. Walenga JM, Bara L. Samama MM, Fareed J. Semin Thromb Haemost 1985; 11:100.
10. Aiach M, Roncato M. Semin Thromb Haemost 1985; 11:108.
11. Holmer E, Söderberg, K. Fribergern P, Sörskog L. Thromb Haemostas 1985; 54:29 (abstract P168).
12. Sié P, Aillaud MF, de Prost D, Droullé C, Forestier F, Guedj P, Juhan-Vague I, Polack B, Potron G, Roncato M, Roussi J, Sampol J, Aiach M. Thromb Haemostast 1987; 58:879.
13. Barrowcliffe TW, Curtis AD, Johnson EA, Thomas DP. Thromb Haemostast 1988; 60:1.
14. Holm HA, Handeland GF, Abildgaard U, Arnesen KE, Gottschalk P, Hoeg V, Aandahl M, Haugen K, Loreum F, Scheel B, Sortland O, Vinje B. Haemostasis 1986; 16(Suppl 2):30.
15. Janvier G, Winnock S, Dugrais G. Haemostasis 1987; 7:49.
16. Levine MN, Planes A, Hirsh J, Goodyear M, Vochelle N, Gent M. Thromb Haemost 1989; 62:940.
17. Aiach M. Thromb Haemost 1991; 65:754 (abstract 307).
18. Nieuwenhuis HK, Albada J, Banga JD, Sixma JJ. Blood 1991; 78:2337.
19. Holmstrom MC, Berglund C, Grandqvist S, Bratt G, Tornebohm E, Lockner D. Thromb Res 1992; 67:49.
20. Hemker HC, Willems GM, Béguin S. Thromb Haemost 1986; 56:9.
21. Hemker HC, Wielders S, Béguin S. In: Fraxiparine: Deuxième symposium international. Données récentes pharmacologiques et cliniques. (Bounameaux H, Samama M, Ten Cate JW, eds.). Stuttgart: Schattauer, 1990:94.
22. Béguin S, Kessels H, Dol F, Hemker HC. Thromb Haemost 1992; 68:136.
23. Walenga JM, Fareed J, Hoppensteadt D. In: Doutremepuich C, ed. Low Molecular Weight Heparins in Clinical Practice. New York: Marcel Dekker, 1992:137.
24. Sorensen JV, Lassen MR, Borris LC, Rahr HB, Jensen HP, Hoppensteadt D, Walenga JA, Fareed J. Blood Coag. Fibrinoly 1992; 3:55.
25. Ireland H, Ryan K, Curtis JR, Lane DA. Thromb Haemost 1991; 65:933 (abstract 845).

4

Deep Venous Thrombosis

An Overview of Diagnosis, Treatment, and Prevention

Samuel Z. Goldhaber

Harvard Medical School and Brigham and Women's Hospital, Boston, Massachusetts

I. INTRODUCTION

Deep venous thrombosis (DVT) is responsible for approximately 200,000 hospitalizations per year in the United States (1). It is diagnosed twice as frequently as pulmonary embolism (PE) and is the underlying cause of both pulmonary embolism (Fig. 1) and chronic venous insufficiency of the legs (Fig. 2). Overall, about one-third of DVTs are recurrent events rather than first episodes (Fig. 3). The clinical significance of calf vein thrombosis is gaining increasing recognition as a cause of recurrent DVT and of chronic venous insufficiency.

Upper extremity venous thrombosis is associated with PE as often as 25% of the time and, therefore, should be managed as a clinically important illness (2). The frequency of this condition appears to be increasing, perhaps because of more widespread utilization of indwelling central venous catheters.

II. DIAGNOSIS

DVT often occurs without any symptoms or signs. When present, however, the major symptoms are leg pain, tenderness, and swelling, and the major signs are leg edema, discomfort in the calf upon forced dorsiflexion of the foot (Homans' sign), venous distention of subcutaneous vessels, discoloration, and a palpable cord (i.e., thrombus). Unfortunately, these clinical features are not specific for DVT, so diagnosis based on physical findings is often incorrect. Therefore, clinical suspicion of DVT should prompt definitive radiological evaluation.

Compression ultrasonography of the legs (3) has revolutionized screening for DVT (Figs. 4 and 5). High-resolution B-mode ultrasonography is sensitive

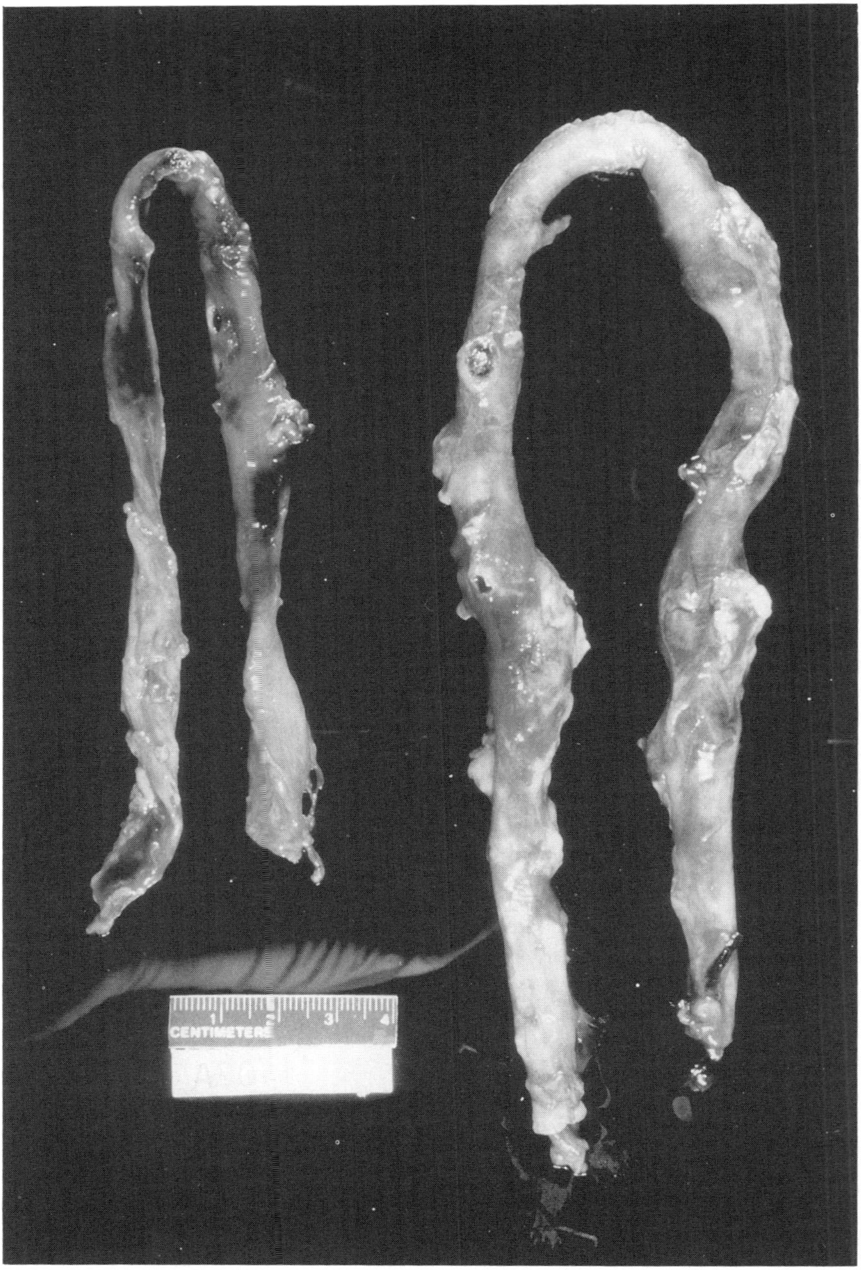

Figure 1 Bilateral DVT involving the external iliac and femoral veins of a 48-year-old woman who died of pulmonary embolism in association with adenocarcinoma of the lung.

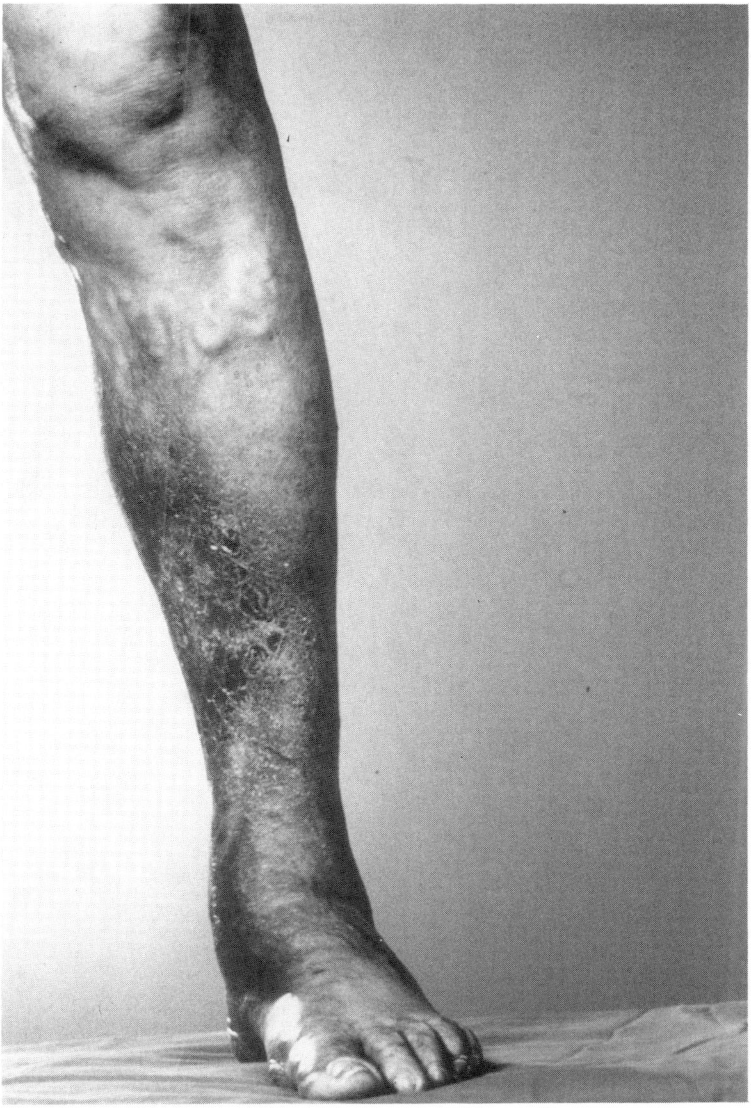

(a)

Figure 2 (a) Patient with moderately severe chronic venous insufficiency, which is indicated by abnormal skin pigmentation, varicosities of the veins (particularly below the knee), and ankle edema. (b) Patient with severe chronic venous insufficiency of the legs manifested by bilateral venous ulcerations, which will require surgical repair. Venous ulcers are typically found on the medial malleolus.

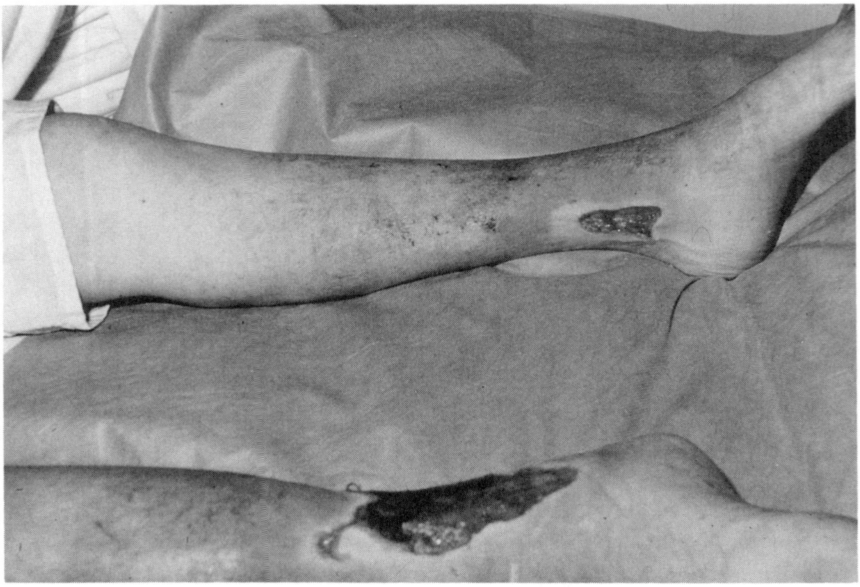

(b)

Figure 2 (Continued)

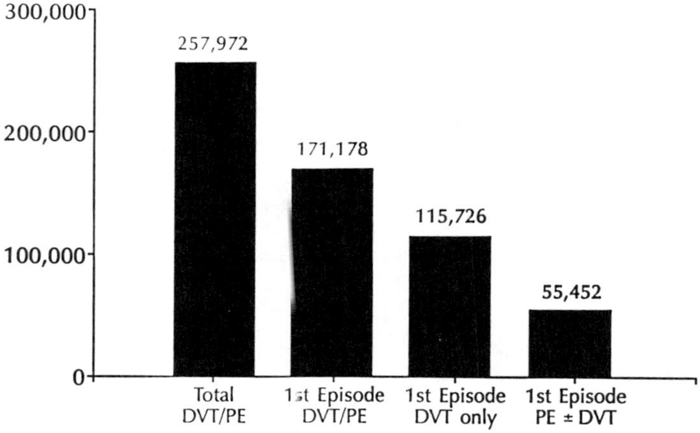

Figure 3 Estimated number of cases of venous thromboembolism in the United States, based on a 15-hospital survey in the Worcester, Massachusetts, area (1).

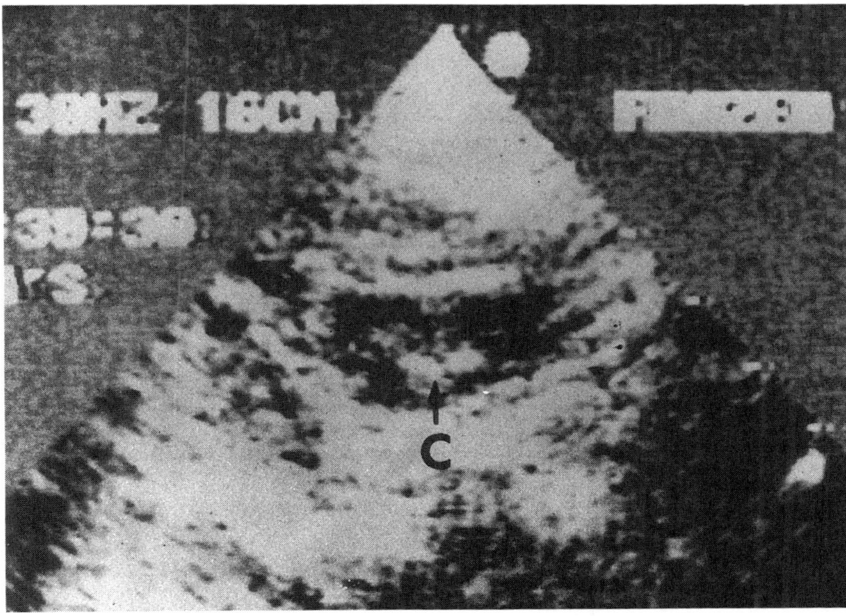

Figure 4 Left common femoral vein thrombus visualized with high-resolution B-mode ultrasonography in a 30-year-old woman. This vein also lacked compressibility. c = clot. (From Goldhaber SZ, Braunwald E. Pulmonary embolism. In: Braunwald E, ed. Heart Disease, 4th ed. Philadelphia: Saunders, 1992:1560, Fig. 48-4.)

and specific for the detection of symptomatic proximal leg DVT, above the trifurcation of the calf veins (4). However, the accuracy of this convenient, noninvasive modality cannot be automatically extrapolated from a population of symptomatic medical patients to other important populations, such as asymptomatic patients who have undergone recent hip surgery (Table 1).

There are probably four situations in which contrast venography should ordinarily be performed for diagnosis of DVT, unless there are compelling contraindications: (1) detection of proximal leg DVT if suspected in high-risk patients with a negative noninvasive examination; (2) workup of suspected isolated calf vein thrombosis; (3) differentiation of chronic venous thrombosis from acute DVT superimposed on chronic disease; and (4) workup of upper extremity thrombosis when the noninvasive examination is nondiagnostic.

Compression ultrasonography, even when combined with color Doppler imaging, may have a sensitivity as low as 38% for detecting asymptomatic proximal leg DVT observed on venography after high-risk orthopedic surgery (5). Therefore, orthopedic surgeons should generally not rely on "negative" noninvasive testing to "rule out" important DVT in their asymptomatic high-

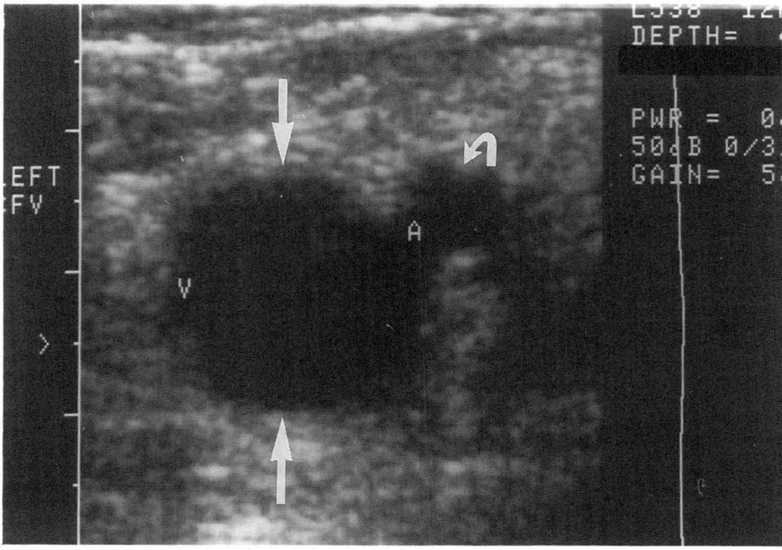

(a)

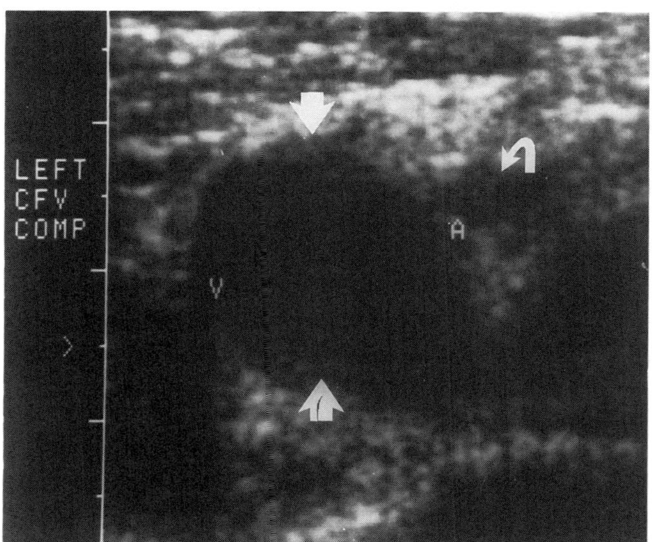

(b)

Figure 5 Loss of compressibility in a venous segment due to acute DVT. V = common femoral vein; A = common femoral artery. (a) Transverse sonogram at the level of the common femoral vein and artery reveals a distended vein (straight arrows) lying medial to the artery (curved arrow). There are no echogenic signals within the lumen of the vein. (b) Transducer has been pressed more vigorously against the skin. Vein (straight arrows) has failed to collapse. This lack of compressibility is diagnostic of DVT. (Reprinted with permission from Ref. 3.)

Table 1 Imaging Tests to Work Up Suspected DVT

Type of DVT	Ultrasound	Venography	MRI
High clinical suspicion, proximal leg	Use to screen	If high clinical suspicion persists despite normal ultrasound	Not necessary
Isolated calf	Use to screen	Necessary	Not necessary
Upper extremity	Use to screen	May be helpful	Often helpful
Recurrence vs. chronic venous insufficiency exacerbation	Use to screen	Usually necessary	May be helpful

risk postoperative patients. These latter patients should probably receive universal prophylaxis with warfarin for at least 1 month (6) after hospital discharge, unless they are at high risk for bleeding complications as outpatients.

With respect to isolated calf vein thrombosis, the accuracy of noninvasive testing has not been validated in any large prospective studies. The technically demanding nature of calf vein ultrasonography cannot be overstated. These small veins are often difficult to identify and follow as they course through the calf. Many patients have anatomical variants such as duplicated venous systems, which make calf vein imaging even more arduous. Therefore, compression ultrasonography is susceptible to inaccuracy.

Third, recurrent DVT can be virtually impossible to distinguish clinically from an acute exacerbation of chronic venous insufficiency without new thrombosis. Although ultrasound may demonstrate signs of chronic DVT such as vein wall thickening or increased echogenicity of intraluminal thrombus, it is often impossible for noninvasive testing to detect acute clot superimposed on chronic thrombus. Venography can at times demonstrate a meniscus suggestive of fresh thrombus and acute, recurrent DVT, as opposed to "webs" that indicate chronic DVT without an acute exacerbation. The distinction is of practical importance. An exacerbation of chronic venous insufficiency does not require hospitalization; usually graduated compression stockings suffice. However, recurrent DVT demands not only hospitalization, but also anticoagulation to a level that is more intense than for a first-time DVT.

Finally, ultrasonography of the upper extremity is more technically demanding than imaging of the proximal leg, partly because the presence of the clavicle and manubrium often precludes compression of the subclavian vein and surrounding venous structures. This is problematic because the principal feature of a positive ultrasound examination is inability to compress the vein lumen in cross-section. To circumvent this difficulty, color and pulsed Doppler can be utilized, along with provocative maneuvers such as inspiration. For example, the normal response of the subclavian vein to deep inspiration is collapse of the wall. When there is no significant change of the vein diameter during inspiration, this lack of response suggests a proximal obstruction within the subclavian vein, the brachiocephalic vein, or the superior vena cava (7).

If venography is not feasible, an alternative is magnetic resonance imaging (MRI). This approach is gaining widespread use for upper extremity thrombosis but, to date, is employed only rarely for leg DVT.

III. TREATMENT

The therapy for DVT should depend on the patient's risk for pulmonary embolism, recurrent DVT, and chronic venous insufficiency (Fig. 6). For large above-calf leg thrombosis and for superior vena caval, subclavian, or axillary vein thrombosis (especially to preserve or restore the patency of a clotted indwelling central venous catheter), thrombolytic therapy should be considered. The latter approach may provide more rapid and complete resolution of the clot than anticoagulation alone (8) (Fig. 7). However, the benefits of accelerated clot lysis must be weighed against the potential risks of increased major bleeding compared with heparin alone (Fig 8).

The venographic appearance of DVT may help to predict whether thrombolysis can successfully dissolve thrombus (9). In a study that compared rt-PA plus heparin versus rt-PA alone versus heparin alone (10), the response to rt-PA plus

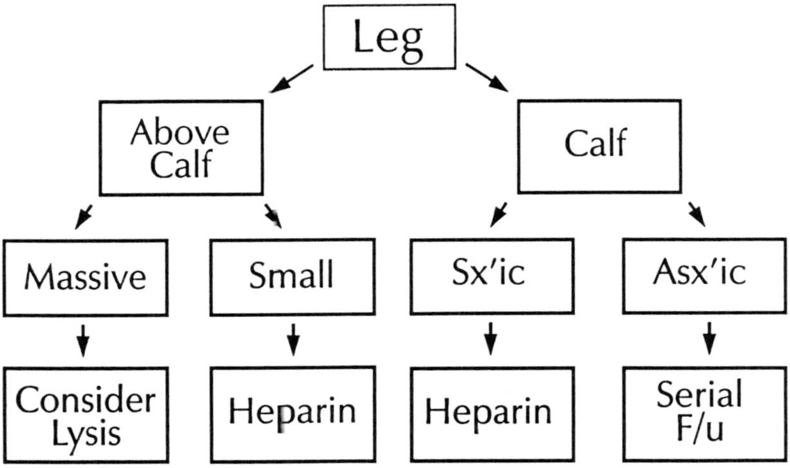

Figure 6 Treatment protocol for leg DVT. Refer to text for details. Sx'ic = symptomatic; Asx'ic = asymptomatic; F/u = follow-up.

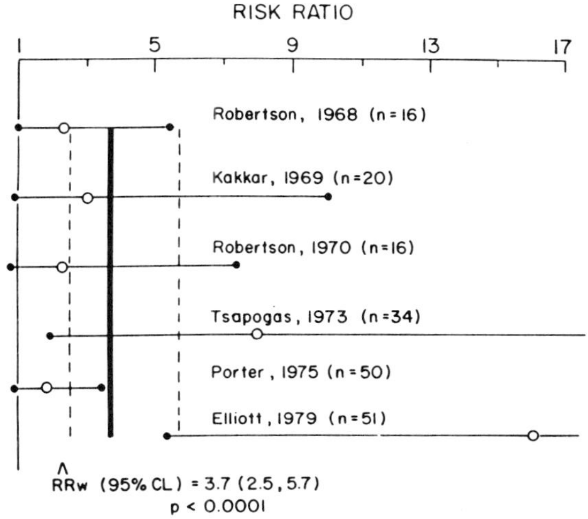

Figure 7 Overview of six randomized trials of streptokinase (SK) versus heparin for acute DVT indicates an overall 3.7 times superior lysis rate (heavy vertical line) for SK versus heparin. A risk ratio greater than 1 indicates a beneficial effect of SK for clot lysis. The pooled risk ratio is statistically significant ($p < 0.001$), with 95% confidence limits (CL) (dashed vertical lines) of 2.5–5.7. In each of the six individual trials, SK achieved superior lysis (open circles), but the lower 95% CL (closed circle, left side of each solid horizontal line) was greater than 1, indicating statistical significance, in only two of six individual trials. (From Brown WD, et al. Chest 1989; 95:276S–78S. Reproduced by permission.)

heparin or rt-PA alone was significantly greater among venous segments showing nonobstructive thrombi than in those showing obstructive thrombi (9).

New thrombolytic regimens are currently being investigated that utilize "bursts" of high concentrations of drug over short periods of time. Our research group has successfully tested urokinase in this setting, with a regimen of 1,000,000 units over 10 min administered 3 times over 24 hr (11). We are now embarking on a trial of recombinant urokinase versus heparin alone. The recombinant form of this thrombolytic agent should theoretically eliminate the rigors that sometimes occurred in association with urokinase prepared from human cell cultures.

For small DVT of the proximal leg, anticoagulation alone may suffice. Patients in this category should ordinarily be hospitalized to receive at least 120 hr of therapeutic levels of heparin while oral anticoagulation with warfarin is initiated. We define therapeutic heparin levels with partial thromboplastin time (PTT) values that are 1.5–2.5 times the control.

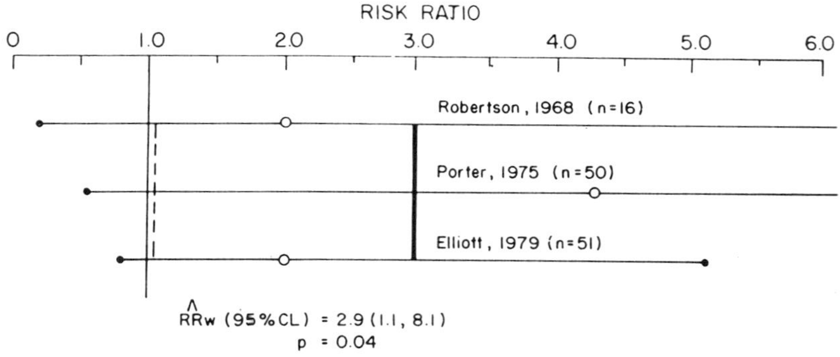

Figure 8 Overview of three trials of streptokinase (SK) versus heparin (three of the trials from Fig. 7 provided inadequate information on bleeding complications) for acute DVT indicates an overall 2.9 increase in the major bleeding rate (heavy vertical line) for SK compared with heparin. A risk ratio greater than 1 indicates more major bleeding complications associated with SK than with heparin. The pooled risk ratio is statistically significant ($p = 0.04$), but the 95% confidence limits are wide, reflecting the small sample size among the individual trials. (From Brown WD, et al. Chest 1989; 95:276S–78S. Reproduced with permission.)

The management of patients with symptomatic isolated calf vein thrombosis is controversial. Some clinicians advocate serial screening without anticoagulation unless the thrombus propagates above the popliteal trifurcation. However, my approach is ordinarily to treat with full-dose anticoagulation, just like patients with small DVT above the calf. Without anticoagulation, as many as 29% of patients with isolated calf vein thrombosis may have recurrent venous thrombosis within the ensuing 3 months (12). In addition, it appears that as many as one-third of patients with isolated calf vein thrombosis may have asymptomatic pulmonary embolism (13–15).

Occasionally, as part of a research protocol, asymptomatic isolated calf vein thrombosis will be detected. The clinical course is usually benign. We educate such patients about symptoms and signs of propagating proximal DVT, and we usually obtain a follow-up ultrasound within several weeks. Ordinarily, we withhold anticoagulation unless the patient appears to be at particularly high risk for venous thrombosis.

A. Anticoagulation

We tend to anticoagulate symptomatic isolated calf vein thrombosis for 3 months, proximal leg or upper extremity thrombosis for 6 months, and recurrent DVT for at least 12 months. To achieve rapid, therapeutic levels of heparinization, we rely on a modification of the heparin nomograms developed at McMaster Univer-

Table 2 Heparin Nomogram

1. Following a bolus of 5000–10,000 units of heparin, a continuous infusion of heparin 25,000 units in 500 ml of D5W or NS is administered, starting at 25 ml/hr (1250 U/hr).
2. Note that 1 ml = 50 units.
3. The PTT is checked 4 hr after initiation of the continuous intravenous infusion.
4. The heparin dose is adjusted according to the following nomogram:

PTT (sec)	HOLD (min)	Rate change (ml/hr)	Repeat PTT (time)
<50	Bolus 2500–5000 U	+4	4–6 hr later
50–59	0	+3	4–6 hr later
60–80	0	0	Next morning
80–90	0	−2	Next morning
90–109	60	−3	4–6 hr later
>110	120	−4	4–6 hr later

Cautionary Note: This nomogram provides a guide to rapid aggressive anticoagulation. It should not be used if patients are at substantial risk of bleeding from heparin or if patients weigh less than 60 kg. Under all circumstances, clinical discretion is advised when utilizing this nomogram.

Source: Modified from the McMaster Nomogram #1 in Arch Intern Med 1991; 151:333–337 and from the McMaster Nomogram #2 in Arch Intern Med 1992; 152:1589–1595.

sity (Table 2) (16, 17). Our conventional approach is to keep patients hospitalized until we have documented: (1) at least 120 hr of therapeutic levels of heparin, and (2) a stable and therapeutic warfarin dose. We initiate warfarin as soon as the heparin has achieved therapeutic levels, and, to ensure consistent bioavailability, we always use the brand Coumadin rather than the generic drug (18). When oral anticoagulation is initiated, the level of protein C may decline, thus creating a thrombogenic potential. By overlapping heparin and oral anticoagulation for at least 5 days, this theoretical procoagulant effect of oral anticoagulation can be counteracted.

The prothrombin time is utilized to adjust the dose of oral anticoagulation. However, it is important that prothrombin time results be reported according to the international normalized ratio (INR) rather than with the prothrombin time ratio or with the prothrombin time expressed in seconds. The reason is that prothrombin time assays are carried out with a variety of thromboplastins that have markedly different sensitivities (19).

The INR is the prothrombin time ratio that would be obtained if the World Health Organization reference thromboplastin were always utilized to perform the prothrombin time test (20). Most available thromboplastins are supplied with a calibration factor known as the international sensitivity index (ISI). By utilizing the ISI, laboratories can express prothrombin time results in terms of the INR. For example, within the United States, a prothrombin time of 18 sec and prothrombin time ratio of 1.5 at one laboratory could be equivalent to a prothrombin time of 22 sec and prothrombin time ratio of 1.8 at another laboratory. The same blood specimen in some European laboratories might yield a prothrombin time of 30 sec and prothrombin time ratio of 2.5. Nevertheless, the INR for this same blood sample would be 3.0 at *all* laboratories, despite the three markedly different prothrombin time ratios and prothrombin times given in this example (19). Thus, to communicate adequately about our patients' anticoagulation to other physicians, visiting nurses, and hospital or commercial laboratories, the common language of the INR is mandatory.

The target INR for oral anticoagulation of patients with a first-time DVT should be 2.0–3.0. For patients who develop recurrent DVT despite an INR of 2.0–3.0, a more intensified anticoagulation regimen with a target INR of 3.0–4.0 should be considered.

Most adjustments in oral anticoagulant dosing are made in the outpatient setting. Traditionally, oral anticoagulants have been adjusted on the basis of the plasma prothrombin time. After the laboratory reported the prothrombin time results, patients would be contacted either to reassure them that their dosing regimen was appropriate or to make dosage adjustments. Unfortunately, it can be quite difficult to explain changes in anticoagulation dosing by telephone. Therefore, we now utilize the Biotrack (Fig. 9) to make in-office assessments of warfarin dosing regimens. The Biotrack provides the prothrombin time result in 2 min by analyzing a drop of whole blood obtained from a fingertip puncture (21).

1. Pregnancy

We do not use warfarin during pregnancy. Instead, we initially treat pregnant patients who have acute DVT by utilizing a continuous intravenous heparin infusion for 5–7 days. We teach self-injection of subcutaneous heparin and prescribe adjusted, high-dose subcutaneous heparin for the remainder of the pregnancy. To monitor the heparin, our target is a midinterval PTT of approximately 1.5–2.0 times control. Although it used to be taught that women taking warfarin postpartum could not breast-feed, it is now evident that breast feeding can be undertaken safely. The level of warfarin in breast milk is so low (approximately 25 ng/ml) that it cannot be detected in the baby's plasma (22, 23).

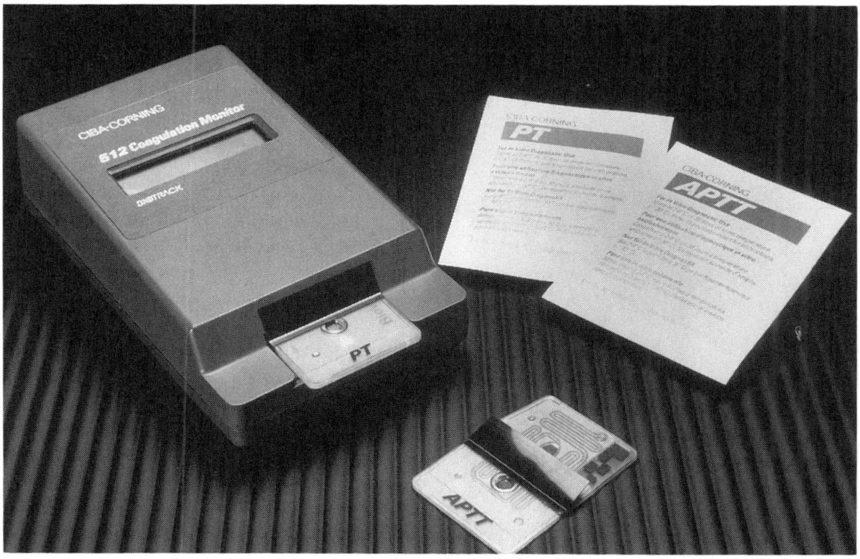

Figure 9 The Ciba Corning Biotrack 512 coagulation monitor employs a laser optical system. The monitor, in conjunction with the appropriate test cartridge, determines the prothrombin time (PT) or partial thromboplastin time (PTT). A drop of fresh whole blood is applied directly to the sample application well of a PT or PTT test cartridge containing a reagent chamber and a reaction path. The blood is drawn by capillary action into the reagent chamber, where it mixes with the chemical activator to initiate coagulation. The blood-reagent mixture moves along the reaction path until a clot forms. The time from application of blood into the test cartridge to cessation of flow is detected by the laser optical system and converted to PT or PTT plasma equivalent. The coagulation monitor reports the PT in seconds and according to the international normalized ratio. The entire assay procedure for PT or PTT values requires less than 2 min.

2. *Cancer*

Anecdotally, patients with cancer and DVT in more than one limb often do not respond to warfarin therapy. Therefore, our usual practice in this group of patients is to maintain continuous intravenous heparin for 5–7 days and then to switch to full-dose adjusted subcutaneous heparin, which is prescribed indefinitely.

B. Inferior Vena Caval Interruption

For patients with proximal leg DVT who cannot tolerate or who fail a trial of anticoagulation, an inferior vena caval filter should be inserted. Percutaneous placement of a bird's nest filter (Fig. 10) or titanium Greenfield filter has the

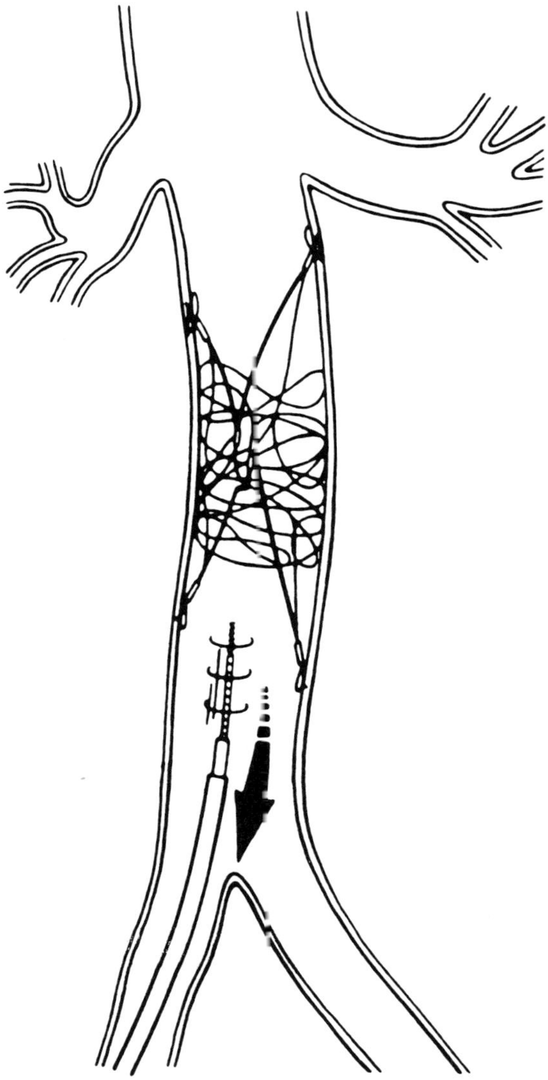

Figure 10 Transfemoral insertion of a bird's nest filter. After successful placement of the filter, the wire guide pusher and empty filter catheter are removed. The introducing sheath is left in place until a venacavogram is obtained. The sheath is then removed, and pressure is applied over the femoral vein insertion site.

advantage of a small sheath size that can minimize the risk of bleeding during and after the procedure (24). The failure rate of these filters is less than 5%, and they have a low rate of thrombogenicity and occlusion.

C. Chronic Venous Insufficiency and Adjunctive Therapy

We prescribe thigh-high graduated compression stockings (GCS), 30–40 mm Hg, to most of our patients with proximal-leg DVT to assist in ambulation (usually after the first 24 hr of hospitalization). The stockings help prevent distention of the vein wall and may mitigate the syndrome of chronic venous insufficiency—most often characterized by leg swelling and discomfort—that the majority of DVT patients will experience. For those patients who do develop the postphlebitic syndrome, preliminary reports indicate potentially dramatic improvement with intermittent pneumatic compression (25).

IV. PREVENTION

The estimated direct cost of diagnosing and treating DVT and PE in the United States is $2.9 billion annually. For every 1,000,000 patients who receive prophylaxis against venous thrombosis, approximately $60 million could be saved in direct health care costs (26). Fortunately, effective mechanical and pharmacological modalities are available to prevent venous thrombosis among most hospitalized patients (27). However, at many institutions, these preventive approaches are underutilized (28).

DVT is easier and less expensive to prevent than to diagnose and to treat. Virtually all hospitalized adult patients, particularly after major surgery, and all women after delivery should receive prophylactic measures against venous thromboembolism. The method of prevention that is selected should be based on an assessment of the patient's level of risk for DVT. Because the risk of DVT continues after hospital discharge, prophylaxis should be continued at home among patients at moderate or high risk for venous thromboembolism, such as those undergoing major knee or hip surgery.

A. Nonpharmacological Prophylaxis

The most commonly used nonpharmacological measures are GCS and intermittent pneumatic compression (IPC) boots (Table 3). GCS for patients confined to bed are usually T.E.D.® stockings with 18 mm Hg compression at the ankle, 14 mm Hg at the calf, 8 mm Hg popliteal, 10 mm Hg at the lower thigh, and 8 mm Hg at midthigh. GCS should be considered as first-line prophylaxis for most hospitalized patients and suffice for prophylaxis among low-risk patients. IPC boots (Fig. 11) provide intermittent inflation of air-filled cuffs that prevent venous stasis in the legs and appear to stimulate the endogenous fibrinolytic system.

GCS and IPC have complementary mechanisms. GCS provide continuous stimulation of linear blood flow velocity and prevent dilation of the venous system in the legs. IPC devices compress the veins more forcefully than GCS, but for a relatively brief period. Vascular compression to prevent venous stasis and low-dose heparin to prevent hypercoagulability can be combined in moderate- or high-risk patients.

B. Fixed-Dose Subcutaneous Heparin

The most comprehensive randomized controlled trial of low-dose heparin (5000 units of subcutaneous heparin 2 hr preoperatively and every 8 hr thereafter for 7 days) as prophylaxis against fatal postoperative PE was organized by Kakkar in the International Multicentre Trial involving 4121 patients (29). Eligible patients were over age 40 and were scheduled to undergo elective major surgery. Of the autopsied subjects, 16 controls died of PE versus only two patients in the heparin group. Although more wound hematomas occurred among heparin-treated patients, the number of deaths due to hemorrhage was not increased among those who received heparin.

Collins and colleagues have reviewed data from 78 randomized controlled trials with 15,598 patients that have confirmed the International Trial Multicentre result (30) There was a 40% reduction in nonfatal PE and 64% reduction in fatal PE among heparin-treated patients. The heparin-treated patients also had about one-third as many DVT as control patients, regardless of whether they had undergone general, urological, elective orthopedic, or traumatic orthopedic surgery. There was no significant difference in fatal hemorrhage between the hepa-

Table 3 Nonpharmacological Approaches to PE Prophylaxis

Modality	Mechanism of action
1. Graduated compression stockings (GCS)	Prevent venous stasis
2. Intermittent pneumatic compression (IPC) boots	(A) Prevent venous stasis; (B) increase endogenous fibrinolytic activity
3. Inferior vena caval (IVC) interruption	Prevents PE by mechanical blocking effect but does not prevent DVT
4. Combined nonpharmacological methods (e.g., GCS + IPC)	Additive or synergistic effect
5. Combined nonpharmacological plus pharmacological approach (e.g., IPC + low-dose heparin)	Additive or synergistic effect

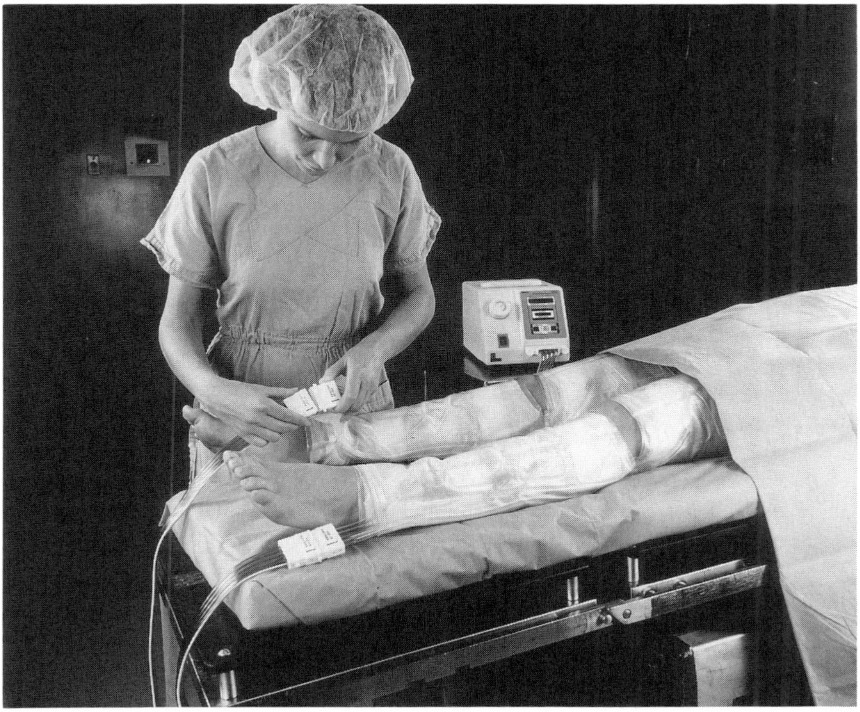

Figure 11 Thigh-high sequential-gradient, intermittent pneumatic compression device.

rin-treated and control groups. Although excessive bleeding was more likely to occur among patients assigned to heparin therapy—especially those who underwent urological procedures—the absolute excess in bleeding was only about 2%.

In 1993, the low-molecular-weight heparin enoxaparin received Food and Drug Administration (FDA) approval for prophylaxis against venous thrombosis following elective total hip replacement. The dose is 30 mg, twice daily, by subcataneous injection for 7–10 days (30a).

C. Universal Adjusted-Dose Warfarin Prophylaxis

Because leg ultrasound is often insensitive for detection of DVT following total hip replacement (31), one approach to preventing venous thrombosis is to utilize 12 weeks of adjusted-dose warfarin for all postoperative patients (32). This strategy has been demonstrated to be safe and cost-effective, especially because no predischarge ultrasonography or venography is required (32).

V. TEAM APPROACH

We have adopted an interdisciplinary team approach to the diagnosis, treatment, and prevention of DVT. Our team includes members of the departments of medicine, radiology, and surgery, as well as both physicians and nurses. We meet periodically to ensure optimal coordination of our efforts and to review ongoing and future management protocols.

REFERENCES

1. Anderson FA Jr, Wheeler HB, Goldberg RJ, Hosmer DW, Patwardhan NA, Jovanovic B, Forcier A, Dalen JE. A population-based perspective of the hospital incidence and case-fatality rates of venous thrombosis and pulmonary embolism: the Worcester DVT Study. Arch Intern Med 1991; 151:933–938.
2. Monréal M, Lafoz E Ruiz J, Valls R, Alastrue A. Upper-extremity deep venous thrombosis and pulmonary embolism. A prospective study. Chest 1991; 99:280–283.
3. Polak JF. Doppler ultrasound of the deep leg veins: a revolution in the diagnosis of deep vein thrombosis and monitoring of thrombolysis. Chest 1991; 99:165S–172S.
4. Lensing AWA, Prandoni P, Brandjes D, Huisman PM, Vigo M, Tomasella G, Krekt J, ten Cate JW, Huisman MV, Büller HR. Detection of deep-vein thrombosis by real-time B-mode ultrasonography. N Engl J Med 1989; 320:342–345.
5. Davidson BL, Elliott CG, Lensing AWA. Low accuracy of color Doppler ultrasound to detect proximal leg vein thrombosis during screening of asymptomatic high-risk patients. Ann Intern Med 1992; 117 (in press).
6. Reis SE, Hirsch DR, Wilson MG, Donovan BC, Goldhaber SZ. A program for the prevention of venous thromboembolism in high risk orthopedic patients. J Arthroplast 1991; 6:S11–S16.
7. Polak JF. Peripheral Vascular Sonography. A Practical Guide. Baltimore: William & Wilkins, 1992:209.
8. Goldhaber SZ, Buring JE, Lipnick RJ. Hennekens CH. Pooled analyses of randomized trials of streptokinase and heparin in phlebographicaly documented acute deep venous thrombosis. Am J Med 1984; 76:393–397.
9. Meyerovitz MF, Polak JF, Goldhaber SZ. Short-term response to thrombolytic therapy in deep venous thrombosis: predictive value of venographic appearance. Radiology 1992; 184:345–348.
10. Goldhaber SZ, Meyerovitz MF, Green D, Vogelzang RL, Citrin P, Heit J, Sobel M, Wheeler HB, Plante D, Kim H, Hopkins A, Tufte M, Stump D, Braunwald E. Randomized controlled trial of tissue plasminogen activator in proximal deep venous thrombosis. Am J Med 1990; 88:235–240.
11. Goldhaber SZ, Polak JF, Feldstein ML, Meyerovitz MF, Creager MA. Efficacy and safety of repeated boluses of urokinase in the treatment of acute deep venous thrombosis. Am J. Cardiol 1994; 73 (in press).
12. Lagerstedt CI, Olsson C-G, Fagher BO, Öqvist BW, Albrechtsson U. Need for long-term anticoagulant treatment in symptomatic calf-vein thrombosis. Lancet 1985; 2:515–518.

13. Doyle DJ, Turpie AGG, Hirsh J, Best C, Kinch D, Levine MN, Gent M. Adjusted subcutaneous heparin or continuous intravenous heparin in patients with acute deep vein thrombosis. Ann Intern Med 1987; 107:441–445.
14. Huisman MV, Büller HR, ten Cate JW, van Royen EA, Vreeken J, Kersten M-J, Bakx R. Unexpected high prevalence of silent pulmonary embolism in patients with deep venous thrombosis. Chest 1989; 95:498–502.
15. Monreal M, Ruiz J, Olazabal A, et al. Deep venous thrombosis and the risk of pulmonary embolism. A systematic study. Chest 1992; 102:677–681.
16. Cruickshank M, Levine MN, Hirsh J, Roberts R, Siguenza M. A standard heparin nomogram for the management of heparin therapy. Arch Intern Med 1991; 151:333–337.
17. Hull R, Raskob G, Rosenbloom D, Lemaire J, Pineo G, Baylis B, Ginsberg J, Panju A, Brill-Edwards P, Brant R. Optimal therapeutic level of heparin therapy in patients with venous thrombosis. Arch Intern Med 1992; 152:1589–1595.
18. Richton-Hewett S, Foster E. Apstein CS. Medical and economic consequences of a blinded oral anticoagulant branch change at a municipal hospital. Arch Intern Med 1988; 148:806–808.
19. Bussey HI, Force RW, Bianco TM, Leonard AD. Reliance on prothrombin time ratios causes significant errors in anticoagulation therapy. Arch Intern Med 1992; 152:278–282.
20. Hirsh J. Substandard monitoring of warfarin in North America. Time for change. Arch Intern Med 1992; 152:257–258.
21. Ansell J, Tiarks C, Hirsh J, McGehee W, Adler D, Weibert R. Measurement of the activated partial thromboplastin time from a capillary (fingerstick) sample of whole blood. A new method for monitoring heparin therapy. Am J Clin Pathol 1991; 95:222–227.
22. Orme ML'E, Lewis PJ, de Swiet M, Serlin MJ, Sibeon R, Baty JD, Breckenridge AM. May mothers given warfarin breast-feed their infants? Br Med J 1977; 1:1564–1565.
23. McKenna R, Cole ER, Vasan U. Is warfarin sodium contraindicated in the lactating mother? J Pediatr 1983; 103:325–327.
24. Grassi CJ, Goldhaber SZ. Interruption of the inferior vena cava for prevention of pulmonary embolism: transvenous filter devices. Herz 1989; 14:182–191.
25. Ginsberg JS, Brill-Edwards P, Kowalchuk G, Hirsh J. Intermittent compression units for the postphlebitic syndrome. A pilot study. Arch Intern Med 1989; 149:1651–1652.
26. Landefeld CS, Hanus P. Economic burden of venous thromboembolism. In: Goldhaber SZ, ed. Prevention of Venous Thromboembolism. New York: Marcel Dekker, 1993:69–86.
27. Goldhaber SZ, Morpurgo M, for the WHO/ISFC Task Force on Pulmonary Embolism. Prevention, diagnosis, and treatment of pulmonary embolism. JAMA 1992 (in press).
28. Anderson FA Jr, Wheeler HB, Goldberg RJ, Hosmer DW, Forcier A, Patwardhan NA. Physician practices in the prevention of venous thromboembolism. Ann Intern Med 1991; 115:591–595.

29. International Multicentre Trial. Prevention of fatal postoperative pulmonary embolism by low doses of heparin. Lancet 1975; 2:45–51.
30. Collins R, Scrimgeour A, Yusuf S, Peto R. Reduction in fatal pulmonary embolism and venous thrombosis by perioperative administration of subcutaneous heparin. Overview of results of randomized trials in general, orthopedic, and urologic surgery. N Engl J Med 1988; 318:1162–1173.
30a. Enoxaparin—A low-molecular-weight heparin. The Medical Letter 1993; 35: 751–776.
31. Davidson BL, Elliott CG, Lensing AWA for the RD Heparin Arthroplasty Group. Low accuracy of color Doppler ultrasound in the detection of proximal leg vein thrombosis in asymptomatic high-risk patients. Ann Intern Med 1992; 117: 735–738.
32. Paiement GD, Wessinger SJ, Hughes R, Harris WH. Routine use of adjusted low-dose warfarin to prevent venous thromboembolism after total hip replacement. J Bone Joint Surg Am 1993; 75:893–898.

5

Interaction of Heparin with Platelets, Including Heparin-Induced Thrombocytopenia

Theodore Earl Warkentin
McMaster University and Hamilton Civic Hospitals, Hamilton, Ontario, Canada

John G. Kelton
McMaster University, Hamilton, Ontario, Canada

I. INTRODUCTION

The interaction of platelets with heparin is of biological and clinical importance for several reasons. First, the specific binding of heparin to platelets results in poorly understood effects on platelet function that may contribute to the bleeding complications of heparin. Second, heparin can initiate an IgG-mediated adverse reaction that results in thrombocytopenia and thrombotic complications (heparin-induced thrombocytopenia). Third, there is growing basic and clinical interest in other sulfated polysaccharide agents with antithrombotic action. These drugs, which include low-molecular-weight heparin (LMWH), heparan sulfate, and dermatan sulfate, generally have lesser interaction with platelets and thus may carry lower risks of bleeding or heparin-induced thrombocytopenia.

A. Structural Determinants of the Interaction of Sulfated Polysaccharides with Platelets

Heparin is a markedly heterogeneous and polydispersed substance extracted from animal tissue. Standard (unfractionated) heparin is obtained from either bovine lung or porcine intestinal mucosa. Several processing steps are required to obtain standard or LMWH products that meet manufacturing requirements. Thus, there can be hundreds or even thousands of different molecular species within a single

Table 1 Relationship Between Sulfated Polysaccharide Structure and Nonimmune and Immune Platelet Interactions

Sulfated polysaccharide	Approximate mean molecular mass (M_r)	Mean sulfate/ disaccharide unit	Ability to bind to (or displace heparin from) platelets	Nonimmune platelet activation	Causes IgG-mediated thrombocytopenia/ thrombosis syndrome?	Cross-reacts with heparin for HIT-IgG
Standard bovine lung heparin	12,000–15,000	2.5	+ + +	+ + +	Yes	Yes
Standard porcine mucosal heparin	12,000–14,000	2.1	+ + +	+ +, + + +	Yes	Yes
Dextran sulfate	Variable	6	+ + + +	+ + +	Unknown (not currently used clinically)	Yes
Pentosan polysulfate	5000	4	+ + + +	+ + +	Yes	Yes
Arteparon® (polysulfated chondroitin sulfate)	7000	≥2		+	Yes	Yes
LMW heparins	4000–6000	≤2	+, + +	+	Yes	Yes

Heparinoid Org 10172 (Orgaran®)	4000–10,000 (contains some high antithrombin-affinity heparan sulfate)	1	0	0	No	No (exception: A subgroup of patients with HIT-IgG will cross-react with Org 10172)
Heparan sulfate		1	0	0	No	No (but see Org 10172)
De-*N*-sulfated heparin	10,000–12,000	1	0	0	No	No
Dermatan sulfate (chondroitin B sulfate)		1	0	0	No	No
Chondroitin A sulfate		1	0	0	No	No
Chondroitin C sulfate		1	0	0	No	No
Pentasaccharide	1400	3.2	0	0	No	No
Dextran	Up to 40,000	0	0	0	No	No

In general, the ability of sulfated polysaccharides to interact with platelets, and to produce various biological effects (including both nonimmune and IgG-mediated activation) is dependent on the degree of sulfation and polysaccharide chain length.

heparin preparation, theoretically resulting in a spectrum of heparin/platelet interactions.

In general, the interaction of heparin and other sulfated polysaccharides with platelets is dependent on their size (number of saccharide units) and degree of sulfation (particularly, N-sulfation) (1). The specific binding of heparin to platelets can lead to different functional consequences, including nonimmune platelet activation as well as the syndrome of IgG-mediated thrombocytopenia and thrombosis that can be initiated by heparin and other highly sulfated polysaccharides. Table 1 compares physical characteristics of several sulfated polysaccharides with some of these platelet effects.

The anticoagulant activities of heparin are critically dependent on the presence of the antithrombin III–binding pentasaccharide. Larger such heparin molecules (at least 18 saccharide units, $M_r > 5400$) possess both antithrombin and anti-Xa anticoagulant activities. Smaller antithrombin-binding heparin molecules have only anti-Xa activity. In contrast, heparin/platelet interactions are not dependent on the antithrombin III–binding characteristics of the heparin (2–6).

II. NONIMMUNE INTERACTIONS OF HEPARIN WITH PLATELETS

Nonimmune heparin/platelet interactions are those that occur between heparin and platelets from all or most normal individuals. In contrast, immune (or idiosyncratic) heparin/platelet interactions are caused by IgG and occur in a minority of patients or volunteers who receive heparin.

We will discuss several aspects of nonimmune heparin/platelet interactions, including: A heparin binding to platelets; B heparin-induced platelet activation; and C effect of heparin on bleeding.

A. Specific Heparin Binding to Platelets

Heparin binds to platelets specifically and reversibly via a single class of binding sites (1, 5–7). There are approximately 3000 heparin-binding sites (5), but this value is affected by differences in heparin size, sulfation, and the degree of platelet activation. For example, approximately 70% more heparin molecules of larger size (M_r 10,000) bind to platelets compared to smaller-sized heparin (M_r 3000) (5). Heparin binding increases markedly following platelet activation (6, 7). Although the predominant binding site(s) on platelets has not been identified, several internal platelet glycoproteins that are released following platelet activation can bind heparin. These include platelet factor 4 (8–11), von Willebrand factor (12), thrombospondin (9, 13), fibronectin (14, 15), vitronectin (16), and histidine-rich glycoprotein (17, 18). Platelet surface GPIb also binds heparin (9, 19), but this may be quantitatively unimportant, as Bernard-Soulier platelets (which lack GPIb) bind normal amounts of heparin (1). Monoclonal antibodies to GPIb, GPIa/IIa, GPIIb/IIIa, and GPIV do not inhibit heparin binding to platelets (6).

The efficiency with which various polysaccharides compete with heparin for platelet binding is dependent on their degree of sulfation and their size (1, 7, 20). Dextran sulfate, pentosan polysulfate, and heparin are more effective competitive inhibitors of the binding of radiolabeled heparin to platelets than are LMW heparins. In contrast, de-N-sulfated heparin, dextran, dermatan sulfate, and a commercial heparinoid preparation (Org 10172) do not compete effectively with heparin for platelet-binding sites.

B. Heparin-Induced Platelet Activation

The effect of heparin on platelet activation can be measured in several ways, including: (1) direct platelet-aggregating effects of heparin; (2) indirect platelet-aggregating effects of heparin, as assessed by measuring the ability of heparin preincubation to augment aggregation initiated by standard platelet agonists; (3) evaluation of platelet responses to agonists using blood obtained from patients or volunteers who received heparin prior to blood drawing; and (4) assays of platelet activation in volunteers or patients given heparin. We will also discuss: (5) the role of heparin size and sulfation in activating platelets; (6) the effects of platelet activation in modulating the anticoagulant activities of heparin; (7) the mechanisms of platelet activation by heparin; and (8) whether these nonimmune effects of heparin could be responsible for mild thrombocytopenia observed in some patients who receive heparin (heparin-*associated* thrombocytopenia).

1. Direct Platelet-Aggregating Effects of Heparin: In Vitro Studies

A large number of studies have evaluated the direct proaggregatory effects of standard and LMWH and other sulfated polysaccharides on platelet aggregation. Using citrated platelet-rich plasma, most studies have shown a consistent—though generally weak—aggregatory effect of heparin in normal volunteers (2, 21–28) and patients (22, 29, 30). The degree of aggregation increases in a dose-dependent manner, between 0.5 and 10 U/ml heparin (4, 27, 28).

2. Indirect Platelet-Aggregating Effects of Heparin (Potentiation of Activation by Other Platelet Agonists

Preincubation of platelets with heparin enhances platelet aggregation by standard platelet agonists, such as adenosine diphosphate, epinephrine, collagen, and arachidonic acid (21, 29–41). These proaggregatory effects are dose-dependent and occur at concentrations of heparin achieved therapeutically (29, 34, 35). The proaggregatory effects of heparin can also be seen using whole blood anticoagulated with either citrate (42–44) or hirudin (44), indicating that the heparin effect can occur at physiological calcium concentrations.

3. *Effects of Heparin on Platelet Aggregation: Ex Vivo Studies*

Both proaggregatory and inhibitory effects of heparin have been reported in humans and animals given heparin. For example, increased spontaneous platelet aggregation (45, 46) as well as potentiation of platelet aggregation to adenosine diphosphate (46–48) has been observed in volunteers and patients who have received heparin. In contrast, platelet aggregation to collagen (46, 49, 50), adenosine diphosphate (49), and epinephrine (49) was inhibited in other studies of platelets obtained from humans given heparin. Inhibition of platelet aggregation to collagen was also observed in studies of animals given heparin (51, 52).

It is possible that the apparent inhibitory effects of heparin could in fact be caused by initial heparin-induced platelet activation, leading to a platelet refractory state (21). Indeed, spontaneous platelet aggregation is a common problem with blood collected into heparin and is a cause of pseudothrombocytopenia (53, 54). However, some of the inhibitory effects of heparin could be due to indirect effects of heparin, such as on inhibiting collagen/platelet interactions (41).

4. *Direct Platelet-Activating Effects of Heparin: In Vivo Studies*

There is debate whether heparin can activate platelets *in vivo*. Early reports indicated that heparin could cause an immediate, transient reduction in the platelet count in animals (55) and humans (56) that usually recovered to normal within 60–120 min. Subsequent human studies using radiolabeled platelets showed that although the platelet count fell transiently following heparin injection, blood radioactivity remained constant (57). These data are consistent with either reversible in vivo aggregation (mild activation) or ex vivo aggregation (artifact). However, acute thrombocytopenia has not generally been observed in more recent studies (46, 47, 49). If platelet activation does occur in vivo following heparin administration, it likely is mild, since no evidence for α-granule release and thromboxane generation was found in a study of humans given heparin (47).

5. *Effects of Polysaccharide Chain Length and Sulfation on Platelet Activation*

There are significant differences in the ability of sulfated polysaccharides to activate platelets. In general, these platelet-activating properties are dependent on saccharide length and sulfation (2, 4, 26, 27, 36–38, 40, 58, 59; see Table 1). Bovine lung heparin is a better potentiator of platelet activation than is porcine mucosal heparin (37, 38, 40), an effect likely related to its greater degree of sulfation (60). Pentosan polysulfate potentiates platelet activation to a similar extent as does porcine mucosal heparin (37). Standard heparins are better platelet activators than are LMWH (4, 27, 36, 37, 38, 40). LMW fractions below 3000 Da have essentially no platelet-activating activity (27).

Certain very large sulfated polysaccharides can activate platelets even more strongly than heparin. For instance, highly sulfated and branched sulfated polysaccharides (e.g., cellulose trisulfuric acid, xylan sulfuric acids) agglutinate human platelets *in vitro* (61, 62), rendering them too toxic for human use. Acidic mucopolysaccharides of molecular weight 30,000–50,000 extracted from sea cucumbers also activate platelets in approximately 90% of normal donors (63). Dextran sulfates activate platelets progressively in a polysaccharide length-dependent fashion (64).

In contrast, low-sulfated polysaccharides (Org 10172, heparan sulfate, dermatan sulfate) have essentially no direct or indirect platelet-aggregating effects (30, 36, 39, 65). The selective removal of N-sulfate groups from standard heparin results in the loss of the platelet proaggregatory effects (66).

6. *Effect of Platelet Activation on Anticoagulant Effects of Heparins*

Platelet activation is associated with release of platelet factor 4 from platelet α-granules and generation of procoagulant platelet-derived microparticles. Both these products of platelet activation can interfere with the anticoagulant effects of heparin (67–71). PF4 is a polypeptide released from the α-granules of activated platelets that strongly binds to heparin and inactivates it (72). However, certain LMWH bind less strongly to PF4 than standard heparin (10, 67, 73) and are more effective inhibitors of thrombin generation in platelet-rich plasma (67) or in the presence of added PF4 (69), compared with standard heparins. These observations have several implications for immune-mediated, heparin-induced thrombocytopenia. First, the release of PF4 and procoagulant microparticles from activated platelets could explain why many patients with heparin-induced thrombocytopenia are "resistant" to heparin therapy; i.e., it is difficult to obtain therapeutic anticoagulant levels despite increasing the rate of heparin infusion (74). Second, the lesser effects of PF4 on inhibiting LMWH anticoagulant activity could help explain why some patients with heparin-induced thrombocytopenia improve on LMWH therapy, even though there is virtual complete cross-reactivity between standard heparin and LMWH for HIT-IgG (discussed subsequently).

7. *Mechanisms of Nonimmune Heparin-Induced Platelet Activation*

The mechanism of nonimmune heparin-induced platelet activation is not well understood. However, it is well established that the heparin-induced platelet aggregation is a metabolically active process (contrast ristocetin-induced platelet agglutination). For the majority of normal volunteers, heparin-induced platelet aggregation is mild, resulting in small platelet aggregates without granule release or thromboxane generation (2, 28). The platelet aggregation is inhibited by calcium chelators and aerobic (antimycin A) or anaerobic (2-deoxyglucose) inhibitors (28). In a minority of normal volunteers, more marked heparin-induced platelet aggregation occurs. The more marked platelet aggregation is accompanied by thromboxane generation (24, 30) and granule secretion (24) and can be inhibited by indomethacin (24, 30) and 13-azaprostanoic acid (thromboxane receptor antagonist) (24). Heparin also antagonizes platelet inhibition mediated by prostacyclin (prostaglandin I_2) (34, 39, 75, 76) or prostaglandin E_1 (34, 77).

There is limited information on the cellular processes of nonimmune heparin-induced platelet activation. Studies have shown that heparin uncouples α_2-adrenoreceptors from the G_i-protein in human platelet membranes (78) and inhibits inositol 1,4,5-trisphosphate binding to its receptor (79). These studies were not performed using intact platelets, and the physiological relevance is uncertain.

8. Nonimmune Heparin-Induced Platelet Activation: Can It Cause Thrombocytopenia?

The observation that heparin has a proaggregatory platelet effect has led some investigators to suggest that nonimmune mechanisms could produce thrombocytopenia in some patients who receive heparin (80–82). Experiments have shown that heparin also can potentiate platelet activation by aggregated IgG and *Staphylococcus aureus* (83), suggesting that nonimmune heparin-induced thrombocytopenia may be more likely to occur in sick patients. Evidence that heparin contributes to an early, mild thrombocytopenia in some patients is suggested by several clinical studies that showed a higher frequency of thrombocytopenia in patients who received heparin compared with those who did not (22, 84, 85), suggesting that heparin could contribute to early thrombocytopenia due to nonimmune platelet-activating mechanisms (Fig. 1).

Chong (86–88) has termed this early, mild thrombocytopenia associated with heparin therapy as type I heparin-induced thrombocytopenia. Type II heparin-induced thrombocytopenia is the corresponding term used to describe IgG-mediated thrombocytopenia (discussed subsequently). We prefer the designations *heparin-associated thrombocytopenia* and *heparin-induced thrombocytopenia* for their descriptive value. As there is no diagnostic test for nonimmune thrombocytopenia caused by heparin, and since many of these thrombocytopenic events are likely caused by other clinical factors that occur during the early hospital period, heparin-*associated* thrombocytopenia has the advantage of not implying causality. On the other hand, heparin-*induced* thrombocytopenia refers to a condition in which the role of heparin is well established, and in which a confirmatory diagnostic test is available.

C. Effect of Heparin on Bleeding Time and Bleeding

Heparin prolongs the bleeding time when administered to normal volunteers (46, 47, 49, 89–91). It is uncertain whether these effects are the result of inhibition

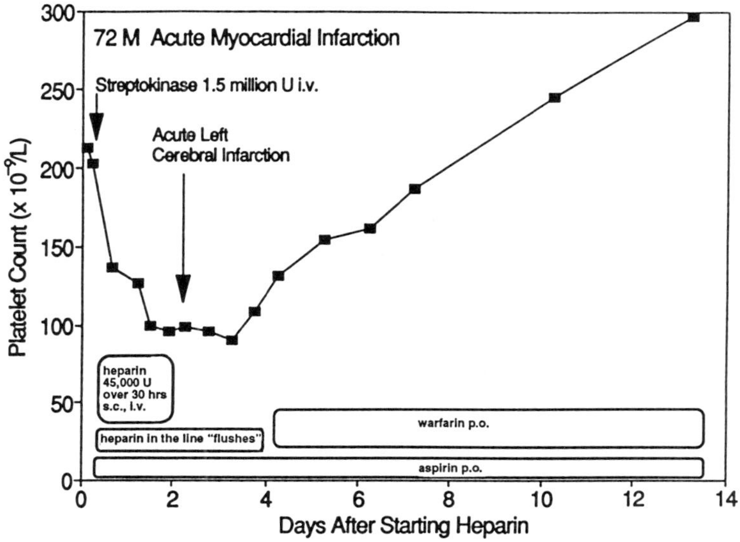

Figure 1 Patient summary: heparin-associated thrombocytopenia. A 72-year-old man developed moderate thrombocytopenia shortly after receiving streptokinase and heparin, which resolved following discontinuation of heparin. The early onset of thrombocytopenia, as well as the negative testing for heparin-induced thrombocytopenia IgG using the platelet ^{14}C-serotonin release assay, suggests that this patient had (nonimmune) heparin-associated thrombocytopenia. Although this patient developed acute cerebral infarction during the period of thrombocytopenia, there are no comparative studies indicating that heparin-associated thrombocytopenia is a prothrombotic disorder, and comorbid explanations for the thrombotic complication are possible (e.g., cardiac source for embolic stroke).

of thrombin-mediated platelet activation (92) or related to the direct effects of heparin on platelets, described previously. Animal studies have shown greater bleeding by standard heparin and pentosan polysulfate, compared with LMWH, ORG 10172, or dermatan sulfate (52, 65, 93, 94).

The bleeding complications of standard heparin and LMWH do not correlate with their anticoagulant effects (3, 95, 96). A series of animal studies demonstrated the role of polysaccharide chain length and extent of sulfation in producing bleeding effects (52, 97, 98). LMWH and dermatan sulfate had equivalent antithrombotic effects as standard heparin, but consistently less hemorrhagic effects (52, 97, 98). Bleeding was greatest when the animals had been given standard heparin and decreased progressively when they were given pentosan polysulfate, LMWH, and dermatan sulfate (52). Increasing the sulfation of low-sulfated polysaccharides such as dermatan sulfate increased their hemorrhagic effects (99).

These animal experiments may have direct relevance to humans. For example, one recent study compared standard heparin with LMWH in over 600 patients undergoing elective hip replacement (100). They observed a similar antithrombotic effect (deep vein thrombosis incidence: standard heparin 19.0%, LMWH 17.1%), but the standard heparin caused more bleeding (9.3% compared to 5.1%). Eriksson et al. (101) also observed less bleeding, together with superior antithrombotic efficacy, using LMWH compared with standard heparin in patients undergoing elective hip surgery. However, a meta-analysis of clinical trials comparing standard with LMWH for postoperative deep vein thrombosis prophylaxis did not find reduced bleeding in the LMWH patients (102).

III. HEPARIN-INDUCED THROMBOCYTOPENIA

Heparin-induced thrombocytopenia is caused by IgG antibodies that develop in patients after 5 or more days of heparin therapy. An important property of the heparin-induced thrombocytopenia IgG (HIT-IgG) is its ability to activate platelets via their Fc receptors. We believe that this property is an important factor in the pathogenesis of both the thrombocytopenia and the paradoxic thrombotic complications that can occur. Heparin-induced thrombocytopenia represents one of the most important "allergic" drug reactions that physicians encounter today, since many affected patients suffer morbidity or death from these thrombotic sequelae.

A. Definition of Immune-Mediated Heparin-Induced Thrombocytopenia

Heparin-induced thrombocytopenia is an *atypical* immune drug-induced thrombocytopenia. Other immune drug-induced thrombocytopenic disorders (e.g., quinine-induced thrombocytopenia) result in clearance of the IgG-sensitized platelets by the reticuloendothelial system. However, *platelet activation* by HIT-IgG, rather than reticuloendothelial clearance, may be the major pathogenic mechanism for accelerated platelet clearance in patients with heparin-induced thrombocytopenia. Thus, a rapid platelet count fall from 700 to 300 $\times$ 10^9 caused by heparin-induced thrombocytopenia can indicate a substantial amount of *in vivo* platelet activation (see Figs. 2 and 3). Indeed, many patients have been described in whom the arterial or venous thrombotic complications coincided with a falling platelet count secondary to heparin-induced thrombocytopenia, even though "thrombocytopenia" did not occur (i.e., the platelet count remained above 150 $\times$ 10^9/L) (103–106). However, if some episodes of heparin-induced thrombocytopenia can produce clinically significant sequelae despite (at times) modest

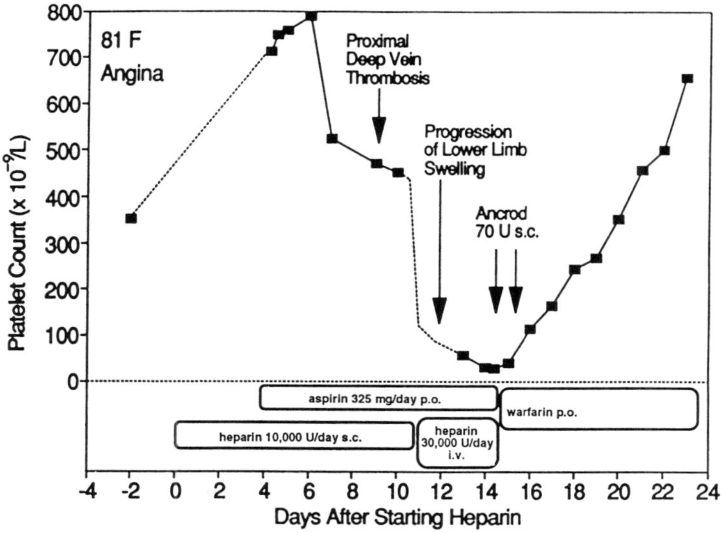

Figure 2 Patient summary: heparin-induced thrombocytopenia and venous thrombosis. An 81-year-old woman developed a drop in the platelet count, from 789 to 454 $\times$ 10^9/L, beginning on day 7 of subcutaneous heparin prophylaxis given for unstable angina. A lower-limb proximal deep vein thrombosis, confirmed by contrast venography, occurred at this time. Full-dose intravenous heparin was commenced, and severe thrombocytopenia (platelet count nadir 26 $\times$ 10^9/L) and progression of lower limb swelling occurred (dose-dependent thrombocytopenia). Heparin-induced thrombocytopenia was confirmed using the platelet ^{14}C-serotonin release assay. The patient recovered uneventfully, following discontinuation of heparin and administration of subcutaneous ancrod and oral warfarin. Note that severe heparin-induced thrombocytopenia occurred, even though the patient had been receiving aspirin for therapy of angina.

''thrombocytopenia,'' there arises a significant diagnostic problem: how can heparin-induced thrombocytopenia be distinguished from other common causes of thrombocytopenia in hospitalized patients, such as hemodilution or septicemia?

In 1986, Sheridan and colleagues reported that the platelet ^{14}C-serotonin release assay is a very sensitive and specific test for HIT-IgG (107), an observation that has been confirmed by several laboratories (87, 108–110). The availability of this test has permitted physicians to determine which patients who develop thrombocytopenia on heparin truly have immune heparin-induced thrombocytopenia. We believe that the diagnostic criteria for *definite* heparin-induced thrombocytopenia must include positive testing using a sensitive and specific assay for this syndrome:

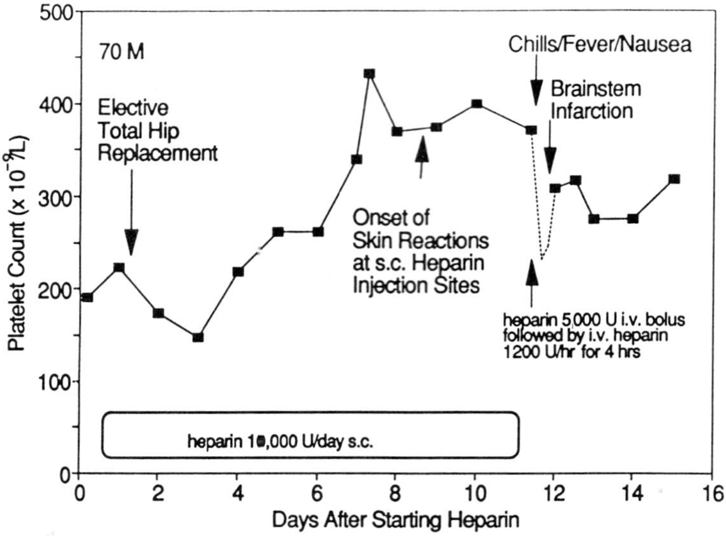

Figure 3 Patient summary: heparin-induced thrombocytopenia, acute systemic reaction, and cerebrovascular accident. A 70-year-old man received subcutaneous heparin prophylaxis for total hip replacement surgery. Beginning on day 8 of heparin therapy, he complained of painful skin reactions at the heparin injection sites, although thrombocytopenia did not occur. On day 11, he was given a 5000-unit intravenous bolus for venogram-confirmed proximal lower limb venous thrombosis. Ten minutes later, he developed chills, fever, and nausea (acute systemic reaction). Intravenous heparin in therapeutic doses was continued for 4 hr, following which the patient developed signs and symptoms of a brain cerebrovascular infarction (later confirmed by magnetic resonance imaging). All heparin was discontinued, and a repeat platelet count was obtained 8 hr later. Only a mild drop in the platelet count was documented (379 to 309 $\times$ 10^9/L); however, a more marked but transient drop in the platelet count cannot be excluded (see Refs. 235 and 254 for examples of the transient nature of the thrombocytopenia in patients with acute systemic reactions following intravenous bolus heparin). Heparin-induced thrombocytopenia was confirmed using the platelet ^{14}C-serotonin release assay.

Definition of heparin-induced thrombocytopenia: A decrease in the platelet count, usually greater than 50%, during or shortly following heparin therapy, that cannot be explained by other clinical factors, in which the presence of HIT-IgG is proven.

B. Incidence of Heparin-Induced Thrombocytopenia

Despite many prospective studies, the frequency of heparin-induced thrombocytopenia remains unknown, for several reasons. First, no prospective studies were performed using the optimal diagnostic test (^{14}C-serotonin release assay). Second, many patients who had "early" thrombocytopenia (within 5 days of beginning heparin treatment), or whose platelet counts initially fell but then recovered on continuing heparin therapy, were included in some studies. It is unlikely these patients had IgG-mediated heparin-induced thrombocytopenia, although heparin may have contributed to the thrombocytopenia by the nonimmune mild platelet-activating properties discussed previously (heparin-associated thrombocytopenia). Third, some patients may have had unrecognized comorbid clinical conditions that explained the thrombocytopenia.

We have used the platelet ^{14}C-serotonin release assay to analyze prospectively collected plasma samples from almost 400 patients who received prophylactic-dose standard or LMWH following elective hip surgery (111). We showed that approximately 7% of patients treated with standard heparin derived from porcine mucosa produced HIT-IgG. The HIT-IgG was first detected between days 5 and 11 (median days 7–8), consistent with a primary immune response. Using a 50% fall in platelet count as a definition of heparin-induced thrombocytopenia in this study, 7/203 (3.4%) patients treated with unfractionated (porcine mucosal) heparin for at least 5 days developed heparin-induced thrombocytopenia in this study. Using a more "standard definition" (platelet count $< 150 \times 10^9$/L), the incidence of heparin-induced thrombocytopenia was 4/203 (2.0%).

1. Incidence of Thrombocytopenia with Different Heparin Preparations

Our meta-analysis of the five prospective studies of thrombocytopenia in patients comparing bovine lung to porcine mucosal heparin showed that the frequency of thrombocytopenia was greater in patients who received bovine lung heparin (112). It is possible that there is a difference in *immunogenicity* between these two heparin preparations, possibly related to the different structural characteristics of these two heparins (Table 1). It is possible that LMWH are less immunogenic than standard heparins (111). "Epidemics" of heparin-induced thrombocytopenia have been reported (113), possibly reflecting the use of a more immunogenic preparation due to manufacturing differences.

2. Incidence of Heparin-Induced Thrombosis

As we have previously noted (112, 114), several patients have developed thrombotic complications during prospective studies of heparin-induced thrombocytopenia. In these studies, if only those patients who developed thrombocytopenia beginning on day 5 or later of heparin therapy are considered as the denominator (i.e., presumed to have IgG-mediated heparin-induced thrombocytopenia), then the risk of heparin-induced thrombosis could be as high as 30% (Table 2). A similar risk of thrombosis was also observed in two large defined-group retrospective studies (Table 3) performed at the University of Missouri–Columbia Health Sciences Center, where daily platelet count measurements and diagnostic testing

Table 2 Estimated Frequency of Heparin-Induced Thrombocytopenia and Heparin-Induced Thrombosis in the Prospective Studies of Intravenous Therapeutic-Dose Heparin

Ref.	Total number of patients studied	Number of patients with early (≤4 days) thrombocytopenia	Number of patients with late (≥5 days) thrombocytopenia	Number of patients with thrombosis (arterial, venous)		
115	43	1	4	0	A-0	V-0
116	104	5	5	0	A-0	V-0
117	43	0	1	1	A-1	V-0
104,[a] 118[a]	211	2	9	3	A-2	V-1
119	143	4	5	1	A-0	V-1
120,121	89	0	2	2	A-1	V-1
122	90	0	1	0	A-0	V-0
123	142	—	9	4	A-2	V-2
124	89	—	2	1	A-0	V-1
22	37	6	3	0	A-0	V-0
125*	120	2	2	2	A-1	V-1
126	131	2	3	0	A-0	V-0
127	94	3	0	0	A-0	V-0
Total	1336	24	46 (3.4%)	14	A-7	V-7

[a] Some of the information for this table was obtained by personal communication (see Ref. 114).

Only prospective studies of therapeutic-dose heparin are analyzed. The platelet count nadir had to be at least below 150 × 10^9/L to be included. Patients who developed thrombocytopenia during the first 4 days of heparin therapy, or whose platelet count returned to baseline despite continuing heparin therapy, are not considered to have heparin-induced thrombocytopenia, as these are unlikely to be IgG-mediated. Heparin-induced thrombosis was defined as any new or progressive thrombosis on heparin therapy that coincided with thrombocytopenia. Whenever there was doubt in the categorization of a thrombocytopenic event, it was arbitrarily included in the heparin-induced thrombocytopenia group, to minimize bias toward overestimating the relative frequency of heparin-induced thrombosis. Two early prospective studies (128, 129) are excluded from this table because day of onset of thrombocytopenia is not indicated, and information regarding thrombotic sequelae is not given. In addition, negative testing for HIT-IgG (130) in one of these studies (128) suggests that the majority of these patients did not have IgG-mediated heparin-induced thrombocytopenia.

Table 3 Frequency of Thrombocytopenia and Thrombosis in Two Large Defined-Group Retrospective Studies

Ref.	Patient population	Number of patients	Number with positive test for heparin-induced thrombocytopenia	Number of patients with thrombotic complications (% of heparin-induced thrombocytopenia patients)
131	Open heart surgery	4261 (10-year study)	82 (1.9%)	31 (38%)
132	Intra-aortic balloon pump	764 (9-year study)	35 (4.5%)	17 (49%)

for heparin-induced thrombocytopenia (platelet aggregation studies) are routinely performed (133). The risk of thrombosis in their study of 169 patients was approximately 20% (133), which is similar to the risk found in our analysis of the prospective studies. The frequency of thrombotic complications is greater in other retrospective studies of heparin-induced thrombocytopenia (Table 4), but this probably reflects worst-case recognition bias.

C. Clinical Characteristics of Heparin-Induced Thrombocytopenia

In recent years, there has been a greater recognition of the clinical characteristics of this unusual drug reaction.

1. Day of Onset and Severity of the Thrombocytopenia

The typical patients with heparin-induced thrombocytopenia develop moderate thrombocytopenia beginning on day 5–12 of heparin therapy (111,134). Table 4 summarizes the platelet count nadirs of several large series of patients with heparin-induced thrombocytopenia (Table 4). In these studies, the mean platelet count ranged between 30 and 55 $\times$ 10^9/L. Rarely, the platelet count can fall to as low as 5–20 $\times$ 10^9/L (137, 143–149). However, this is uncommon and is in contrast to other more typical drug-induced thrombocytopenic disorders (e.g., quinine-induced thrombocytopenia), where the platelet count almost invariably is below 20 $\times$ 10^9/L (150). Indeed, the platelet count nadirs seen in patients

Table 4 Platelet Count Nadirs in Large (Minimum 10 Patients) Retrospective Studies of Heparin-Induced Thrombocytopenia

Ref.	Number of patients	Patients with arterial or venous thrombosis complicating heparin-induced thrombocytopenia	Mean platelet count ($\times 10^{-9}$/L)	Median platelet count ($\times 10^{-9}$/L)
135	22	16 (73%)	32	25
136	12	7 (58%)	44	51
137	62	38 (61%)	—	—
138	25	25 (100%)	44	32
139	23	23 (100%)	31	19
105	16	10 (63%)	53	—
133	169	30 (18%)	56	—
140	21	13 (62%)	47	44
141	10	10 (100%)	32	33
142	53	37 (70%)	49	—
Total	391[a]	201 (~50%)[a]	49	—

[a] Totals exclude Ref. 135, since these patients are included in Ref. 137.

The mean platelet count is approximately 50 × 10^9/L in this compilation of large retrospective studies of heparin-induced thrombocytopenia.

Note: The % thrombotic complications varies widely (18–100%), because some studies selected only patients with thrombotic complications.

with heparin-induced thrombocytopenia resemble more closely those seen in patients with septicemia-induced thrombocytopenia, another disorder that may be characterized by platelet activation.

It remains unknown what factors are the most important in determining the severity of the thrombocytopenia. Some of the causative factors could include the dose of heparin given, interpatient variability in the number or function of platelet Fc receptors, the titer of the HIT-IgG, the baseline platelet count, and megakaryocyte responsiveness to the thrombocytopenia.

2. *Dose and Route of Heparin*

Heparin-induced thrombocytopenia can be caused by heparin given by any route and at any dose. For example, patients have been reported in whom severe heparin-induced thrombocytopenia occurred in patients receiving small amounts of heparin given as ''flushes'' to maintain intravascular catheters (105, 151–157). However, in some patients there is evidence for dose-dependent thrombocytopenia (see Fig. 2; see in particular Ref. 158). Further evidence for dose-dependent thrombocytopenia is suggested by the observation that the incidence of thrombocytopenia is higher in the prospective studies of therapeutic-dose compared with prophylactic-dose heparin (112, 114). Many patients have been reported who developed moderate thrombocytopenia and venous thrombotic complications while receiving prophylactic-dose heparin, only to develop more severe thrombocytopenia and progression of thrombosis when the heparin dose was increased (136, 159–165).

3. *Other Sulfated Polysaccharides Implicated as Causes of Thrombocytopenia and Thrombosis*

Recently, it has been recognized that sulfated polysaccharides other than heparin can cause a syndrome of thrombocytopenia and paradoxic thrombosis. Use of heparin to treat thrombotic complications in these patients leads to continuing or progressive thrombocytopenia and thrombosis. The implicated drugs are: LMWH (166–172), pentosan polysulfate (173–186), and an antiarthritic polysulfated chondroitin sulfate preparation known as Arteparon® (187–189). Conversely, there have been many instances of patients with heparin-induced thrombocytopenia treated with LMWH in which persistent or recurrent thrombocytopenia occurred, accompanied by thrombotic compications in some instances (190–195).

Standard heparin, LMWH, pentosan polysulfate, and Arteparon® share common structural features—they are all high-sulfated, nonbranching, polysaccharide chains of 10 or more saccharide units. Moreover, these substances show virtually 100% cross-reactivity with standard heparin for HIT-IgG. Using sensitive assays, HIT-IgG activates platelets equally well in the presence of LMWH, pentosan polysulfate, Arteparon®, or dextran sulfate (187, 189, 196–198).

4. *Thrombotic, Hemorrhagic, and Other Sequelae of Heparin-Induced Thrombocytopenia*

Arterial and venous thrombotic complications are responsible for most of the morbidity and mortality associated with this syndrome. Less commonly, fatal hemorrhagic events occur. Recently, acute systemic reactions caused by administration of heparin bolus therapy to patients who have HIT-IgG have been recognized.

5. *Arterial Thrombosis*

The occurrence of unexpected multiple arterial thrombi, beginning between days 7 and 15 of heparin therapy, was first reported in 10 patients by Weismann and Tobin in 1958 (199). Subsequently, Roberts and colleagues reported 14 similar patients (200–202). The recognition that thrombocytopenia was an inherent feature in these patients with apparent heparin-induced thrombosis occurred almost 20 years later (74, 135, 158, 161, 164).

The most common arterial thrombotic complications include lower limb arterial thrombosis (often leading to gangrene and lower limb loss), thrombotic cerebrovascular accidents, and myocardial infarction (see References cited in Table 4). However, many other arterial thromboses with serious sequelae have been reported, including upper limb arterial thrombosis (203, 204), renal artery thrombosis (resulting in renal failure) (161), paraplegia secondary to distal aortic or spinal artery thrombosis (82, 148, 158, 205, 206), ischemic lumbosacral plexopathy (207), thrombosis of left or right ventricular or atrial chambers (186, 208–211), arterial graft occlusions (137, 151, 212), arteriovenous fistulae used for hemodialysis (213, 214), and prosthetic valve thrombosis (215).

6. *Pathological and Angiographic Features of the Thrombi*

Heparin-induced thrombocytopenia is sometimes called the "white clot syndrome" (151), as the arterial thrombi are usually pale in appearance, reflecting their platelet-rich nature (141, 151, 162, 191, 192, 199, 216); however, variegated thrombi with both pale and red components have been observed (216). The thrombi can be adherent to the endothelial surface (217, 218) and angiographically appear as lobulated excrescences within the vessels (162). Large or medium-sized arteries usually are involved (*macro*vascular thrombosis). This is in contrast to thrombotic thrombocytopenic purpura, which is characterized by *micro*vascular thrombosis consisting of platelet-rich hyaline thrombi.

7. *Venous Thrombosis*

Many patients have been reported who have developed venous thrombosis and pulmonary embolism following onset of heparin-induced thrombocytopenia (113, 119, 136–140, 145–147, 163, 168, 175, 212, 217–219). Sometimes, the temporal relationship between the two events suggests causality. Other times, the relationship is more obscure. For example, many of these complications occur in patients who are receiving heparin because of their increased risk for venous thrombosis. However, many patients have been reported in whom the venous thrombosis progressed to gangrene, leading to limb amputation (138, 141, 148, 151, 212, 220–223). Further, pale, platelet-rich thrombi have been removed from large veins of some patients with severe venous thrombotic complications (141, 216). Other, unusually severe venous thrombotic complications that have occurred in patients with heparin-induced thrombocytopenia include thrombosis of cerebral veins (including dural sinus and cavernous sinus thrombosis) (136, 183, 224–227) and venous thrombosis of upper limb veins (141, 223). In some patients, platelet-rich "white clots" have been observed in the pulmonary arteries, possibly indicating *in situ* pulmonary artery thrombosis rather than true embolism (147, 217–219). Heparin-induced thrombocytopenia and malignancy were the two risk factors identified for recurrent venous thromboembolism in a large retrospective analysis of heparin treatment for venous thrombosis (228).

8. Skin Necrosis

There are many reports of patients who have developed painful, erythematous dermal lesions at the sites of standard or LMWH injections, which sometimes progress to necrosis (106, 109, 164, 229–235). Although not all these patients are thrombocytopenic, we postulate that the skin lesions represent a localized form of heparin-induced thrombocytopenia (235). These patients are at risk for thrombocytopenia and other thrombotic reactions if the heparin dose is increased (231, 235).

Patients have also been reported in whom skin necrosis complicated heparin-induced thrombocytopenia caused by heparin administered via the intravenous route (236–239). In some of the patients, warfarin may have played a role in the dermal necrosis (239).

9. Bilateral Adrenal Hemorrhage

One of the few characteristic "hemorrhagic" manifestations of heparin-induced thrombocytopenia is bilateral adrenal hemorrhage (192, 240–248), although unilateral adrenal hemorrhage has been observed on some occasions (249). Adrenal vein thrombosis has been found in several of these patients (240, 245), suggesting that the adrenal hemorrhage is secondary to infarction of the glands. Hemorrhagic necrosis of the adrenal glands also occurs in certain other prothrombotic disorders (e.g., Waterhouse-Friderichsen syndrome of meningococcemia, disseminated intravascular coagulation, and bilateral adrenal hemorrhage in children; antiphospholipid antibody syndrome) (250, 251). Both acute and chronic adrenal insufficiency syndromes have been reported, and physicians should consider this complication in patients with possible heparin-induced thrombocytopenia who develop unexplained hypotension, hyponatremia, or abdominal pain.

10. Patient-Dependent Factors in Thrombotic Complications

Several studies suggest that patient-dependent factors "localize" thrombotic complications in heparin-induced thrombocytopenia (104, 138, 142, 252, 253). For example, it was observed that lower limb thrombosis occurred at sites of vessel injury (e.g., following angiography) in 19 of 25 patients with heparin-induced thrombosis (138). Recently, we observed that heparin-induced thrombocytopenia was more likely to be complicated by venous thrombosis in postoperative patients receiving heparin prophylaxis, whereas arterial thrombotic complications were more likely to occur in patients hospitalized with preexisting cardiovascular disease (142).

11. Acute Systemic Reactions

Recently, it has been reported that patients who develop HIT-IgG following heparin exposure can have an abrupt fall in the platelet count and an acute systemic reaction following intravenous bolus heparin administration. These patients develop fever chills, hypertension and tachycardia, diaphoresis, flushing, and other symptoms (235). Cardiac or respiratory arrest has occurred in some patients following heparin bolus therapy as well (158, 159, 231). It is important to recognize this syndrome promptly, as continued use of heparin can result in life-threatening sequelae. An abrupt platelet count fall coinciding with transient global amnesia has also been reported in two patients with heparin-induced thrombocytopenia following intravenous heparin bolus use (254). These complications of bolus heparin therapy could be caused by inflammatory mediators produced as a consequence of marked *in vivo* platelet activation of abrupt onset.

12. Disseminated Intravascular Coagulation (DIC)

DIC has been reported in some patients with severe heparin-induced thrombocytopenia (143, 163, 165, 188, 192, 226, 255–259). Only rarely are red cell fragments observed (165, 255). Sometimes, the fibrinogen falls immediately after the heparin is stopped (143), suggesting competing roles of heparin in promoting (i.e., via platelet activation) and inhibiting (i.e., via thrombin inhibition) the DIC. We have observed several patients with heparin-induced thrombocytopenia, in whom the platelet count fell further, immediately after the heparin therapy was discontinued.

13. Heparin Resistance

The inability to readily achieve therapeutic levels of anticoagulation in patients who develop heparin-induced thrombocytopenia has been observed in some patients (74, 137). Possible explanations for this phenomenon include release of the heparin-neutralizing substance, platelet factor 4, from the activated platelets (67–69) or procoagulant effects of platelet-derived microparticles (70, 71).

14. Bleeding Complications

Bleeding complications are relatively uncommon in heparin-induced thrombocytopenia. In a series of 169 patients with heparin-induced thrombocytopenia reported by Laster and colleagues, 30 patients developed thrombotic complications, whereas only eight patients had bleeding events (133). Serious bleeding complications have included intracranial hemorrhage (133, 137, 151), retroperitoneal hemorrhage (260), and gastrointestinal hemorrhage (133).

15. Children and Neonates

Heparin-induced thrombocytopenia has been observed in children (133, 211, 261). In addition, one group (using citrated platelet aggregation studies) reported that heparin-induced thrombocytopenia and thrombosis can occur in neonates receiving heparin in the newborn intensive care unit (262). If confirmed by more specific assays for heparin-induced thrombocytopenia, this study would have important implications for neonatal patients.

16. Risk of Reexposure to Heparin in Patients with Heparin-Induced Thrombocytopenia

The risk of thrombocytopenia and thrombosis is high in patients with a recent history of heparin-induced thrombocytopenia, in whom HIT-IgG can still be detected (213). However, the HIT-IgG usually disappears within several weeks of the episode of heparin-induced thrombocytopenia (133, 263). For these patients, the risk of recurrence of HIT-IgG and thrombocytopenia following reexposure to heparin is unknown. Recently, a patient developed fatal recurrence of heparin-induced thrombocytopenia when given a course of heparin 6 years following an initial episode of heparin-induced thrombocytopenia (264).

17. Delayed Onset and Prolonged Thrombocytopenia

Rarely, a brief exposure to heparin, ranging from a single injection to a few days of use, can result in onset of thrombocytopenia and thrombosis that begins several days after the exposure to heparin has ceased (188, 265, 266). Recovery may take several weeks in these patients. In other patients in whom thrombocytopenia begins during heparin treatment, the platelet count can remain reduced for more than a week after the heparin is stopped (145, 165). The explanation for the persistence of the thrombocytopenia is unknown, but could involve formation of an autoreactive, platelet-activating IgG.

D. Pathogenesis of Heparin-Induced Thrombocytopenia

Several aspects of the pathogenesis of heparin-induced thrombocytopenia will be considered: (1) IgG-mediated platelet activation; (2) role of platelet Fc receptor; (3) platelet microparticle generation; (4) endothelial activation; (5) the identity of the putative antigen; (6) the role of platelet membrane glycoproteins.

1. Heparin-Induced Thrombocytopenia Is Caused by IgG that Activates Platelets in the Presence of Heparin

Evidence for the role of IgG in the pathogenesis of heparin-induced thrombocytopenia was first provided by Rhodes et al. (267). These physicians described two patients with heparin-induced thrombocytopenia complicated by myocardial infarction. Sera and purified IgG from these patients produced aggregation of normal donor platelets in the presence of therapeutic concentrations of heparin (267). Over the next 10 years, several other groups confirmed these findings (82, 144, 145, 161, 268–271). The HIT-IgG are potent platelet activators and result in platelet granule release (107, 161, 271, 272) and thromboxane generation (82, 271–273).

2. *Platelet Activation by IgG Occurs via the Platelet $Fc_{\gamma}II$ Receptors*

Platelets bear a 40-kDa receptor for the Fc component of IgG (Fc_{γ}RIIA, CD32) (274–276). The critical role of these receptors in the pathogenesis of heparin-induced thrombocytopenia was first shown in 1988. Platelet activation by sera or purified IgG from patients with heparin-induced thrombocytopenia could be progressively inhibited by increasing concentrations of human or goat Fc, as well as patient, but not control, $F(ab')_2$ (277). In addition, the monoclonal antibody IV.3, which recognizes and blocks access to the Fc_{γ}II receptors, completely blocked platelet activation by HIT-IgG (277). The critical role for the Fc_{γ}II receptors has been confirmed by other investigators (196, 278–280). Despite the role of the platelet Fc receptors, there is no evidence that soluble IgG/heparin immune complexes are formed; it appears that the pathogenic immune complex is formed on the platelet surface microenvironment (*in situ* immune complex).

Various murine monoclonal antibodies reactive with certain platelet epitopes can result in potent platelet activation (281). This suggests that heparin-induced thrombocytopenia could be a prototypic model for other disorders in which platelet activation occurs via IgG that interacts with the platelet Fc_{γ}II receptors. Recent work indicates that intracellular tyrosine phosphorylation of the Fc_{γ}II receptors may be related to the functional activity of these receptors (282).

3. *Role of Fc Receptor Variability*

It is possible that Fc_{γ}II receptor variability explains some of the marked differences in severity of thrombocytopenia and clinical outcomes observed in this syndrome. For example, platelets from different individuals exhibit considerable variability in their response to IgG immune complexes (283, 284) or to HIT-IgG (284). Recently, increased platelet Fc receptor number and reactivity to HIT-IgG was observed in a subset of heparin-induced thrombocytopenia patients with severe disease (285). Previously, other investigators had shown that the ability to detect HIT-IgG could be increased by a few weeks if—following recovery from the thrombocytopenia—the patient's own platelets were used for diagnostic testing (105, 268, 286); sometimes, only autologous platelets were activated by patient plasma (151). Taken together, these observations suggest an important pathogenic role for platelet Fc receptor function in heparin-induced thrombocytopenia.

4. *Role of Procoagulant Platelet-Derived Microparticles*

As discussed earlier, venous thrombosis, venous gangrene, pulmonary embolism, and disseminated intravascular coagulation can occur in some patients with heparin-induced thrombocytopenia. A plausible pathogenic explanation for these findings are our observations that HIT-IgG can cause platelets to generate platelet-derived microparticles with procoagulant activity (287, 288). Recently, we have observed circulating platelet-derived microparticles with procoagulant activity in patients with severe heparin-induced thrombocytopenia (289).

5. *Role of Endothelial Activation*

The pathological finding of adherent platelet-rich thrombi adherent to endothelial cells in some patients with severe heparin-induced thrombocytopenia suggests a possible role for endothelial activation in this syndrome. Endothelial cells also carry certain sulfated polysaccharides, including heparan sulfate (290). Structurally, heparan sulfate closely resembles heparin, but is less highly epimerized and N- and O-sulfated than heparin (291). Cines and colleagues have reported that heparan sulfate can cross-react with heparin for the HIT-IgG (154). They demonstrated that HIT-IgG resulted in tissue factor expression on the surface of cultured endothelial cells in the absence of added heparin (154). Furthermore, these effects could be nullified by preincubation of the serum with heparin-treated platelets or by heparin/heparan sulfate–coated beads or following treatment of the endothelial cells with heparinase.

6. *What Is the Antigen in Heparin-Induced Thrombocytopenia?*

Despite the important role of heparin in initiating and sustaining this syndrome, a number of investigators have been unable to demonstrate directly in vitro an interaction between the HIT-IgG and heparin (145, 187, 198, 257). This has led to suggestions that a complex between heparin and a platelet component could be responsible for formation of the antigen (145).

Several recent observations suggest that the role of heparin in producing this syndrome is immunologically less specific than initially believed. First, as discussed previously, other highly sulfated polysaccharides can produce an IgG-mediated syndrome characterized by thrombocytopenia and thrombosis (LMW heparin, Arteparon®, pentosan polysulfate). Second, there is both *in vivo* and *in vitro* evidence for cross-reactivity among these and other highly sulfated polysaccharides with heparin for HIT-IgG (20, 189, 196, 198). Third, high levels of both high (107, 277) and low (20) sulfated polysaccharides will inhibit the platelet activation caused by these IgG. Fourth, de-N-sulfation of heparin nullifies its platelet interactions, including (1) its specific binding to platelets (20), (2) its nonimmune proaggregatory effects (66), and (3) its ability to support activation of platelets by HIT-IgG (20). These various observations suggest that the "immunogenicity" of heparin and other highly sulfated polysaccharides could relate to a "carrier" role; i.e., they localize (and perhaps modify the antigenic structure) of another antigenic moiety to the platelet surface.

Recent studies suggest that the α-granule protein, platelet factor 4 (PF4), may comprise the antigen recognized by HIT-IgG. PF4 is a cationic glycoprotein that binds strongly to heparin (9, 10, 72, 73). Recently, Amiral and colleagues showed that recombinant or natural PF4, complexed with heparin, could be used as an immunological target for an ELISA that they reported to be sensitive and specific for the diagnosis of heparin-induced thombocytopenia (292).

The formation of an antigenic complex between a negatively charged polysaccharide (i.e., heparin) and a protein such as PF4 has a clinicopathological parallel: increasing evidence suggests that the antigen target for antiphospholipid (lupus anticoagulant) antibodies is a complex between negatively charged phospholipids and β_2-glycoprotein I (apolipoprotein H) (293–295). Indeed, a recent study suggested that anticardiolipin antibodies are present in a subset of patients with heparin-induced thrombocytopenia (296), indicating that some immunological cross-reactivity could exist between phospholipid/β_2-glycoprotein I and heparin/PF4 complexes.

7. *Role of Platelet Surface Glycoproteins*

As yet, no role for integral membrane glycoproteins (other than the Fc receptor) has been implicated in the pathogenesis of heparin-induced thrombocytopenia. Both Bernard-Soulier (GP Ib/IX complex deficiency) and Glanzmann's thrombasthenia (GP IIb/IIIa complex deficiency) platelets can be readily activated by HIT-IgG (273, 277, 278, 280, 297).

E. Diagnostic Testing

Although a large number of assays for heparin-induced thrombocytopenia have been reported, tests of platelet activation are most frequently used.

1. *Tests of Platelet Activation: Platelet Aggregation Studies*

In many centers, platelet aggregation studies, using patient plasma and normal donor platelets in citrated plasma, are used to diagnose heparin-induced thrombocytopenia. Unfortunately, this assay has very low sensitivity (approximately 50%) (108, 110, 298). As discussed previously, heparin can result in aggregation of normal donor platelets, and therefore other platelet-activating factors in patient plasma may be augmented by heparin, thus resulting in false-positive results (low specificity). In our view, these assays are unsatisfactory for the diagnosis of heparin-induced thrombocytopenia. The sensitivity can be increased by using several platelet donors (299, 300).

2. *Tests of Platelet Activation: Platelet ^{14}C-Serotonin Release Assay*

In 1986, Sheridan and colleagues reported a new assay for heparin-induced thrombocytopenia (107). This technique uses normal donor platelets that are radiolabeled, washed, and then resuspended in divalent cation-containing buffer. These investigators observed a characteristic pattern for heparin-induced thrombocytopenic sera—^{14}C-serotonin release at therapeutic heparin concentrations that was inhibited at high heparin concentrations (107). Subsequent studies have shown that sensitivity for the ^{14}C-serotonin release can be increased by selecting platelet donors with optimal reactivity to Fc receptor stimuli and by including weakly positive heparin-induced thrombocytopenia sera controls to be sure that the platelets selected can react to weak heparin-induced thrombocytopenia sera (284). Other groups have confirmed that the ^{14}C-serotonin release assay is more sensitive than aggregation studies using citrated PRP (87, 108, 110). Provided that the donor platelets are washed and resuspended in buffer as per the serotonin release assay, other platelet activation end-points can be used, including aggregation of the washed platelets (108) and flow cytometric detection of platelet-derived microparticles (301).

3. *Other Tests for Heparin-Induced Thrombocytopenia: Indirect Immunofluorescence Assays for Platelet-Associated IgG*

Assays have been developed for heparin-induced thrombocytopenia that make use of non-platelet-activation-dependent end-points, such as various tests for platelet-associated IgG. Using indirect immunofluorescence, an increase in platelet-associated IgG can be shown in the presence of heparin and patient serum or plasma in some patients (178, 187, 302). However, the increase in fluorescence is often weak, suggesting that these assays may not be very sensitive for HIT-IgG. Indeed, indirect immunofluorescence was less sensitive than platelet aggregation assays in one study (302).

4. *Other Tests for Heparin-Induced Thrombocytopenia: ELISAs*

The enzyme-linked immunosorbent assay (ELISA) technique has been adapted for use as a diagnostic test for heparin-induced thrombocytopenia (292, 303, 304). For example, washed and formalin-fixed platelets have been used as a "target" for HIT-IgG in the presence of various concentrations of heparin (303, 304). Recently, Amiral and colleagues reported that recombinant or naturally obtained PF4, complexed with heparin, could be used as a target for HIT-IgG (292). None of these assays have been compared directly with the ^{14}C-serotonin release assay.

F. Treatment of Heparin-Induced Thrombocytopenia

1. *General Approach*

For most patients with heparin-induced thrombocytopenia, discontinuation of heparin therapy will result in an increase in the platelet count within 24–48 h and recovery to above 150×10^9/L within 4–5 days. Platelet transfusions should not be given, both because bleeding complications are uncommon, and because thrombotic complications can occur following platelet transfusions (147, 268). For patients with a confirmed venous or arterial thrombosis, alternate anticoagulant therapy should be used (discussed subsequently). It is uncertain whether patients who develop heparin-induced thrombocytopenia during heparin prophylaxis (e.g., postoperative patients) and who are asymptomatic should receive alternate anticoagulation or platelet inhibitors when heparin-induced thrombocytopenia is diagnosed, or whether these patients should only be monitored carefully for thromboembolic complications. Some physicians prescribe aspirin in this situation (305).

2. *Ancrod*

Ancrod (Arvin®, Knoll Pharmaceuticals) is a rapidly acting anticoagulant that has been used for the treatment of heparin-induced thrombocytopenia (306, 307). Derived from the venom of the Malayan pit viper (*Agkistrodon rhodostoma*), ancrod cleaves fibrinopeptide A from fibrinogen, producing an unstable monomer that is removed by the reticuloendothelial system (308–310). We administer ancrod intravenously, giving 70 units for an average-sized adult over 6–12 h. Although ancrod can be given subcutaneously, there may be greater delays before achieving a target fibrinogen value, and immunological ancrod resistance may occur more quickly. Following achievement of the target fibrinogen level (0.5–0.75 g/L), further ancrod administration is based on the fibrinogen concentrations. Recently, we have been giving ancrod by constant infusion (conveniently prepared as 70 units ancrod mixed with 100 cc normal saline and administered using infusion pump), adjusting the dose twice daily depending on the fibrinogen levels.

There are several laboratory issues relating to the measurement of fibrinogen when ancrod therapy is used. First, coagulation instruments that utilize optical endpoints can overestimate the clottable fibrinogen value, because these instruments can also detect the fibrin/fibrinogen monomers. Thus, we perform assays for clottable fibrinogen (e.g., Clauss assay). We have also used the 10-unit thrombin clotting time to estimate the fibrinogen levels. This is done by determining a standard curve relationship between the clottable fibrinogen and the thrombin times, using the laboratory's own methods for these assays. The thrombin time has the advantage of being easier to perform than the Clauss fibrinogen assay. In general, fibrinogen and thrombin time assays are among the least well standardized in coagulation testing, so the physician using ancrod should communicate carefully with the laboratory regarding coagulation testing in these patients. Second, it is possible that *ex vivo* degradation of fibrinogen by ancrod can occur, particularly if there are delays before testing the sample. Some investigators recommend adding antivenom to the plasma sample prior to analysis to avoid this potential problem. Third, the low fibrinogen levels on ancrod usually prolong the prothrombin time (PT). Thus, for patients receiving warfarin, factor assays may be needed to monitor warfarin anticoagulation. We aim for a target prothrombin level of 0.20–0.30 (normal, 1.0) on warfarin before discontinuing ancrod therapy.

We usually give ancrod for several days, waiting until the platelet count has returned to near-normal levels, before starting the warfarin. Side effects are uncommon and can include inflammation at the injection site (particularly when given subcutaneously). The risk of bleeding appears to be low (306, 311). Resistance to the drug, presumably mediated by antiancrod antibodies, can occur in patients who are receiving the drug for 4–6 weeks (306, 312).

3. ORG 10172 (Lomoparan®, also known as Orgaran®)

ORG 10172 is a mixture of sulfated glycosaminoglycans derived from animal intestinal mucosa and consists of 84% heparan sulfate (approximately 5% with high antithrombin affinity), 12% dermatan sulfate, and 4% chondroitin sulfate (65). Unlike ancrod, which anticoagulates by removing the final substrate of coagulation (fibrinogen), ORG 10172 will inhibit coagulation proximally (inhibition of thrombin and Xa) (65). A theoretical advantage of ORG 10172 is its ability to inhibit platelet activation by HIT-IgG *in vitro* (198, 313). However, there is a major potential disadvantage of ORG 10172—approximately 10% of HIT-IgG sera will cross-react with ORG 10172 (313, 314), and in these patients the treatment could produce thrombotic complications. Although ORG 10172 has been used successfully in many patients (197, 198, 313–318), larger experience is needed before broad recommendations can be made.

4. High-Dose Intravenous Immunoglobulin G (IVIgG)

In theory, high-dose IVIgG could inhibit platelet activation by HIT-IgG by blocking access to the platelet Fc receptors. There are a few reports indicating benefit to this therapy (319–321; see Fig. 4). Greater experience is required to determine the indications for this novel therapy in patients with heparin-induced thrombocytopenia.

5. Plasmapheresis

Plasmapheresis has been used to treat patients with heparin-induced thrombocytopenia (322–325). Reduction in HIT-IgG can be demonstrated following pheresis, but thrombotic sequelae are not necessarily prevented (325).

6. Antithrombin III Concentrates

Antithrombin III concentrates have been used to treat severe heparin-induced thrombocytopenia with disseminated intravascular coagulation (256).

7. Aspirin/Dipyridamole/Dextran/Iloprost

Many physicians use one or more antiplatelet agents, such as aspirin, dipyridamole, dextran, and iloprost, in the management of patients with heparin-induced thrombocytopenia (138, 151, 212, 213, 305, 326). *In vitro* studies show that

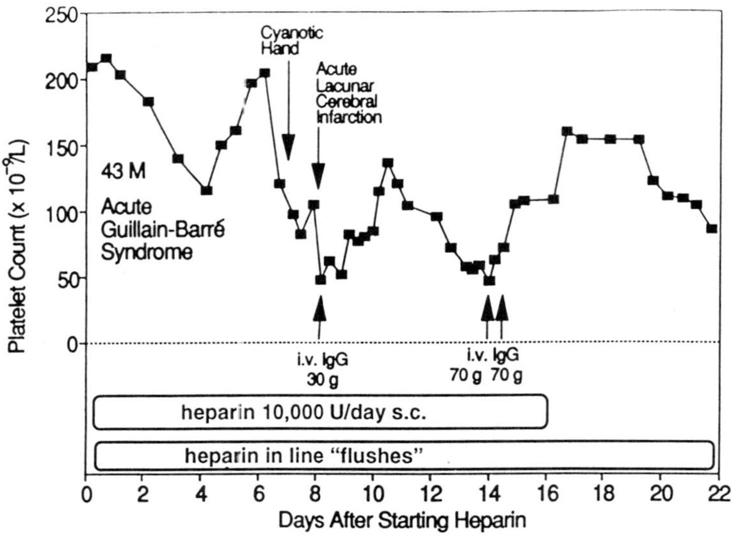

Figure 4 Patient summary: heparin-induced thrombocytopenia, with response to high-dose intravenous gamma globulin. A 43-year-old man with acute demyelinating polyradiculoneuropathy (Guillain-Barré syndrome) developed abrupt-onset thrombocytopenia on day 7 of subcutaneous heparin prophylaxis, together with unilateral hand cyanosis and new neurological signs suggesting cerebrovascular infarction (subsequently confirmed by computed-tomography brain scan). The patient received two courses of high-dose intravenous gamma globulin, given for treatment of Guillain-Barré syndrome. On both occasions, improvement in the platelet counts occurred. Heparin-induced thrombocytopenia was confirmed using the platelet ^{14}C-serotonin release assay.

aspirin can reduce reactivity to HIT-IgG (138, 145, 273). Clinical benefit to aspirin has been observed in some instances (214, 327, 328). *In vitro*, dextran reduces heparin-mediated platelet aggregation (329). Iloprost can completely block platelet aggregation by HIT-IgG (330) and has been used in the treatment of heparin-induced thrombocytopenia (168). In general, we believe that these are second-line treatments for heparin-induced thrombocytopenia and can never be used as an alternative to discontinuing the heparin.

8. *Special Maneuvers in Selected Patients: Thrombectomy, Embolectomy, Greenfield Filters, and Thrombolytic Therapy*

Some patients with heparin-induced arterial or venous thrombosis benefit from limb-salvaging maneuvers, such as thrombectomy or embolectomy (151, 221). Placement of Greenfield vena cava filters has been used to reduce the risk of pulmonary embolism, but may be associated with thrombosis of the filter and inferior vena cava (221, 331). Thrombolytic therapy is effective in some patients with arterial or venous thrombotic complications (192, 215, 223, 258, 332–334).

9. Low-Molecular-Weight Heparin

There is virtually 100% cross-reactivity between LMWH and standard heparin for HIT-IgG (198). In addition, there are several reports of persistent or recurrent thrombocytopenia, along with progressive or new thromboembolic events, in HIT patients treated with LMWH (190–195). Accordingly, LMWH cannot generally be recommended as a treatment for heparin-induced thrombocytopenia.

It is possible that some LMWH preparations can be developed that do not cross-react with HIT-IgG. For example, the synthetic pentasaccharide synthesized by Choay et al. (335) did not cross-react with HIT-IgG in one study (41). Moreover, short-chain-sulfated oligosaccharides do not interact with PF4 (10). However, the pentasaccharide has not been used for the treatment of heparin-induced thrombocytopenia. The lesser effects of PF4 on inhibiting LMWH anticoagulant activity could help explain why some patients with heparin-induced thrombocytopenia improve on LMWH therapy (163, 193–195, 336), even though there is virtual complete cross-reactivity between standard heparin and LMWH for HIT-IgG.

10. Avoid Further Heparin Exposure

Heparin is a commonly used drug in hospitalized patients. Thus, physicians must be very careful to ensure that patients are not inadvertently exposed to further heparin following the diagnosis of heparin-induced thrombocytopenia. This can occur in many ways, including use during central line insertion, administration of heparin "flushes" to maintain intravascular catheters, "routine" use during cardiac catheterization and other angiographic procedures, in combination with other medications (e.g., prothrombin complex concentrates) (198), and so forth. In addition, heparin-induced thrombocytopenia can be caused by the heparin that is bound to certain pulmonary artery catheters (337, 338) and some filters used during cardiopulmonary bypass.

G. Future Anticoagulation of a Patient with a Past History of Heparin-Induced Thrombocytopenia

Anticoagulation of a patient with a past history of heparin-induced thrombocytopenia poses major dilemmas for physicians. The issue is confounded by the fact that sometimes the previous diagnosis of heparin-induced thrombocytopenia was tenuous. Usually, the HIT-IgG has disappeared, so the laboratory is unhelpful in assessing a previous diagnosis of heparin-induced thrombocytopenia. Sometimes, the history is convincing for heparin-induced thrombocytopenia. The patients may require future anticoagulation for a number of reasons, including recurrence of a deep vein thrombosis, requirement for anticoagulation during a procedure such as cardiopulmonary bypass surgery, or hemodialysis. The most important principle in the management of these patients is to avoid heparin reexposure, if at all possible. If the patient requires an anticoagulant with rapid onset of action, we prefer to use ancrod.

1. *Management of a Patient with a Recent or Previous History of HIT Who Requires Cardiopulmonary Bypass Surgery*

Not infrequently, patients with a previous history of heparin-induced thrombocytopenia require heart surgery. Different approaches to the management of these patients have been advocated. Since the HIT-IgG has a relatively short half-life, some physicians have felt it acceptable to use heparin only for the heart operation, provided the disappearance of the HIT-IgG is documented by sensitive *in vitro* testing. No preoperative (e.g., during heart catheterization) or postoperative (e.g., deep vein thrombosis prophylaxis; catheter ''flushes'') heparin is used. Anecdotal experience with this approach has been successful (286). However, this approach could be dangerous for certain rare patients in whom severe heparin-induced thrombocytopenia could be initiated by this recurrent exposure to heparin.

If heart surgery is urgently required, and the patient has a detectable HIT-IgG, then two approaches have been used. First, an alternate anticoagulant, such as ancrod, can been used. A group in Toronto, Canada (339) has used ancrod in several patients in whom heparin could not be given for heart surgery. The risk of bleeding appears to be greater than with typical cardiopulmonary bypass using conventional heparin anticoagulation. Other physicians have used the heparinoid ORG 10172 to provide anticoagulation in patients with heparin-induced thrombocytopenia who required heart surgery (317, 340, 341). The inability of protamine to reverse its anticoagulant effects can make treatment of postoperative bleeding difficult, however (340). A second approach is to administer heparin along with one or more antiplatelet agents. These have included aspirin and dipyridamole (342, 343) or iloprost (330, 344, 345), a prostacyclin analog. The potential risk of such an approach was shown in one report (338), in which a patient who received heparin and iloprost together uneventfully during heart surgery developed fatal thrombotic complications during the postoperative phase that appeared to have been related to ''heparin rebound'' following the surgery.

2. *Management of Patients Who Require Hemodialysis*

Uremic patients can develop heparin-induced thrombocyotpenia following exposure to heparin during hemodialysis. Characteristic thrombotic complications in this patient population include clot formation in the extracorporeal circuit (328, 346–348) and occlusion of the arteriovenous fistula (213, 214). Heparin-free hemodialysis (e.g., frequent saline flushing technique or use of alternate anticoagulants) can be used to treat these patients (349, 346–348). Aspirin can prevent recurrent thrombocytopenia and thrombosis in some patients who continue to receive heparin during hemodialysis (214, 327, 328).

H. Prevention of Heparin-Induced Thrombocytopenia and Thrombotic Complications

1. Frequent Platelet Count Monitoring

We recommend daily platelet counts in all patients who are receiving heparin in doses of 10,000 units/day, or higher. Because the risk of thrombocytopenia does not begin to rise until day 5 or later of heparin therapy, some physicians recommend performing daily platelet counts beginning at that time (350). In our experience, the platelet count frequently fluctuates for many patients during the early phase of hospitalization (surgical dilution, administration of blood products and fluids, admission diagnosis of septicemia, etc.), rendering it difficult to interpret later platelet count values if early ones are not known. Another problem is that patients may have previously been exposed to heparin, and thrombocytopenia may occur earlier than 5 days.

2. Increased Awareness and Earlier Recognition of the Syndrome

Heparin-induced thrombocytopenia should be considered immediately in any patient who develops a thrombotic complication while receiving heparin therapy. An immediate platelet count should be ordered and compared with previous values. If an unexplained platelet count fall is found, a presumptive diagnosis of heparin-induced thrombocytopenia should be made, with alternate anticoagulant therapy introduced pending confirmation of the diagnosis by laboratory testing.

3. Avoid Heparin Flushes

Heparin-induced thrombocytopenia can be initiated or sustained by the small doses of heparin used to "flush" intravascular catheters (105, 151–157). We have observed patients who have developed HIT-IgG following a single exposure to heparin via catheter flushes used during an operative procedure (235). Heparin should not be used to flush indwelling intermittent-injection venous catheters ("hep-locks"), as there are no advantages over saline flushes (351–355). Heparin does appear to improve the longevity of radial and umbilical artery catheters, however (356–358).

4. Early Use of Warfarin for Deep Vein Thrombosis

Several studies have shown that commencement of warfarin anticoagulation can begin very soon after heparin treatment for deep vein thrombosis (359–361). In one study, this approach reduced the incidence of heparin-induced thrombocytopenia (361).

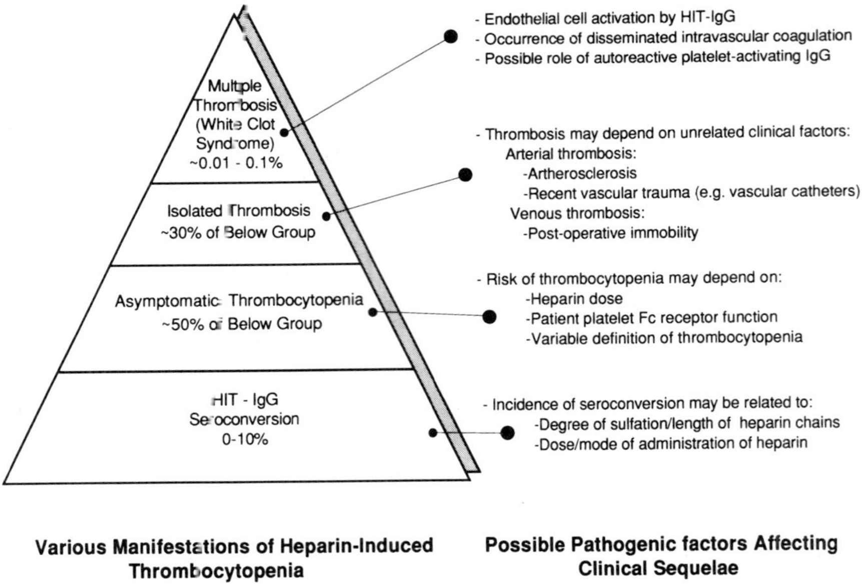

Figure 5 Iceberg model of heparin-induced thrombocytopenia. The spectrum of heparin-induced thrombocytopenia varies from asymptomatic heparin-dependent IgG seroconversion; to thrombocytopenia without sequelae; to isolated venous or arterial thrombosis; to disseminated arterial and/or venous thrombosis (''white clot syndrome''). Possible pathogenic factors that determine the wide spectrum of HIT-IgG seroconversion and clinical sequelae are shown.

IV. OVERVIEW AND FUTURE CONSIDERATIONS

Heparin-induced thrombocytopenia is a relatively common complication of heparin therapy that is caused by heparin-dependent IgG that activates platelets via their Fc receptors. The clinical manifestations of heparin-induced thrombocytopenia are wide, ranging from asymptomatic heparin-dependent IgG seroconversion to disseminated arterial and/or venous thrombosis. Figure 5 shows the ''iceberg model'' of heparin-induced thrombocytopenia, summarizing the potential role of different pathogenic factors in determining the clinical outcome for these patients.

The interaction of sulfated polysaccharides with platelets is responsible for several clinically relevant effects of these drugs, especially heparin-induced thrombocytopenia. The recognition that the extent of N-sulfation and increasing polysaccharide chain length is responsible for many of the undesirable effects of heparin treatment is one reason for the increasing interest in LMWH and other less sulfated polysaccharide agents. It is possible that some LMWH will be less likely to induce heparin-induced thrombocytopenia. However, reducing chain length and sulfation potentially can reduce certain of the anticoagulant effects of these agents. The challenge for both basic and clinical investigators is to identify those agents with the optimal therapeutic efficacy.

ACKNOWLEDGMENTS

Studies described in this chapter were supported by a grant from the Heart and Stroke Foundation of Ontario. Dr. Warkentin was a research fellow of the Heart and Stroke Foundation of Canada.

REFERENCES

1. Horne MK III. Heparin binding to normal and abnormal platelets. Thromb Res 1988; 51:135–144.
2. Salzman EW, Rosenberg RD, Smith MH, Lindon JN, Favreau L. Effect of heparin and heparin fractions on platelet aggregation. J Clin Invest 1980; 65:64–73.
3. Ockelford PA, Carter CJ, Cerskus A, Smith CA, Hirsh J. Comparison of the in vivo hemorrhagic and antithrombotic effects of a low antithrombin-III affinity heparin fraction. Thromb Res 1982; 27:679–690.
4. Brace LD, Fareed J. Heparin-induced platelet aggregation: dose/response relationships for a low molecular weight heparin derivative (PK 10169) and its subfractions. Thromb Res 1986; 42:769–782.
5. Horne MK III, Chao ES. The effect of molecular weight on heparin binding to platelets. Br J Haematol 1990; 74:306–312.
6. Horne MK III, Chao ES. Heparin binding to resting and activated platelets. Blood 1989; 74:238–243.
7. Sobel M, Adelman B. Characterization of platelet binding of heparins and other glycosaminoglycans. Thromb Res 1988; 50:815–826.
8. George JN, Onofre AR. Human platelet surface binding of endogenous secreted factor VIII-von Willebrand factor and platelet factor 4. Blood 1982; 59:194.
9. Gogstad GO, Solum NO, Krutnes MB. Heparin-binding platelet proteins demonstrated by crossed affinity immunoelectrophoresis. Br J Haematol 1983; 53:563–573.
10. Lane DA, Denton J, Flynn AM, Thunberg L, Lindahl U. Anticoagulant activities of heparin oligosaccharides and their neutralization by platelet factor 4. Biochem J 1984; 218:725–732.
11. Capitanio AM, Niewiarowski S, Rucinski B, Tuszynski GP, Cierniewski CS, Hershock D, Kornecki E. Interaction of platelet factor 4 with human platelets. Biochim Biophys Acta 1985; 839:161–173.
12. Fujimura Y, Titani K, Holland LZ, Roberts JR, Kostel P, Ruggeri ZM, Zimmerman TS. A heparin binding domain of human von Willebrand factor. Characterization and localization to a tryptic fragment extending from amino acid residue val-449 and lys-728. J Biol Chem 1987; 262:1734–1739.

13. Dixit VM, Grant GA, Santoro SA, Frazier WA. Isolation and characterization of a heparin-binding domain from the amino terminus of platelet thrombospondin. J Biol Chem 1984; 259:10100.
14. Stathakis N, Mosesson M. Interactions among heparin, cold insoluble globulin and fibrinogen in formation of the heparin precipitable fraction of plasma. J Clin Invest 1977; 60:855–860.
15. Gold LI, Frangione B, Pearlstein E. Biochemical and immunological characterization of three binding sites on human plasma fibronectin with different affinities for heparin. Biochemistry 1983; 22:4113.
16. Preissner KT, Muller-Berghaus G. Neutralization and binding of heparin by S protein/vitronectin in inhibition of factor Xa by antithrombin III. J Biol Chem 1987; 262:12247–12253.
17. Lijnen HR, Collen D. Interaction of heparin with histidine-rich glycoprotein. Ann NY Acad Sci 1989; 556:181–185.
18. Lerch PG, Nydegger UE, Kuyas C, Haeberli A. Histidine-rich glycoprotein binding to activated human platelets. Br J Haematol 1988; 70:219–224.
19. Wolf H, Glassl H, Nowack H, Wick G. Identification of binding site for heparin and other polysulfated glycosaminoglycans on human thrombocytes. Int Arch Allergy Appl Immunol 1986; 80:231.
20. Greinacher A, Michels I, Mueller-Eckhardt C. Heparin associated thrombocytopenia: immune complexes are bound to platelets by the negative charge of highly sulfated oligosaccharides. Blood 1992; 80(Suppl 1):62a (abstract).
21. Eika C. Platelet refractory state induced by heparin. Scand J Haematol 1972; 9:665–672.
22. Nelson JC, Lerner RG, Goldstein R, et al. Heparin-induced thrombocytopenia. Arch Intern Med 1978; 138:548.
23. McLean MR, Hause LL. Heparin-induced aggregation of normal human platelets. Thromb Haemost 1981; 46:570 (letter).
24. Brace LD, Fareed J. An objective assessment of the interaction of heparin and its fractions with human platelets. Semin Thromb Hemost 1985; 11:190–198.
25. Brace LD, Issleib S, Fareed J. Heparin-induced platelet aggregation is inhibited by antagonists of the thromboxane pathway. Thromb Res 1985; 39:533–539.
26. Brace LD, Fareed J, Tomeo J, Issleib S. Biochemical and pharmacological studies on the interaction of PK 10169 and its subfractions with human platelets. Haemostasis 1986; 16:93–103.
27. Brace LD, Fareed J. Heparin-induced platelet aggregation. II. Dose/response relationships for two low molecular weight heparin fractions (CY 216 and CY 222). Thromb Res 1990; 59:1–14.
28. Chong BH, Ismail F. The mechanism of heparin-induced platelet aggregation. Eur J Haematol 1989; 43:245–251.
29. Mims JA, Sarji KE, Kleinfelder JS, Eurenius K. Heparin-induced platelet aggregation in burn patients. Thromb Res 1977; 1:291–299.
30. Mikhailidis DP, Barradas MA, Jeremy JY, Gracey L, Wakeling A, Dandona P. Heparin-induced platelet aggregation in anorexia nervosa and in severe peripheral vascular disease. Eur J Clin Invest 1985; 15:313–319.

31. Thomson C, Forbes CD, Prentice CRM. The potentiation of platelet aggregation and adhesion by heparin *in vitro* and *in vivo*. Clin Sci Mol Med 1973; 45:485–494.
32. Hammerschmidt DE. Thrombocytopenia during heparin therapy. N Engl J Med 1976; 295:1200 (letter).
33. Ellison N, Edmunds LH Jr, Colman RW. Platelet aggregation following heparin and protamine administration. Anesthesiology 1978; 48:65–68.
34. MacIntyre DE, Handin RI, Rosenberg R, Salzman EW. Heparin opposes prostanoid and non-prostanoid platelet inhibitors by direct enhancement of aggregation. Thromb Res 1981; 22:167–175.
35. Mohammad SF, Anderson WH, Smith JB, Chuang HYK, Mason RG. Effects of heparin on platelet aggregation and release and thromboxane A_2 production. Am J Pathol 1981; 104:132–141.
36. Fabris F, Fussi F, Casonata A, Visentin L, Randi M, Smith MR, Girolami A. Normal and low molecular weight heparins: interaction with human platelets. Eur J Clin Invest 1983; 13:135–139.
37. Dunn F, Soria J, Soria C, Thomaidis A, Tobelem G, Caen JP. Fibrinogen binding on human platelets. Influence of different heparins and of pentosane polysulfate. Thromb Res 1983; 29:141–148.
38. Dunn FW, Soria C, Thomaidis A, Soria J, Dupuy E, Bellucci S, Tobelem G. Interactions of platelets with standard heparin and low molecular weight fractions. Nouv Rev Fr Hématol 1984; 26:249–253.
39. Mikhailidis DP, Barradas MA, Mikhailidis AM, Magnani H, Dandona P. Comparison of the effect of a conventional heparin and a low molecular weight heparinoid on platelet function. Br J Clin Pharmacol 1984; 17:43–48.
40. Barradas MA, Mikhailidis DP, Epemolu O, et al. Comparison of the platelet pro-aggregatory effect of conventional unfractionated heparins and a low molecular weight heparin fraction (CY 222). Br J Haematol 1987; 67:451–457.
41. Messmore HL, Jr, Griffin B, Fareed J, Coyne E, Seghatchian J. In vitro studies of the interaction of heparin, low molecular weight heparin and heparinoids with platelets. Ann NY Acad Sci 1989; 556:217–232.
42. Chen J, Karlberg K-E, Sylvén C. Heparin and low molecular weight heparin but not hirudin stimulate platelet aggregation in whole blood from acetylsalicylic acid treated healthy volunteers. Thromb Res 1991; 63:319–329.
43. Chen J, Sylvén C. Heparin potentiation of collagen-induced platelet aggregation is related to the GPIIb/GPIIIa receptor and not to the GPIb receptor, as tested by whole blood aggregometry. Thromb Res 1992; 66:111–120.
44. Chen J, Karlberg K-E, Sylvén C. Heparin enhances platelet aggregation irrespective of anticoagulation with citrate or with hirudin. Thromb Res 1992; 67:253–262.
45. Lecrubier C, Conard J, Horellou MH, Kher A, Samama M. Spontaneous platelet aggregation in heparin-treated patients. Acta Haematol 1984; 71:63–65.
46. Heinrich D, Görg T, Schulz M. Effects of unfractionated and fractionated heparin on platelet function. Haemostasis 1988; 18 (Suppl 3):48–54.
47. Ljungberg B, Beving H, Egberg N, Johnsson, H, Vesterqvist O. Immediate effects of heparin and LMW heparin on some platelet and endothelial derived factors. Thromb Res 1988; 51:209–217.

48. Berglund U, Wallentin L. Influence on platelet function by heparin in men with unstable coronary artery disease. Thromb Haemost 1991; 66:648–651.
49. Heiden D, Mielke CH Jr, Rodvien R. Impairment by heparin of primary haemostasis and platelet [^{14}C]5-hydroxytryptamine release. Br J Haematol 1977; 36:427.
50. Gillett MPT, Besterman EMM. Effects of heparin derived from different tissues on plasma-phospholipids and platelet aggregation. Lancet 1973; 2:1204–1205.
51. Rowsell HC, Glynn MF, Mustard JF, Murphy EA. Effect of heparin on platelet economy in dogs. Am J Physiol 1967; 213:915–922.
52. Fernandez F, N'guyen P, Van Ryn J, Ofosu FA, Hirsh J, Buchanan MR. Hemorrhagic doses of heparin and other glycosaminoglycans induce a platelet defect. Thromb Res 1986; 43:491–495.
53. Copley AL, Robb TP. Studies on platelets. II. The effect of heparin on the platelet count in vitro. Am J Clin Pathol 1942; 12:416–423.
54. Beattie RB, Dallaway P, Oakland M, Whittle MJ. Blood-sample-bottle anticoagulant and fetal and adult platelet counts. Lancet 1993; 341:111 (letter).
55. Fidlar E, Jaques LB. The effect of commercial heparin on the platelet count. J Lab Clin Med 1948; 33:1410–1423.
56. Gollub S, Ulin AW. Heparin-induced thrombocytopenia in man. J Lab Clin Med 1962; 59:430.
57. Davey MG, Lander H. Effect of injected heparin on platelet levels in man. J Clin Pathol 1968; 21:55–59.
58. Holmer E, Lindahl U, Bäckström G, Thunberg L, Sandberg H, Soderstrom G, Andersson LO. Anticoagulant activities and effects on platelets of a heparin fragment with high affinity for antithrombin. Thromb Res 1980; 18:861–869.
59. Westwick J, Scully MF, Poll C, Kakkar VV. Comparison of the effects of low molecular weight heparin and unfractionated heparin on activation of human platelets in vitro. Thromb Res 1986; 42:435–447.
60. Casu B, Johnson EA, Mantovani M, Mulloy B, Oreste P, Pescador R, Prino G, Torri G, Zoppetti G. Correlation between structure, fat-clearing and anticoagulant properties of heparins and heparan sulphates. Arzneim-Forsch/Drug Res 1983; 33:135–142.
61. Piper J. Influence of synthetic polysaccharid sulfuric acid esters on the thrombocytes in vivo and in vitro. Acta Physiol Scand 1945; 9:28–38.
62. Astrup T. The toxicity of synthetic heparin substitutes. Scand J Clin Lab Invest 1953; 5:137–142.
63. Ling J-Z, Lian E-Y Aggregation of human platelets by acidic mucopolysaccharides extracted from Stichopus japonicus Selenka. Thromb Haemost 1988; 59:435–439.
64. Walton KW. Observations on the effects of a series of dextran sulphates of varying molecular weight on the formed elements of the blood in vitro. Br J Pharmacol 1953; 8:340–347.
65. Meuleman DG. Orgaran (Org 10172): its pharmacological profile in experimental models. Haemostasis 1992; 22:58–65.
66. Mastacchi R, Barbanti M, Fantuz M, Bianchini P. Structural determinants of the heparin platelet-proaggregating effect. IRCS Med Sci 1986; 14:1013–1014.
67. Béguin S, Mardiguian J, Lindhout T, Hemker HC. The mode of action of low

molecular weight heparin preparation (PK10169) and two of its major components on thrombin generation in plasma. Thromb Haemost 1989; 61:30–34.
68. Béguin S, Wielders S, Lormeau JC, Hemker HC. The mode of action of CY216 and CY222 in plasma. Thromb Haemost 1992; 67:33–41.
69. Padilla A, Gray E, Pepper DS, Barrowcliffe TW. Inhibition of thrombin generation by heparin and low molecular weight (LMW) heparins in the absence and presence of platelet factor 4 (PF4). Br J Haematol 1992; 82:406–413.
70. Bode AP, Eick L. Lysed platelets shorten the activated coagulation time (ACT) of heparinized blood. Am J Clin Pathol 1989; 91:430–434.
71. Bode AP, Castellani WJ, Hodges ED, Yelverton S. The effect of lysed platelets on neutralization of heparin in vitro with protamine as measured by the activated coagulation time (ACT). Thromb Haemost 1991; 66:213–217.
72. Zucker MB, Katz IR. Platelet factor 4: production, structure, and physiologic and immunologic action. Proc Soc Exp Biol Med 1991; 198:693–702.
73. Stuckey JA, St. Charles R, Edwards BFP. A model of the platelet factor 4 complex with heparin. Proteins 1992; 14:277–287.
74. Rhodes GR, Dixon RH, Silver D. Heparin induced thrombocytopenia: eight cases with thrombotic-hemorrhagic complications. Ann Surg 1977; 186:752.
75. Saba HJ, Saba SR, Blackburn CA, Hartmann RC, Mason RG. Heparin neutralisation of PGI_2: effects upon platelets. Science 1979; 205:499–501.
76. Eldor A, Weksler BB. Heparin and dextran sulphate antagonize PGI_2 inhibition of platelet aggregation. Thromb Res 1979; 16:617–628.
77. Reches A, Eldor A, Salomon Y. Heparin inhibits PGE_1-sensitive adenylate cyclase and antagonizes PGE_1 anti-aggregating effect in human platelets. J Lab Clin Med 1979; 93:638.
78. Willuweit B, Aktories K. Heparin uncouples α_2-adrenoceptors from the G_i-protein in membranes of human platelets. Biochem J 1988; 249:857–863.
79. Rao GHR, Fareed J, White JG. Influence of heparins on inositol 1,4,5-trisphosphate-induced calcium mobilization in permeabilized human platelets. Biochem Med Metab Biol 1991; 45:171–180.
80. Bell WR. Heparin-associated thrombocytopenia and thrombosis. J Lab Clin Med 1988; 111:600–605.
81. Mikhailidis DP, Barradas MA, Jeremy JY, Dandona P. Heparin-associated thrombocytopenia and thrombosis. J Lab Clin Med 1989; 113:655–656 (letter).
82. Chong BH, Pitney WR, Castaldi PA. Heparin-induced thrombocytopenia: association of thrombotic complications with heparin-dependent IgG antibody that induces thromboxane synthesis and platelet aggregation. Lancet 1982; 2:1246–1249.
83. Chong BH, Castaldi PA. Platelet proaggregating effect of heparin: possible mechanism for non-immune heparin-associated thrombocytopenia. Aust NZ J Med 1986; 16:715–716.
84. Blauhut B, Kramar H, Vinazzer H, Bergmann H. Substitution of antithrombin III in shock and DIC: a randomized study. Thromb Res 1985; 39:81–89.
85. Balduini CL, Noris P, Bertolino G, Previtali M. Heparin modifies platelet count and function in patients who have undergone thrombolytic therapy for acute myocardial infarction. Thromb Haemost 1993; 69:522–523 (letter).

86. Chong BH. Heparin-induced thrombocytopenia. Blood Rev 1988; 2:108–114.
87. Chong BH, Berndt MC. Heparin-induced thrombocytopenia. Blut 1989; 58:53–57.
88. Chong BH. Heparin-induced thrombocytopenia. Aust NZ J Med 1992; 22:145–152.
89. Borchgrevink CF. The mechanism of the prolonged bleeding time provoked by dextran sulphate or by excessive doses of heparin. Acta Med Scand 1961; 170:365–373.
90. Kelton JG. Heparin-induced thrombocytopenia. Haemostasis 1986; 16:173.
91. Schulman S, Johnsson H. Heparin, DDAVP and the bleeding time. Thromb Haemost 1991; 65:242–244.
92. Sié P, Fernandez F, Caranobe C, Gabaig AM, Boneu B. Inhibition of thrombin-induced platelet aggregation and serotonin release by antithrombin III and heparin cofactor II in the presence of standard heparin, dermatan sulfate and pentosan polysulfate. Thromb Res 1982; 35:231–236.
93. Barrowcliffe TW, Merton RE, Gray E, Thomas DP. Heparin and bleeding: an association with lipoprotein lipase. Thromb Haemost 1988; 60:434–436.
94. Ljungberg B, Johnsson H. In vivo effects of a low molecular weight heparin fragment on platelet aggregation and platelet dependent hemostasis in dogs. Thromb Hameost 1988; 60:232–235.
95. Hirsh J. In vivo effects of low molecular weight heparins on experimental thrombosis and bleeding. Haemostasis 1986; 16:82–86.
96. Hirsh J. Overview of low molecular weight heparins and heparinoids: basic and clinical aspects. Aust NZ J Med 1992; 22:487–495.
97. Carter CJ, Kelton JG, Hirsh J, Cerskus A, Santos AV, Gent M. The relationship between the hemorrhagic and antithrombotic properties of low molecular weight heparin in rabbits. Blood 1982; 59:1239–1245.
98. Cade JF, Buchanan MR, Boneu B, Ockelford P, Carter C, Cerskus AL, Hirsh J. A comparison of the antithrombotic and haemorrhagic effects of low molecular weight heparin fractions: the influence of the method of preparation. Thromb Res 1984; 36:613–625.
99. Van Ryn-McKenna J, Ofosu FA, Hirsh J, Buchanan MR. Antithrombotic and bleeding effects of glycosaminoglycans with different degrees of sulfation. Br J Haematol 1989; 71:265–269.
100. Levine MN, Hirsh J, Gent M, Turpie AG, Leclerc J, Powers PJ, Jay RM, Neemeh J. Prevention of deep vein thrombosis after elective hip surgery. A randomized trial comparing low molecular weight heparin with standard unfractionated heparin. Ann Intern Med 1991; 114:545–551.
101. Eriksson BI, Kalebo J, Anthmyr BA, Wadenvik I, Tengborn L, Risberg B. Prevention of deep vein thrombosis and pulmonary embolism after total hip replacement. J Bone Joint Surg 1991; 73A:484–493.
102. Nurmohamed MT, Rosendaal FR, Büller HR, et al. Low-molecular-weight heparin versus standard heparin in general and orthopaedic surgery: a meta-analysis. Lancet 1992; 340:152–156.
103. Phelan BK. Heparin-associated thrombosis without thrombocytopenia. Ann Intern Med 1983; 99:637–638.
104. Ramirez-Lassepas M, Cipolle RJ, Rodvold KA, Seifert RD, Strand L, Taddeini L, Cusulos M. Heparin-induced thrombocytopenia in patients with cerebrovascular disease. Neurology 1984; 34:736–740.

105. Kappa JR, Fisher CA, Berkowitz HD, Cottrell ED, Addonizio VP Jr. Heparin-induced platelet activation in sixteen surgical patients: diagnosis and management. J Vasc Surg 1987; 5:101–109.
106. Kearsley JH, Jeremy RW, Coates AS. Leucocytoclastic vasculitis and skin necrosis following subcutaneous heparin calcium. Aust NZ J Med 1982; 12:288–289.
107. Sheridan D, Carter C, Kelton JG. A diagnostic test for heparin-induced thrombocytopenia. Blood 1986; 67:27–30.
108. Greinacher A, Michels I, Kiefel V, Mueller-Eckhardt C. A rapid and sensitive test for diagnosing heparin-associated thrombocytopenia. Thromb Haemost 1991; 66:734.
109. Stricker H, Lämmle B, Furlan M, Sulzer I. Heparin-dependent in vitro aggregation of normal platelets by plasma of a patient with heparin-induced skin necrosis: specific diagnosis for a rare side effect. Am J Med 1988; 85:721–724.
110. Favaloro EJ, Bernal-Hoyos E, Exner T, Koutts J. Heparin-induced thrombocytopenia: laboratory investigation and confirmation of diagnosis. Pathology 1992; 24:177–183.
111. Warkentin TE, Levine MN, Roberts RS, Gent M, Horsewood P, Kelton GJ. Heparin-induced thrombocytopenia is more common with unfractionated heparin than with low molecular weight heparin. Thromb Haemost 1993; 69:911 (abstract).
112. Warkentin TE, Kelton JG, Heparin-induced thrombocytopenia. Progr Hemost Thromb 1991; 10:1–34.
113. Stead RB, Schafer AI, Rosenberg RD, Handin RI, Josa M, Khuri SF. Heterogeneity of heparin lots associated with thrombocytopenia and thromboembolism. Am J Med 1984; 77:185–188.
114. Warkentin TE, Kelton JG. Heparin and platelets. Hematol/Oncol Clin North Am 1990; 4:243–264.
115. Ansell J, Slepchuk N Jr, Kumar R, Lopez A, Southard L, Deykin D. Heparin induced thrombocytopenia: a prospective study. Thromb Haemost 1980; 43:61–65.
116. Ansell JE, Price JM, Shah S, Beckner RR. Heparin-induced thrombocytopenia. What is its real frequency? Chest 1985; 88:878–882.
117. Bailey RT, Ursick JA, Heim KL, Hilleman DE, Reich JW. Heparin-associated thrombocytopenia: a prospective comparison of bovine lung heparin, manufactured by a new process, and porcine intestinal heparin. Drug Intell Clin Pharm 1986; 20:374–378.
118. Cipolle RJ, Rodvold KA, Seifert R, Clarens R, Ramirez-Lassepas M. Heparin-associated thrombocytopenia: a prospective evaluation of 211 patients. Ther Drug Monit 1983; 5:205–211.
119. Gallus AS, Goodall KT, Beswick W, Chesterman CN. Heparin-associated thrombocytopenia: case report and prospective study. Aust NZ J Med 1980; 10:25–31.
120. Green D, Martin GJ, Shoichet SH, DeBacker N, Bomalaski JS, Lind RN. Thrombocytopenia in a prospective, randomized, double-blind trial of bovine and porcine heparin Am J Med Sci 1984; 288:60–64.
121. Green D. Heparin-induced thrombocytopenia. Med J Aust 1986; 144(Suppl): HS37–HS39.
122. Holm HA, Eika C, Laake K. Thrombocytes and treatment with heparin from porcine mucosa. Scand J Haematol 1980; 36(Suppl):81–84.

123. Kakkasseril JS, Cranley JJ, Panke T, Grannan K. Heparin-induced thrombocytopenia: a prospective study of 142 patients. J Vasc Surg 1985; 2:382–384.
124. Monreal M, Lafoz E, Salvador R, Roncales J, Navarro A. Adverse effects of three different forms of heparin therapy: thrombocytopenia, increased transaminases, and hyperkalemia. Eur J Clin Pharmacol 1989; 37:415–418.
125. Powers PJ, Cuthbert D, Hirsh J. Thrombocytopenia found uncommonly during heparin therapy. JAMA 1979; 241:2396–2397.
126. Powers PJ, Kelton JG, Carter CJ. Studies on the frequency of heparin-associated thrombocytopenia. Thromb Res 1984; 33:439–443.
127. Rao AK, White GC, Sherman L, Colman R, Lan G, Ball AP. Low incidence of thrombocytopenia with porcine mucosal heparin. A prospective study. Arch Intern Med 1989; 149:1285–1288.
128. Bell WR, Tomasulo PA, Alving BM, Duffy TP. Thrombocytopenia occurring during the administration of heparin. A prospective study in 52 patients. Ann Intern Med 1976; 85:155–160.
129. Bell WR, Royall RM. Heparin-associated thrombocytopenia: a comparison of three heparin preparation. N Engl J Med 1980; 303:902–907.
130. Alving BM, Shulman NR, Bell WR, Evatt BL, Tack KM. In vitro studies of heparin-associated thrombocytopenia. Thromb Res 1977; 11:827–834.
131. Walls JT, Curtis JJ, Silver D, Boley TM, Schmaltz RA, Nawarawong W. Heparin-induced thrombocytopenia in open heart surgical patients: sequelae of late recognition. Ann Thorac Surg 1992; 53:787–791.
132. Walls JT, Boley TM, Curtis JJ, Silver D. Heparin induced thrombocytopenia in patients undergoing intra-aortic balloon pumping afteropen heart surgery. ASAIO J. 1992; 38:M574–M576.
133. Laster J, Cikrit D Walker N, Silver D. The heparin-induced thrombocytopenia syndrome: an update. Surgery 1987; 102:763–770.
134. King DJ, Kelton JG. Heparin-associated thrombocytopenia. Ann Intern Med 1984; 100:535.
135. Kapsch DN, Adelstein EH, Rhodes GR, Silver D. Heparin-induced thrombocytopenia, thrombosis, and hemorrhage. Surgery 1979; 86:148–155.
136. Van der Weyden MB, Hunt H, McGrath K, Fawcett T, Fitzmaurice A, Sawers RJ, Rosengarten DS. Delayed-onset heparin-induced thrombocytopenia. A potentially malignant syndrome. Med J Aust 1983; 2:132.
137. Silver D, Kapsch DN, Tsoi EKM. Heparin-induced thrombocytopenia, thrombosis, and hemorrhage. Ann Surg 1983; 198:301–306.
138. Makhoul RG, Greenberg CS, McCann RL. Heparin-associated thrombocytopenia and thrombosis: a serious clinical problem and potential solution. J Vasc Surg 1986; 4:522–528.
139. Chang JC. White clot syndrome associated with heparin-induced thrombocytopenia: a review of 23 cases. Heart Lung 1987; 16:403.
140. Glock Y, Szmil E, Boudjema B, Boccalon H, Fournial G, Cerene AL, Puel P. Cardiovascular surgery and heparin induced thrombocytopenia. Int Angiol 1988; 7:238–245.
141. Stanton PE Jr, Evans JR, Lefemine AA, Vo NM, Rannick GA, Morgan CV Jr., Hinton PJ, Read M. White clot syndrome. South Med J 1988; 81:616–620.

142. Boshkov LB, Warkentin TE, Hayward C, Andrew M, Kelton JG. Heparin-induced thrombocytopenia and thrombosis: clinical and laboratory studies. Br J Haematol 1993; 84:322–328.
143. Natelson EA, Lynch EC, Alfrey CP Jr, Gross JB. Heparin-induced thrombocytopenia. An unexpected response to treatment of consumption coagulopathy. Ann Intern Med 1969; 71:1121–1125.
144. Fratantoni JC, Pollet R, Gralnick HR. Heparin-induced thrombocytopenia: confirmation of diagnosis with in vitro methods. Blood 1975; 45:395–401.
145. Green D, Harris K, Reynolds N, Roberts M, Patterson R. Heparin immune thrombocytopenia: evidence for a heparin-platelet complex as the antigenic determinant. J Lab Clin Med 1978; 91:167–175.
146. Cottingham JK, Wheelock JB. Heparin-associated thrombocytopenia: a complications of low-dose heparin prophylaxis. Milit Med 1989; 154:242–244.
147. Van Damme H, Damas P, David JL, Limet R. Heparin-induced thrombocytopenia: a case report. Angiology 1990; 41:1075–1081.
148. Obadia JF, Lancon JP, Becker F, David M, Etievent P. Thrombopénie induites par l'héparine. Attitude pratique face aux complications vasculaires. Ann Chir 1991; 45:729–734.
149. Thomas D, Block AJ. Thrombocytopenia, cutaneous necrosis, and gangrene of the upper and lower extremities in a 35-year-old man. Chest 1992; 102:1578–1580.
150. Kelton JG, Meltzer D, Moore J, Giles AR, Wilson WE, Barr R, Hirsh J, Neame PB, Powers PJ, Walker I, Bianchi F, Carter CJ. Drug-induced thrombocytopenia is associated with increased binding of IgG to platelets both in vivo and in vitro. Blood 1981; 58:524–529.
151. Towne JB, Bernhard VM, Hussey C, et al. White clot syndrome. Peripheral vascular complications of heparin therapy. Arch Surg 1979; 114:372.
152. Doty JR, Alving BM, McDonnell DE, Ondra SL. Heparin-associated thrombocytopenia in the neurosurgical patient. Neurosurgery 1986; 19:69–72.
153. Heeger PS, Backstrom JT. Heparin flushes and thrombocytopenia. Ann Intern Med 1986; 105:143 (letter).
154. Cines DB, Tomaski A, Tannenbaum S. Immune endothelial-cell injury in heparin-associated thrombocytopenia. N Engl J Med 1987; 316:581–589.
155. Rizzoni WE, Miller K, Rick M, Lotze MT. Heparin-induced thrombocytopenia and thromboembolism in the postoperative period. Surgery 1988; 103:470–476.
156. Rama BN, Haake RE, Bander SJ, Ghasem-Zadeh A, Gorla C. Heparin-flush associated thrombocytopenia-induced hemorrhage: a case report. Nebr Med J 1991; 76:392–394.
157. Brushwood DB. Hospital liable for allergic reaction to heparin used in needle flush. Am J Hosp Pharm 1992; 49:1491–1492.
158. Baird RA, Convery FR. Arterial thromboembolism in patients receiving systemic heparin therapy. A complication associated with heparin-induced thrombocytopenia J Bone Joint Surg 1977; 59A:1061–1064.
159. Ansell JE, Clark WP Jr, Compton CC. Fatal reactions associated with intravenous heparin. Drug Intell Clin Pharm 1986; 20:74–75.
160. Barber FA, Burton WC, Guyer R. The heparin-induced thrombocytopenia and thrombosis syndrome. Report of a case. J Bone Joint Surg 1987; 69A:935–937.

161. Cimo PL, Moake JL, Weinger RS, Ben-Menachem Y, Khalil KG. Heparin-induced thrombocytopenia: association with a platelet-aggregating factor and arterial thromboses. Am J Hematol 1979; 6:125–133.
162. Lindsey SM, Maddison FE, Towne JB. Heparin-induced thrombocytopenia: angiographic features. Radiology 1979; 131:771–774.
163. Vitoux JF, Mathieu JF, Roncato M, et al. Heparin-associated thrombocytopenia treatment with low molecular weight heparin. Thromb Haemost 1986; 55:37.
164. White PW, Sadd JR, Nensel RE. Thrombotic complications of heparin therapy. Including six cases of heparin-induced skin necrosis. Ann Surg 1979; 190:595.
165. Zalcberg JR, McGrath K, Dauer R, Wiley JS. Heparin-induced thrombocytopenia with associated disseminated intravascular coagulation. Br J Haematol 1983; 54:655–660.
166. Ball A, L'Hullier AM, Dreyfuss L, Porte JL, Barthel JC. Thrombopénie à la Fraxiparine, une observation. Presse Méd 1989; 18:1254–1255 (letter).
167. Tardy B, Page Y, Tardy-Pncet B, Comtet C, Zeni F, Bertrand JC. Thrombopénie induite par une héparine de bas poids moléculaire. Therapie 1990; 45:453 (letter).
168. Metz D, N'Guyen P, Chapoutot L, Graciet J, Taupin JM, Grentzinger A, Elaerts J, Bajolet A. Embolie pulmonaire massive révelant une thrombopénie induite par héparine de bas poids moléculaire succès thérapeutique d'une prostacyline. Ann Cardiol Angéiol 1991; 40:619–621.
169. Mohr VD, Lenz J. Heparin-assoziierte Thrombocytopenia, Thrombose und Embolie. Unerwünschte Wirkung der Thromboemboliepropylaxe mit dem niedermolekularen Heparin Enoxaparin? Chirurg 1991; 62:686–690.
170. Wattrisse G, Lecoutre D, Groux-Pante C. Thrombopénie induite par une héparine de bas poids moléculaire. Cah Anesth 1990; 38:175–177.
171. Wattrisse G, Lecoutre D, Groux-Pante C. Étude prospective non contrôlée de l'efficacité et de la tolérance d'une héparine de bas poids moléculaire (tédelparine) dans la prophylaxie thromboembolique en chirurgie traumatologique du col du fémur. J Mal Vasc 1991; 16:367–371.
172. Lévy G, Lévy PY, Jamet M, Toroyan P. Thrombopénie induite par une héparine de bas poids moléculaire au cours d'un traitement hypotenseur et diurétique: coincidence ou relation? Ann Fr Anesth Réanim 1991; 10:586–588.
173. Gouault-Heilmann M, Payen D, Contant G, Intrator L, Huet Y, Schaeffer A. Thrombocytopenia related to synthetic heparin analogue therapy. Thromb Haemost 1985; 54:557 (letter).
174. Maiza D, Derlon A, Khayat MC, Coulhon JP, Leporrier M. Rôle du polysulfate de pentosane dans le déclanchement de deux accidents thrombopéniques. Presse. Méd 1985; 14:1289–1290.
175. Vitoux JF, Roncato M, Hourdebaigt P, Aiach M, Fiessinger J-N. Heparin-induced thrombocytopenia and pentosan polysulfate: treatment with a low molecular weight heparin despite in vitro platelet aggregation. Thromb Hemost 1985; 55:294–295 (letter).
176. Bayle J, Chichmanian RM, Caramella A, et al. Les thrombopénies allergiques induites par les héparines ou le polysulfate de pentosane. Thérapie 1986; 41:339–343.
177. Borg JY, Fléchet B, Legendre M, Toulemonde F, Piguet H, Monconduit M. Severe heparin and pentosan polysulphate-induced thrombocytopenias: clinical aspects—in

vitro effects of pentosan polysulfate, low molecular weight (LMW) heparins and oligosaccharides. Thromb Res 1986; (Suppl. VI):96 (abstract).
178. Follea G, Hamandjian I, Trzeciak MC, Nedey C, Streichenberger R, Dechavanne M. Pentosane polysulfate associated thrombocytopenia. Thromb Res 1986; 42:413–418.
179. Le Querrec A, Derlon A, Tobelem G, Thomas M. Pentosane polysulfate like heparin may induce severe thrombocytopenia. Thromb Res 1986; (Suppl. VI):90 (abstract).
180. Manchon ND, Flechet B, Borg JY, Cotard-Guillem I, Bercoff E, Bourreille J. Démonstration du rôle du polysulfate de pentosane à l'origine d'un accident thrombopénique. Presse Méd 1986; 15:1930–1931.
181. Papazian L, Alazia M, Levy G, François G. Thromboses artérielles et veineuses multiples associées à une thrombopénie. Rôle du polysulfate de pentosane et des héparines. Presse Méd 1986; 15:1246–1247 (letter).
182. Dalger J, Dussarat GV, Dumoulin M. Infarctus myocardique compliquant une thrombopénie induite par le polysulfate de pentosane. Ann Cardiol Angéiol 1988; 37(4):191–193.
183. Jacquin V, Salama J, Le Roux G, Delaporte P. Thromboses veineuses cérébrales et des membres supérieurs associées à une thrombopénie, induites par le polysulfate de Pentosane. Ann Med Interne 1988; 139:194–197.
184. Meyer P, Couzi G, Bavle J, Blanc P, Gibelin P, Camous JP, Morand P. Thromboses coronaires disséminées et thrombopénies induites par le polysulfate de pentosane. Arch Mal Coeur 1988; 81:913–919.
185. Paille F, Boccaccini A, De Korwin JD, Schmidt C, Laprevote MC, Schmitt J, Royer RJ. Thrombopénie sous héparine de bas poids moléculaire après traitement par pentosane polysulphate. Therapie 1988; 43:322–323 (letter).
186. Leclercq C, de Place C, Rioux C, Mabo P, Paillard F, Daubert JC. Infarctus du myocarde et thrombose biventriculaire massive au cours d'une thrombopénie induite par le pentosane polysulfate et l'héparine. Arch Mal Coeur 1990; 83:117–120.
187. Wolf H, Nowack H, Wick G. Detection of antibodies interacting with glycosaminoglycans polysulfate in patients treated with heparin or other polysulfated glycosaminoglycans. Int Arch Allergy Appl Immunol 1983; 70:157–163.
188. Van Aken WG. Thrombocytopenia (and consumption coagulopathy) induced by heparin. A case report. Scand J Haematol 1980; 25(Suppl 36):85–90.
189. Greinacher A, Michels I, Schäfer M, Kiefel V, Mueller-Eckhardt C. Heparin-associated thrombocytopenia in a patient treated with polysulphated chondroitin sulphate: evidence for immunological crossreactivity between heparin and polysulphated glycosaminoglycan. Br J Haematol 1992; 81:252–254.
190. Horellou MH, Conard J, Lecrubier C, Samama M, Roque-D'Orbcastel O, de Fenoyl O, DiMaria G, Bernadou A, Persistent heparin induced thrombocytopenia despite therapy with low molecular weight heparin. Thromb Haemost 1984; 51:134 (letter).
191. Benhamou AC, Gruel Y, Barsotti J, et al. The white clot syndrome or heparin associated thrombocytopenia and thrombosis (WCS or HATT): (26 cases). Int Angio 1985; 4:303–310.
192. Leroy J, Leclerc MH, Delahousse B, et al. Treatment of heparin-associated thrombocytopenia and thrombosis with low molecular weight heparin (CY 216). Semin Thromb Hemost 1985; 11:326–329.
193. Gouault-Heilmann M, Huet Y, Adnot S, Contant G, Bonnet F, Intrator L, Payen

D, Levent M. Low molecular weight heparin fractions as an alternative therapy in heparin-induced thrombocytopenia. Haemostasis 1987; 17:134–140.
194. Reuter HD. Niedermolekulares Heparin in der Therapie der heparininduzierten Thrombozytopenia. Med Klin 1987; 82:115–118.
195. Warkentin TE, Kelton JG. Heparin-induced thrombocytopenia Annu Rev Med 1989; 40:31–44.
196. Anderson GP. Insights into heparin-induced thrombocytopenia. Br J Haematol 1992; 80:504–508.
197. Greinacher A, Drost W, Michels I, Leitl J, Gottsmann M, Kohl HG, Glaser M, Mueller-Eckhardt C. Heparin associated thrombocytopenia successfully treated with the heparinoid Org 10172 in a patient showing cross-reaction to LMW heparins. Ann Haematol 1992; 64:40–42.
198. Greinacher A, Michels I, Mueller-Eckhardt C. Heparin-associated thrombocytopenia: the antibody is not heparin specific. Thromb Haemost 1992; 67:545–549.
199. Weismann RE, Tobin RW. Arterial embolism occurring during systemic heparin therapy. Arch Surg 1958; 76:219–227.
200. Roberts B, Rosato FE, Rosato EF. Heparin—a cause of arterial emboli? Surgery 1964; 55:803.
201. Barker CF, Rosato FE, Roberts B. Peripheral arterial embolism. Surg Gynecol Obstet 1966; 123:22–26.
202. Kaupp HA, Roberts B. Arterial embolization during subcutaneous heparin therapy. Case report. J Cardiovasc Surg 1972; 13:210–212.
203. Arthur CK, Isbister JP, Aspery EM. The heparin induced thrombosis–thrombocytopenia syndrome (H.I.T.T.S.): a review. Pathology 1985; 17:82–86.
204. Krueger SK, Andres E, Weinand E. Thrombolysis in heparin-induced thrombocytopenia with thrombosis. Ann Intern Med 1985; 103:159 (letter).
205. Maurin N, Biniek R. Bohndorf K, Heintz B, Kierdorf H, Schulte-Bockholt A. Heparininduzierte thrombozytopenie und Thrombose with spinaler Ischämie. Internist 1991; 32:431–434.
206. Meagher AP, Lord RSA, Graham AR, Hill DA. Acute aortic occlusion presenting with lower limb paralysis. J Cardiovasc Surg 1991; 32:643–647.
207. Jain A. Ischemic lumbosacral plexus neuropathy secondary to possible heparin-induced thrombosis following aortoiliac bypass. Arch Phys Med Rehabil 1986; 67:680 (abstract).
208. Commeau P, Grollier G, Charbonneau P, et al. Thrombopénie immuno-allergique induite par l'héparine responsable d'une thrombose intraventricularie gauche. Thérapie 1986; 41:345–347.
209. Guittard M, Pradalier A, Vincent D, Dry J. Thrombose intraventriculaire droite et thrombopénie à l'héparine. Presse Méd 1988; 17:871 (letter).
210. Dion D, Dumesnil JG, LeBlanc P. In situ right ventricular thrombus secondary to heparin induced thrombocytopenia. Can J Cardiol 5:308–310.
211. Oriot D, Wolf M, Wood C, Brun P, Sidi D, Devictor D, Tchernia G, Huault G. Thrombopénie sévère induite par l'héparine chez un nourrisson porteur d'une myocardite aiguë. Arch Fr Pediatr 1990; 47:357–359.
212. AbuRahma AF, Boland JP, Witsberger T. Diagnostic and therapeutic strategies of white clot syndrome. Am J Surg 1991; 162:175–179.

213. Laster J, Elfrink R, Silver D. Reexposure to heparin of patients with heparin-associated antibodies. J Vasc Surg 1989; 9:677–682.
214. Hall AV, Clark WF, Parbtani A. Heparin-induced thrombocytopenia in renal failure. Clin Nephrol 1992; 38:86–89.
215. Bernasconi F, Metivet F, Estrade G, Garnier D, Donatien Y. Thrombose d'une prosthèse valvulaire mitrale au cours d'une thrombopénie induite par l'héparine. Traitement fibrinolytique. Presse Méd 1988; 17:1366.
216. Tanner JR, Downs AR. White clot syndrome: a rare complication of heparin therapy. Can J Surg 1986; 29:122–124.
217. Warkentin TE, Hayward CPM, Kelton JG. High frequency and wide spectrum of clinical sequelae in heparin-induced thrombocytopenia. Blood 1991; 78(Suppl 1):343a (abstract).
218. Garcia JH, Barton JC, Shin MS, Henderson HM. Isolated thrombocytopenia in a 56-year-old man with mitral stenosis. Ala J Med Sci 1986; 23:67–73.
219. Gouault-Heilmann M, Huet Y, Contant G, Payen D, Bloch G, Rapin M. Cardiopulmonary bypass with a low-molecular-weight heparin fraction. Lancet 1983; 2:1374 (letter).
220. Battey PM, Salam AA. Venous gangrene associated with heparin-induced thrombocytopenia. Surgery 1985; 97:618.
221. Sobel M, Adelman B, Szentpetery S, et al. Surgical management of heparin-associated thrombocytopenia. Strategies in the treatment of venous and arterial thromboembolism. J Vasc Surg 1988; 8:395–401.
222. Cohen DJ, Briggs R, Head HD, Acher CW. Phlegmasia cerulea dolens and its association with hypercoagulable states: case reports. Angiology 1989; 40:498–508.
223. Mehta DP, Yoder EL, Appel J, Bergsman KL. Heparin-induced thrombocytopenia and thrombosis: reversal with streptokinase. A case report and review of literature. Am J Hematol 1991; 36:275–279.
224. Calhoun BC, Hesser JW. Heparin-associated antibody with pregnancy: discussion of two cases. Am J Obstet Gynecol 1987; 156:964–966.
225. Stevenson MM. Thrombocytopenia during heparin therapy. N Engl J Med 1976; 295:1200–1201 (letter).
226. Buge A, Poisson M, Vidhaillet M, Chamouard JM, Duyckaerts C, Vincent D. Thrombopénie et coagulation intravasculaire disséminée au cours d'un traitement par l'héparine: deux cas avec complications neurologiques. Rev Neurol (Paris) 1988; 144:289–294.
227. Kyritsis AP, Williams EC, Schutta HS. Cerebral venous thrombosis due to heparin-induced thrombocytopenia. Stroke 1990; 21:1503–1505.
228. Gallus AS, Goodall KT, Tillett J, Jackaman J, Wycherley A. The relative contributions of antithrombin III during heparin treatment, and of clinically recognisable risk factors, to early recurrence of venous thromboembolism. Thromb Res 1987; 46:539–553.
229. Ulrich PJ, Manoharan A. Heparin-induced skin reaction. Med J Aust 1984; 140:287–289.
230. Tuneu A, Moreno A, de Moragas JM. Cutaneous reactions secondary to heparin injections. J Am Acad Dermatol 1985; 12:1072–1077.

231. Platell CFE, Tan EGC. Hypersensitivity reactions to heparin: delayed onset thrombocytopenia and necrotizing skin lesions. Aust NZ J Surg 1986; 56:621–623.
232. Fowlie J, Stanton PD, Anderson JR. Heparin-associated skin necrosis. Postgrad Med J 1990; 66:573–575.
233. Manoharan A. Heparin-induced skin reaction with low molecular-weight heparin. Eur J Haematol 1992; 48:234 (letter).
234. Ojeda E, del Carmen Perez M, Mataix R, Arbelo A, Jimenez S, Campo C, Balda I. Skin necrosis with a low molecular weight heparin. Br J Haematol 1992; 82:620.
235. Warkentin TE, Soutar RL, Panju A, Ginsberg JS. Acute systemic reactions to intravenous bolus heparin therapy: characterization and relationship to heparin-induced thrombocytopenia. Blood 1992; 80 (Suppl 1):160a (abstract).
236. Kelly RA, Gelfand JA, Pincus SH. Cutaneous necrosis caused by systemically administered heparin. JAMA 1981; 246:1582–1583.
237. Levine LE, Bernstein JE, Soltani K, Medenica MM, Yung CW. Heparin-induced cutaneous necrosis unrelated to injection sites. A sign of potentially lethal complications. Arch Dermatol 1983; 119:400–403.
238. Hartman AR, Hood RM, Anagnostopoulos CE. Phenomenon of heparin-induced thrombocytopenia associated with skin necrosis. J Vasc Surg 1988; 7:781–784.
239. Celoria GM, Steingart RH, Banson B, Friedmann P, Rhee SW, Berman JA. Coumarin skin necrosis in a patient with heparin-induced thrombocytopenia—a case report. Angiology, 1988; 39:915–920.
240. Arthur CK, Grant SJB, Murray WK, Isbister JP, Stiel JN, Lauer CS. Heparin-associated acute adrenal insufficiency. Aust NZ J Med 1985; 15:454–455.
241. Findling JW, Korducki JM, Lahiri PK, et al. Bilateral adrenal hemorrhage associated with heparin-induced thrombocytopenia. Wisc Med J 1987; 86:2.
242. Cheng TC. Thrombocytopenia associated with minidose heparin therapy. Postgrad Med 1981; 70(6):73–74, 76, 78.
243. Chadenas D, Walle T, Dutilleux PH, Rousseau A, Pariente EA, Emy P, Pinsard D, Maze A, Vaugier GL. Hématome bilatéral des surrénales sous héparine. Une observation exceptionnelle. Presse Méd 1986; 15:1334 (letter).
244. Granry JC, Houet JF, Delhumeau A. Hematomes des surrénales et héparine. Ann Fr Anesth Reanim 1989; 9:650–655.
245. Delhumeau A, Houet JF, Bourrier P, et al. Thrombopénies à l'héparine compliquées d'hématome des surrénales et d'insuffisance surrénalienne aiguë. Ann Fr Anesth Reanim 1989; 8:656–658.
246. Ernest D, Fisher MM. Heparin-induced thrombocytopaenia complicated by bilateral adrenal haemorrhage. Intens Care Med 1991; 17:238–240.
247. Souid F, Pourria JL, Le Roux G, Hoang P. Adrenal haemorrhagic necrosis related to heparin-associated thrombocytopenia. Crit Care Med 1991; 19:297–299.
248. Bleasel JF, Rasko JEJ, Rickard KA, Richards G. Acute adrenal insufficiency secondary to heparin-induced thrombocytopenia-thrombosis syndrome. Med J Aust 1992; 157:192–193.
249. Eichinger S, Kyrle PA, Brenner B, et al. Thrombocytopenias associated with low-molecular-weight heparin. Lancet 1991; 337:1425–1426.
250. McKay DG. Late manifestations of intravascular coagulation-tissue necrosis. In:

McKay DG, ed. Disseminated Intravascular Coagulation. An Intermediary Mechanism of Disease. New York: Harper & Row, 1965:392–471.
251. Carette S, Jobin F. Acute adrenal insufficiency as a manifestation of the anticardiolipin syndrome? Ann Rheum Dis 1989; 48:430–431.
252. Lefemine AA. Complications of heparin-induced thrombocytopenia. Am Surg 1982; 48:202–206.
253. Atkinson JLD, Sundt TM Jr. Kazmier FJ, Bowie EJW, Whisnant JP. Heparin-induced thrombocytopenia and thrombosis in ischemic stroke. Mayo Clin Proc 1988; 63:353–361.
254. Warkentin TE, Hirte HW, Anderson DR, Wilson WEC, O'Connell GJ, Lo RC. Transient global amnesia caused by heparin-induced thrombocytopenia (submitted).
255. Klein HG, Bell WR. Disseminated intravascular coagulation during heparin therapy. Ann Intern Med 1974; 80:477–481.
256. Gouault-Heilmann M, Contant G, Pochmalicki G, Jan F. Coagulation intravasculaire disséminée induite par l'héparine. Traitement par l'association héparine de bas poids moléculaire et concentrés d'antithrombine III. Presse Méd 1984; 13:1393–1394.
257. Sandler RM, Seifer DB, Morgan K, et al. Heparin-induced thrombocytopenia and thrombosis: detection and specificity of a platelet-aggregating IgG. Am J Clin Pathol 1985; 83:760.
258. Fiessinger JN, Aiach M, Roncato M, Debbure C, Gaux J-C. Critical ischemia during heparin-induced thrombocytopenia. Treatment by intra-arterial streptokinase. Thromb Res 1984; 33:235–238.
259. Desmet G, Louwagie A, Criel A, Hidayat M, Van Hoof A. Heparin-induced thrombocytopenia with dissseminated intravascular coagulation and white clot syndrome: a case report. Acta Clin Belg 1988; 43:419–422.
260. Lynch DM, Howe SE. Heparin-associated thrombocytopenia: antibody binding specificity to platelet antigens. Blood 1985; 66:1176–1181.
261. Potter C, Gill JC, Scott JP, McFarland JG. Heparin-induced thrombocytopenia in a child. J Pediatr 1992; 121:135–138.
262. Spadone D, Clark F, James E, Laster J, Hoch J, Silver D. Heparin-induced thrombocytopenia in the newborn. J Vasc Surg 1992; 15:306–312.
263. Boshkov LB, Warkentin TE, Hayward C, Andrew M, Kelton JG. Heparin-induced thrombocytopenia and thrombosis: clinical and laboratory studies. Blood 1990; 76(Suppl 1):447a.
264. Gruel Y, Lang M, Darnige L, Pacouret G, Dreyfus X, Leroy J, Charbonnier B. Fatal effect of re-exposure to heparin after previous heparin-associated thrombocytopenia and thrombosis. Lancet 1990; 336:1077 (letter).
265. Castaman G, Ruggeri M, Girardello R, Rodeghiero F. An unusually prolonged case of heparin-induced thrombocytopenia and disseminated intravascular coagulation. Haematologica 1992; 77:174–176.
266. Pfueller SL, David R, Firkin BG, Bilston RA, Cortizo WF, Raines G. Platelet aggregating IgG antibody to platelet surface glycoproteins associated with thrombosis and thrombocytopenia. Br J Haematol 1990; 74:336–341.
267. Rhodes GR, Dixon RH, Silver D. Heparin induced thrombocytopenia with thrombotic and hemorrhagic manifestations. Surg Gynecol Obstet 1973; 136:409–416.

268. Babcock RB, Dumper CW, Scharfman WB. Heparin-induced immune thrombocytopenia. N Engl J Med 1976; 295:237–241.
269. Trowbridge AA, Caraveo J, Green JB III, et al. Heparin-related immune thrombocytopenia. Studies of antibody-heparin specificity. Am J Med 1978; 65:277.
270. Cines DB, Kaywin P, Bina M, Tomaski A, Schreiber AD. Heparin-associated thrombocytopenia. N Engl J Med 1980; 303:788–795.
271. Chong BH, Grace CS, Rozenberg MC. Heparin-induced thrombocytopenia: effect of heparin platelet antibody on platelets. Br J Haematol 1981; 49:531–540.
272. Kappa JR, Fisher CA, Addonizio VP Jr. Heparin-induced platelet activation: the role of thromboxane A_2 synthesis and the extent of platelet granule release in two patients. J Vasc Surg 1989; 9:574–579.
273. Chong BH, Castaldi PA. Heparin-induced thrombocytopenia: further studies of the effects of heparin-dependent antibodies on platelets. Br J Haematol 1986; 64:347–354.
274. Rosenfeld SI, Looney RJ, Leddy JP, Phipps DC, Abraham GN, Anderson CL. Human platelet Fc receptor for immunoglobulin G. Identification as a 40,000-molecular-weight membrane protein shared by monocytes. J Clin Invest 1985; 76:2317.
275. Kelton JG, Smith JW, Santos AV, Murphy WG, Horsewood P. The platelet IgG Fc receptor. Am J Hematol 1987; 25:299.
276. Keller MA, Cassel DL, Surrey S, Schwartz E, Schreiber AD, Rappaport EF, McKenzie SE. FcγRIIA is the platelet Fc receptor. Blood 1992; 80(Suppl):55a (abstract).
277. Kelton JG, Sheridan D, Santos A, Smith J, et al. Heparin-induced thrombocytopenia: laboratory studies. Blood 1988; 72:925–930.
278. Chong BH, Fawaz I, Chesterman CN, Berndt MC. Heparin-induced thrombocytopenia: mechanism of interaction of the heparin-dependent antibody with platelets. Br J Haematol 1989; 73:235–240.
279. Chong BH, Castaldi PA, Berndt MC. Heparin-induced thrombocytopenia: effect of rabbit IgG, and its Fab and Fc fragments on antibody-heparin-platelet interaction. Thromb Res 1989; 55:291–295.
280. Adelman B, Sobel M, Fujimura T, Ruggeri ZM, Zimmerman TS. Heparin-associated thrombocytopenia: observations on the mechanism of platelet aggregation. J Lab Clin Med 1989; 113:204–210.
281. Horsewood P, Hayward CPM, Warkentin TE, Kelton JG. The investigation of the mechanisms of monoclonal antibody-induced platelet activation. Blood 1991; 78:1019–1026.
282. Mitchell M, Huang MM, Indik Z, Chien P, Brugge JS, Schreiber AD. Structure-function relationships of the Fcγ receptor, FcγRIIA, in transmission of a phagocytic signal. Blood 1992; 80(Suppl):159a (abstract).
283. Myllylä G. Aggregation of human blood platelets by immune complexes in the sedimentation pattern test. Scand J Haematol 1973; (Suppl 19):1–56.
284. Warkentin TE, Hayward CPM, Smith CA, Kelly PM, Kelton JG. Determinants of donor platelet variability when testing for heparin-induced thrombocytopenia. J Lab Clin Med 1992; 120:371–379.
285. Chong BH, Pilgrim RL, Cooley MA, Chesterman CN. Increased expression of

platelet IgG Fc receptors in immune heparin-induced thrombocytopenia. Blood 1993; 81:988–993.
286. Olinger GN, Hussey CV, Olive JA, Malik MI. Cardiopulmonary bypass for patients with previously documented heparin-induced platelet aggregation. J Thorac Cardiovasc Surg 1984; 87:673–677.
287. Warkentin TE, Santos AV, Hayward CPM, Horsewood P, Kelton JG. Platelet-derived microparticles are produced by heparin-induced thrombocytopenia sera and other platelet Fc receptor stimuli. Blood 1991; 78(Suppl 1):343a (abstract).
288. Warkentin TE, Santos AV, Hayward CPM, Boshkov LK, Kelton JG. Heparin-but not quinine/quinidine-induced thrombocytopenia sera produce procoagulant platelet-derived microparticles: an explanation for the differing clinical syndromes. Br J Haematol 1992; (Suppl):18 (abstract).
289. Warkentin TE, Hayward CPM, Santos AV, Kelton JG. Platelet-derived microparticles are found *in vivo* in patients with heparin-induced thrombocytopenia. Thromb Haemost; 69:912 (abstract).
290. Marcum JA, Rosenberg RD. Role of endothelial cell surface heparin-like polysaccharides. Ann NY Acad Sci 1989; 556:81–94.
291. Conrad HE. Structure of heparan sulfate and dermatan sulfate. Ann NY Acad Sci 1989; 556:18–28.
292. Amiral J, Bridey F, Dreyfus M, Vissac AM, Fressinaud E, Wolf M, Meyer D. Platelet factor 4 complexed to heparin is the target for antibodies generated in heparin-induced thrombocytopenia. Thromb Haemost 1992; 68:95–96 (letter).
293. McNeil HP, Simpson RJ, Chesterman CN, Krilis SA. Antiphospholipid antibodies are directed against a complex antigen that includes a lipid-binding inhibitor of coagulation: β_2-glycoprotein I (apolipoprotein H). Proc Natl Acad Sci USA 1990; 87:4120–4124.
294. Galli M, Comfurius P, Maassen C, et al. Anticardiolipin antibodies (ACA) directed not to cardiolipin but to a plasma protein cofactor. Lancet 1990; 335:1544–1547.
295. Jones JV, James H, Tan MH, Mansour M. Antiphospholipid antibodies require β_2-glycoprotein I (apolipoprotein H) as cofactor. J Rheumatol 1992; 19:1397–1402.
296. Gruel Y, Rupin A, Watier H, Vigier S, Bardos P, Leroy J. Anticardiolipin antibodies in heparin-associated thrombocytopenia. Thromb Res 1992; 67:601–606.
297. Makhoul RG, Devine DV, Brenckman WD Jr, McCann RL, Greenberg CS. Evidence for the involvement of platelet glycoproteins other than GP Ib in heparin-associated thrombocytopenia and thrombosis. Thromb Res 1987; 45:421–425.
298. Kelton JG, Sheridan D, Brain H, Powers PJ, Turpie AG, Carter CJ. Clinical usefulness of testing for a heparin-dependent platelet-aggregating factor in patients with suspected heparin-associated thrombocytopenia. J Lab Clin Med 1984; 103:606–612.
299. Pfueller SL, David R. Different platelet specificities of heparin-dependent platelet aggregating factors in heparin-associated immune thrombocytopenia. Br J Haematol 1986; 64:149–159.
300. Salem HH, Van der Weyden MB. Heparin induced thrombocytopenia. Variable platelet-rich plasma reactivity to heparin dependent platelet aggregating factor. Pathology 1983; 15:297–299.

301. Warkentin TE, Santos AV, Hayward CPM, Horsewood P, Kelton JG. Importance of platelet preparation in diagnostic testing for heparin-induced thrombocytopenia. Blood 1991; 78 (suppl 1):344a (abstract).
302. Silberman S, Kovarik P. Heparin-induced thrombocytopenia: use of indirect immunofluorescence. Ann Clin Lab Sci 1987; 17:106–110.
303. Howe SE, Lynch DM. An enzyme-linked immunosorbent assay for the evaluation of thrombocytopenia induced by heparin. J Lab Clin Med 1985; 105:554–559.
304. Gruel Y, Rupin A, Darnige L, Moalic-Reverdiau P, Poumier-Gaschard P, Binet C, Bardos P, Leroy J. Specific quantification of heparin-dependent antibodies for the diagnosis of heparin-associated thrombocytopenia using an enzyme-linked immunosorbent assay. Thromb Res 1991; 62:377–387.
305. Greinacher A, Mueller-Eckhardt C. Therapie der Heparin-assoziierten Thrombozytopenia. Dtsch Med Wochenschr 1991; 116:1483–1484.
306. Demers C, Ginsberg JS, Brill-Edwards, P, Panju A, Warkentin TE, Anderson DR, Turner C, Kelton JG. Rapid anticoagulation using ancrod for heparin-induced thrombocytopenia. Blood 1991; 78:2194–2197.
307. Cole CW, Bormanis J. Ancrod: a practical alternative to heparin. J Vasc Surg 1988; 8:59–63.
308. Bell WR, Bolton G, Pitney WR. The effect of Arvin on blood coagulation factors. Br J Haematol 1968; 15:589–602.
309. Edgar W, Prentice CRM. The proteolytic actions of ancrod on human fibrinogen and polypeptide chains. Thromb Res 1973; 2:85–96.
310. Bell WR, Pitney WR, Goodwin JF. Therapeutic defibrination in the treatment of thrombotic disease. Lancet 1968; 1:490–493.
311. Latallo ZS. Retrospective study on complications and adverse effects of treatment with thrombin-like enzymes—a multicentre trial. Thromb Haemost 1983; 50:604–609.
312. Pitney WR, Bray C, Holt PJL, Bolton G. Acquired resistance to treatment with Arvin. Lancet 1969; 1:79–81.
313. Chong BH, Ismail F, Cade J, Gallus AS, Gordon S, Chesterman CN. Heparin-induced thrombocytopenia: studies with a new low molecular weight heparinoid, Org 10172. Blood 1989; 73:1592–1596.
314. Chong BH, Magnani HN. Orgaran in heparin-induced thrombocytopenia. Haemostasis 1992; 22:85–91.
315. Harenberg J, Zimmermann R, Schwarz F, et al. Treatment of heparin-induced thrombocytopenia with thrombosis by new heparinoid. Lancet 1983; 1:986.
316. Kiers L, Grigg LE, Cade JF, et al. Use of Org 10172 in the treatment of heparin-induced thrombocytopenia and thrombosis. Aust NZ J Med 1986; 16.
317. Rowlings PA, Mansberg R, Rozenberg MC, Evans S, Murray B. The use of a low molecular weight heparinoid (Org 10172) for extracorporeal procedures in patients with heparin dependent thrombocytopenia and thrombosis. Aust NZ J Med 1991; 21:52–54.
318. Ortel TL, Gockerman JP, Califf RM, et al. Parenteral anticoagulation with the heparinoid Lomoparan (Org 10172) in patients with heparin induced thrombocytopenia and thrombosis. Thromb Haemost 1992; 67:292–296.

319. Frame JN, Mulvey KP, Phares JC, Anderson MJ. Correction of severe heparin-associated thrombocytopenia with intravenous immunoglobulin. Ann Intern Med 1989; 111:946–947.
320. Warkentin TE, Levine MN, Roberts RS, Gent M, Horsewood P, Kelton JG. Heparin-induced thrombocytopenia is more common with unfractionated heparin than with low molecular weight heparin. Thromb Haemost 1993; 69:911 (abstract).
321. Prull A, Nechtwatal R, Riedel H, Maurer W. [The therapy of the heparin-induced thrombosis-thrombocytopenia syndrome with immunoglobulins]. Dtsch Med Wochenschr 1992; 117:1838–1842.
322. Vender JS, Matthew EB, Silverman IM, Konowitz H, Dau PC. Heparin-associated thrombocytopenia: alternative managements. Anesth Analg 1986; 65:520–522.
323. Nand S, Robinson JA. Plasmapheresis in the management of heparin-associated thrombocytopenia with thrombosis. Am J Hematol 1988; 28:204–206.
324. Bouvier JL, Lefebre P, Villain P, Elias A, Durand JM, Juhan I, Serradimigni A. Treatment of serious heparin-induced thrombocytopenia by plasma exchange: report on 4 cases. Thromb Res 1988; 51:335–336.
325. Brady J, Riccio JA, Yumen OH, Makary AZ, Greenwood SM. Plasmapheresis. A therapeutic option in the management of heparin-associated thrombocytopenia with thrombosis. Am J Clin Pathol 1991; 96:394–397.
326. Gruel Y, Lermusiaux P, Lang M, Darnige L, Rupin A, Delahousse B, Guilmot JL, Leroy J. Usefulness of antiplatelet drugs in the management of heparin-associated thrombocytopenia and thrombosis. Ann Vasc Surg 1991; 5:552–555.
327. Janson PA, Moake JC, Carpinito G. Aspirin prevents heparin-induced platelet aggregation in vivo. Br J Haematol 1983; 53:166–168.
328. Matsuo T, Yamada T, Chikahira Y, Kadowaki S. Effect of aspirin on heparin-induced thrombocytopenia (HIT) in a patient requiring hemodialysis. Blut 1989; 59:393–395.
329. Sobel M, Adelman B, Greenfield LJ. Dextran 40 reduces heparin-mediated platelet aggregation. J Surg Res 1986; 40:382–387.
330. Kappa JR, Fisher CA, Todd B, Stenach N, Bell P, Campbell F, Ellison N, Addonizio VP. Intraoperative management of patients with heparin-induced thrombocytopenia. Ann Thorac Surg 1990; 49:714–723.
331. Stewart JR, Greenfield LJ. Transvenous vena caval filtration and pulmonary embolectomy. Surg Clin North Am 1982; 62:411–430.
332. Cohen JI, Cooper MR, Greenberg CS. Streptokinase therapy of pulmonary emboli with heparin-associated thrombocytopenia. Arch Intern Med 1985; 145:1725–1726.
333. Clifton GD, Smith MD. Thrombolytic therapy in heparin-associated thrombocytopenia with thrombosis. Clin Pharm 1986; 5:597–601.
334. Delagardelle C, Harf C, Dondelinger RF, Goffette P, Beissel J, Pesch C, Welter R. Traitement par thrombolyse locale d'une thrombose artérielle massive par thrombopénie induite par l'héparine. Arch Mal Coeur 1990; 83:113–115.
335. Choay J, Petitou M, Lormeau JC, Sinaÿ P, Casu B, Gatti G. Structureactivity relationship in heparin: a synthetic pentasaccharide with high affinity for antithrombin III and eliciting high anti-factor Xa activity. Biochem Biophys Res Commun 1983; 116:492–499.

336. Grau E, Fontcuberta J, Martinez R, Latorre J, Felez J, Rutllant ML. Thrombopénie sévère précoce induite par l'héparine de bas poids moléculaire. Nouv Rev Fr Hematol 1985; 27:385–387.
337. Laster J, Silver D. Heparin-coated catheters and heparin-induced thrombocytopenia. J Vasc Surg 1988; 7 667–672.
338. Moberg PO, Geary VM, Sheikh FM. Heparin-induced thrombocytopenia: a possible complication of heparin-coated pulmonary artery catheters. J Cardiothorac Anesth 1990; 4:226–228.
339. Zulys VJ, Teasdale SJ, Michel ER, Skala RA, Keating SE, Viger JR, Glynn MFX. Ancrod (Arvin®) as an alternative to heparin anticoagulation for cardiopulmonary bypass Anesthesiology 1989; 71:870–877.
340. Doherty DC, Ortel TL, De Bruijn N, Greenberg CS, Van Trigt P III. "Heparin-free" cardiopulmonary bypass: first reported use of heparinoid (Org 10172) to provide anticoagulation for cardiopulmonary bypass. Anesthesiology 1990; 73:562–565.
341. Marshall LR, Cannell PK, Herrmann RP. Successful use of the APTT in monitoring of the anti-factor Xa activity of the heparinoid Organon 10172 in a case of HITS requiring open heart surgery. Thromb Haemost 1992; 67:587 (letter).
342. Makhoul RG, McCann RL, Austin EH, Greenberg CS, Lowe JE. Management of patients with heparin-associated thrombocytopenia and thrombosis requiring cardiac surgery. Ann Thorac Surg 1987; 43:617–621.
343. Smith JP, Walls JT, Muscato MS, McCord ES, Worth ER, Curtis JJ, Silver D. Extracorporeal circulation in a patient with heparin-induced thrombocytopenia. Anesthesiology 1985; 62:363–365.
344. Addonizio VP Jr, Fisher CA, Kappa JR, Ellison N. Prevention of heparin-induced thrombocytopenia during open heart surgery with iloprost (ZK36374). Surgery 1987; 102:796–807.
345. Kraenzler EJ, Starr NJ. Heparin-associated thrombocytopenia: management of patients for open heart surgery. Case reports describing the use of iloprost. Anesthesiology 1988; 69:964–967.
346. Matsuo T, Chikahira Y, Yamada T, Nakao K, Ueshima S, Matsuo O. Effect of synthetic thrombin inhibitor (MD805) as an alternative drug on heparin induced thrombocytopenia during hemodialysis. Thromb Res 1988; 52:165–171.
347. Matsuo T, Yamada T, Yamanashi T, Ryo R. Anticoagulant therapy with MD805 of a hemodialysis patient with heparin-induced thrombocytopenia. Thromb Res 1990; 58:663–666.
348. Matsuo T, Kario K, Chikahira Y, Nakao K, Yamada T. Treatment of heparin-induced thrombocytopenia by use of argatroban, a synthetic thrombin inhibitor. Br J Haematol 1992; 82:627–629.
349. Leehey DJ, Kanak RJ, Messmore HL, Nawab ZM, Popli S, Ing TS. Heparin-associated thrombocytopenia in maintenance hemodialysis patients. Int J Artif Organs 1987; 10:390–392.
350. Greinacher A, Mueller-Eckhardt C. Diagnostik der Heparin-assoziierten Thrombozytopenie. Dtsch Med Wochenschr 1991; 116:1479–1482.
351. Epperson EL. Efficacy of 0.9% sodium chloride injection with and without heparin for maintaining indwelling intermittent injection sites. Clin Pharm 1984; 3:626–629.

352. Hamilton RA, Plis JM, Clay C, Sylvan L. Heparin sodium versus 0.9% sodium chloride injection for maintaining patency of indwelling intermittent infusion devices. Clin Pharm 1988; 7:439–443.
353. Garrelts JC, LaRocca J, Ast D, Smith DF Jr, Sweet DE. Comparison of heparin and 0.9% sodium chloride injection in the maintenance of indwelling intermittent i.v. devices. Clin Pharm 1989; 8:34–39.
354. Goode CJ, Titler M, Rakel B, et al. A meta-analysis of effects of heparin flush and saline flush: quality and cost implications. Nurs Res 1991; 40:324–330.
355. Garrelts JC. White clot syndrome and thrombocytopenia: reasons to abandon heparin i.v. lock flush solution. Clin Pharm 1992; 11:797–799.
356. Bedford RF, O'Brien TE. Comparison of bovine lung and porcine intestinal heparin for arterial thrombosis in man. Am J Hosp Pharm 1977; 34:936–939.
357. Rajani K, Goetzman BW, Wennberg RP, Turner E, Abildgaard C. Effect of heparinization of fluids infused through an umbilical artery catheter on catheter patency and frequency of complications. Pediatrics 1979; 63:552–556.
358. Butt W, Shann F, McDonnell G, Hudson I. Effect of heparin concentration and infusion rate on the patency of arterial catheters. Crit Care Med 1987; 15:230–232.
359. Gallus A, Jackaman J, Tillett J, Mills W, Wycherley A. Safety and efficacy of warfarin started early after submassive venous thrombosis or pulmonary embolism. Lancet 1986; 2:1293–1296.
360. Hull RD, Raskob GE, Hirsh J, et al. Heparin for 5 days as compared with 10 days in the initial treatment of proximal venous thrombosis. N Engl J Med 1990; 322:1260–1264.
361. Mohiuddin SM, Hilleman DE, Destache CJ, Stoysich AM, Gannon JM, Sketch MH Sr. Efficacy and safety of early versus late initiation of warfarin during heparin therapy in acute thromboembolism. Am Heart J 1992; 123:729–732.

6

Interactions Between Glycosaminoglycans and Endothelial Cells

Gérard Tobelem
INSERM 348, Hôpital Lariboisière, Paris, France

I. INTRODUCTION

Proteoglycans are proteins that carry large carbohydrates, the glycosaminoglycans. The glycosaminoglycans exist in four main forms: heparan sulfate and heparin, chondroitin sulfate and dermatan sulfate, keratan sulfate, and hyaluronic acid. Hyaluronic acid is made as a free glycosaminoglycan devoid of sulfate. Although proteoglycans constitute a minor component of vascular tissue, they have been shown to influence vascular cell biology, including nonthrombogenic properties, cell adhesion, cell migration, cell-cell interactions, and cell growth. Heparin, a highly charged molecule produced virtually only by mast cells, is an effective anticoagulant that has been used as an effective antithrombotic agent in human beings for about 50 years. Exogenous heparin interacts with the vascular endothelium. During the last few years, studies on these interactions made it possible to define the consequences for heparin and endothelium biology.

II. ENDOGENOUS GLYCOSAMINOCLYCANS IN VASCULAR TISSUE

A. Distribution

Glycosaminoglycans are widely distributed in human tissues and body fluids. These macromolecules are synthesized by most cells and are found in the plasma membrane, in intracellular structures, or throughout the extracellular matrix. They exhibit a peculiar structural variability according to the tissue and species of origin. Their diversity derives from the number of different protein cores.

Polydispersity of proteoglycan families also results from posttranslational modifications. Families of proteoglycans identified in blood vessels include proteoglycans containing chondroitin sulfate, dermatan sulfate, and heparan sulfate (1, 2).

Proteoglycans are actively synthesized by endothelial cells in culture; some of them are hydrophobic and associated with plasma membrane. Vascular endothelial cells synthesize and secrete both heparan sulfate and dermatan sulfate proteoglycans. A variety of heparan sulfate proteoglycans differing in size and in ability to interact with other molecules are synthesized by cultured endothelial cells. For instance, a high-molecular-weight subclass exhibits hydrophobic properties and interacts specifically with antithrombin III (3). A significant proportion of the heparan sulfate proteoglycans synthesized by the endothelium are deposited in arterial basement membrane.

Proteoglycans secreted by cultured cells can be found in conditioned media. This secretion may account for the presence of glycosaminoglycans in human plasma (4, 5). The most abundant glycosaminoglycan in plasma is a single species of undersulfated chondroitin sulfate associated with a single protein. The high-charge fraction consists of heparan sulfate, chondroitin sulfate, and keratan sulfate (type I) in association with several plasma proteins. Glycosaminoglycans in plasma are not covalently linked to plasma proteins. Complex formation with proteins has occurred through lectin-type and/or ionic-type binding. No endogenous heparin has been found in plasma (4), although other authors have described a procedure to extract endogenous heparin from human plasma and detected it in significant amounts (6).

High-charge fractions of glycosaminoglycans have been found in plasma as high-molecular-weight complexes, while urinary high-charge heparan sulfate and chondroitin sulfate have been found protein-free (4). The plasma higher-molecular-weight glycosaminoglycans may, therefore, have probably been depolymerized to smaller units before being filtered and eliminated in urine.

High levels of circulating high-charge glycosaminoglycans (heparan sulfate/dermatan sulfate) with anticogulant activity have been reported in plasma of cancer patients treated with suramine (7) and of patients with hematological malignancies (8).

B. Anticoagulant Activity

Heparin-like molecules located in close proximity to the vascular endothelium may be involved in enhancing the function of antithrombin III and account for some of the nonthrombogenic properties of blood vessels (9). Heparin and heparan sulfate are related molecules from the large family of heterogeneous proteoglycans. Heparin differs from heparan sulfate in that it is more highly charged, it appears to occur entirely in mast cells, and it is an effective anticoagulant.

Heparin is richer in *N*- and *O*- sulfate and iduronic acid. However, both heparin and heparan sulfate contain anticoagulant and nonanticoagulant species (1).

Perfusion of rat hindlimbs with purified thrombin and antithrombin III confirmed that endogenous heparin-like molecules associated with the vascular endothelium enhanced circulating antithrombin III action, as shown by measurement of the rate of enzyme-inhibitor complex formation (10). Anticoagulant-active heparan sulfates were synthesized in vitro by capillary endothelial cells derived from the epididymal fatpads of mouse as well as rats (10, 11). Cloned bovine aortic macrovascular endothelial cells synthesized anticoagulant heparan sulfate chains (12). Only a small proportion of the total heparan sulfate proteoglycans synthesized by aortic and microvascular endothelial cells (1% and 10%, respectively) accounted for antithrombin III binding and anticoagulant activity. Iduronic acid containing tri- and disulfated disaccharides and tetra- and penta-sulfated tetrasaccharides typical of heparin was found in heparan sulfate proteoglycans of rabbit endothelial cells in culture (13). Endothelial cell surface proteoglycans are capable of binding not only antithrombin III, but also thrombin (14).

Purification of anticoagulantly active heparan sulfate proteoglycan and anticoagulantly inactive compound from cell surface and media of cloned rat fatpad microvascular endothelial cells showed that the active material represented about 5% of inactive heparan sulfate proteoglycans. Total heparan sulfate isolated from the cell-associated fraction constitutes about 10% of that from culture media (5). Active heparan sulfate proteoglycans bear mainly active heparan sulfate chains with small amounts of inactive glycosaminoglycan and chondroitin sulfate. Inactive heparan sulfate proteoglycans bear mainly inactive heparan sulfate chains. Active and inactive heparan sulfate chains seem therefore to be segregated on two different species of protein core. Active and inactive glycosaminoglycans exhibit molecular masses of 25–30 kDa. Active heparan sulfate derived from endothelial cells was enriched in the minimal pentasaccharide sequence required for antithrombin III–binding site. Active and inactive heparan sulfates exhibited the same relative overall distribution of the monosulfated and disulfated disaccharides. However, active heparan sulfate exhibited about nine glucuronsyl 3-*O*-sulfated glucosamine groups per chain, whereas inactive heparan sulfate had 3 glucuronsyl 3-*O*-sulfated glucosamine groups per chain. Direct isolation of the antithrombin-binding site of active compound showed a single site with two to three glucuronyl 3-*O*-sulfated glucosamine residues. After isolation of the core proteins of active and inactive heparan sulfate proteoglycans, three major components with molecular weights of 50, 30, and 25 kDa, respectively, were demonstrated. The 25-kDa component appeared to be a proteolytic degradation product of the 30-kDa species. Molecular cloning and expression of two distinct cDNAs encoding the three proteoglycan components made it possible to define a new core protein ryudocan (15). The rat ryudocan cDNA encoded a novel 202-amino-acid protein with a predicted molecular mass of 21,948 Da that corresponds to the 30-kDa component. Ryudocan is likely to play a role in maintaining blood fluidity. The rat syndecan cDNA encoded a known 313-amino-acid protein with a predicted molecular mass of 33,168 Da that corresponds to the 50-kDa component.

III. HEPARINS AND VASCULAR ENDOTHELIAL CELLS

Binding of heparin by vascular endothelium has been shown after intravenous administration (16) and after incubation of vessel fragments with heparin solutions (17). Binding of heparin has also been reported using vascular endothelium in culture (18). These interactions of heparin with endothelial cells have been implicated as a possible indirect mechanism of antithrombotic action (19). Our group (20–27) has established the characteristics of binding of different heparins and the consequences of this binding for heparins (Fig. 1).

A. Characteristics of Binding of Heparins to Endothelial Cells

Unfractionated heparin (UH) and low-molecular-weight fragments or fractions of heparin (LMWH) can bind to cultured human endothelial cells (20). The binding is a slow, saturable process that requires hours to reach equilibrium. A high ratio of specific binding was found with different labeled ligands: ^{125}I heparin, ^{3}H-acetylated heparin, or ^{35}S heparin. From the Scatchard plot of experimental data obtained from the ^{35}S heparin saturation curve, two groups of binding sites were found for human umbilical vein endothelial cells: low-affinity binding sites with a K_d of 1.37 ± 0.13 μM and high-affinity binding sites with a K_d of 0.12 ± 0.14 μM with a relatively large number of copies $1.16 \pm 0.07 \times 10^7$ molecules/cell (21). Similar results were shown with ^{35}S-heparin-labeled ligand (24) or with unlabeled ligand in competition experiments with ^{125}I heparin. Different binding affinities were found according to human endothelial cells from different sources. The K_d values were 0.025 μM and 0.35 μM for microvascular endothelial cells (25) and adult saphenous vein endothelial cells (27), respectively. Microvascular endothelial cells had therefore much greater affinity for heparin. In regard to the large surface of the microvascular endothelium, this is probably of great importance for heparin-endothelial cells interactions. Binding to endothelial cells was strongly dependent on M_r and degree of sulfation of heparins (Table 1). LMWH fractions or fragments had much lower affinity for endothelium (21, 24). The analysis of molecular weight distribution of the bound heparin molecules demonstrated a selective binding of high-molecular-weight chains from polydisperse UH or LMWH preparations (24). Chondroitin sulfate, dermatan sulfate, and purified heparan fraction I did not compete for the binding

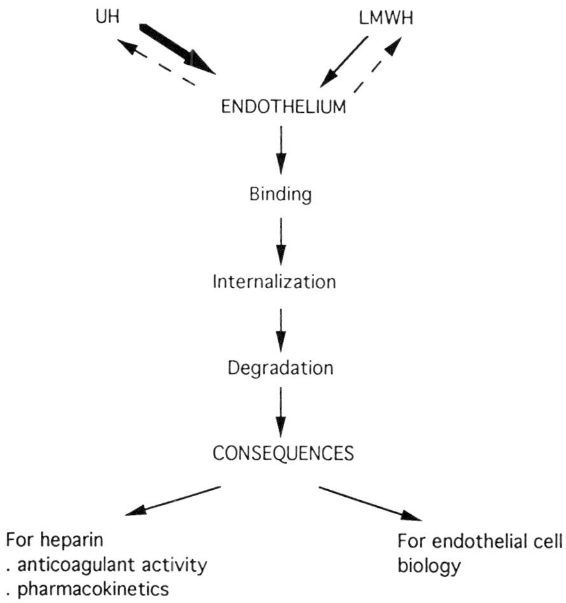

Figure 1 Schematic representation of the interactions of heparins with vascular endothelium. UH = unfractionated heparin; LMWH = low-molecular-weight heparin fragments or fractions.

of ^{125}I heparin, suggesting that binding sites could be specific for heparins. Antithrombin III at concentrations higher than 10 nM added in the incubation medium inhibited heparin binding. This observation strengthened the hypothesis that affinity for endothelium might also depend on affinity for antithrombin III. However, glycosaminoglycans with a higher degree of sulfation, such as heparan sulfate fraction IIa, additionally sulfated dermatan sulfate, hypersulfated UH, or LMWH (CY 216; CY 222), had a much higher affinity for endothelial cells than the parent compounds (Table 1). Moreover, highly sulfated heparinoids having a different polysaccharide backbone, such as pentosan polysulfate or other anionic polyelectrolytes devoid of anticoagulant activity, were able to compete with heparin binding (21). Since oversulfation yields compounds with high affinity for endothelium and low antithrombin III–dependent anticoagulant activity, these two properties of heparin can be dissociated. It must be mentioned, however, that for an equal degree of sulfation, the I_{50} was still dependent on molecular weight (Table 1). Therefore, endothelial binding sites are not specific receptors for heparins, but rather acceptor sites for anionic polyelectrolytes.

Table 1 Competition of Labeled-Heparin Binding to Endothelial Cells by Low-Molecular-Weight Heparin Fractions, Polyanions, and Other Sulfated Derivatives

Compound	M_r	Degree of sulfation (OSO_3/COO)	Anticoagulant activity in vitro APTT	Anti-Xa	Affinity for endothelium [I_{50} (μM)]
Unfractionated heparin	15,000	2.16	144	165	0.17
		3.01	60	35	0.025
CY 216	4,500	2.1	26	224	15.0
		2.5	22	30	0.15
CY 222	2,500	2.1	12	250	>100
Enoxaparin	4,500	2.24	28	66	10.0
Dermatan sulfate	30,000	2.24	2	6	0.02
Pentosan polysulfate	4,700	5.6			0.13
Polystyrene sulfate	31,000	3.18			0.52
	4,000	5.0			6.0

B. Endocytosis and Degradation of Heparins by Endothelial Cells

Temperature dependence of binding reversibility suggested that endocytosis of a fraction of bound heparin occurred. This phenomenom was confirmed by the addition of histone, a basic protein known to stimulate endocytosis of heparin, which increased irreversible heparin binding (23). Furthermore, undissociable bound heparin was not sensitive to heparinase treatment. Endocytosis of heparin has been also reported using other cell types, such as macrophages (28), hamster ovary cells (29), or smooth muscle cells (30).

A fraction of bound heparin was slowly released into the medium and exhibited low anticoagulant activity (21), suggesting that internalized heparin might be degraded by the endothelium. The gel filtration pattern of heparin bound to the endothelial cell surface after incubation at 4°C confirmed a selection of higher-molecular-weight chains (24). After incubation for 5 hr at 37°C, the molecular weight distribution of bound fractions was significantly shifted to the lower-molecular-weight domain. This shift occurring at 37°C suggested a depolymerization of heparin as a consequence of binding to endothelial cells. To localize the intracellular degradation, the same experiments were performed in the presence of chloroquine, a compound known to inhibit lysosomal hydrolases (23). Binding and internalization of heparin were not changed by chloroquine, and the shift in molecular weight distribution was completely prevented. Degradation of exogenous glycosaminoglycans by human endothelial cells has been reported by another group who described a new catabolism pathway (31). These authors showed that incorporation of exogenous glycosaminoglycans (heparin, heparan sulfate, pentosan polysulfate) occurred not only into the endothelial cellular fraction, but also into the subcellular matrix. Only a small proportion of labeled compound was present in the cells at any one time; most glycosaminoglycans present in the supernatant at 24 hr had been catabolyzed, degradation products being therefore readily exported. This group confirmed that dermatan sulfate, the least sulfated glycosaminoglycan, was not found in cellular or subcellular matrix. The degradation process of glycosaminoglycans taken up by the cells appeared to involve initial complete desulfation. Similar desulfation before depolymerization had been reported after injection of ^{125}I heparin into healthy volunteers (32). The metabolism of heparin by cultured endothelial cells seems to be relevant to a catabolic process occurring in the whole organism. These authors concluded that if lysosomal exoenzymes are essential for the catabolism of endogenous glycosaminoglycans, exogenous glycosaminoglycans could first be desulfated before being depolymerized.

Internalization and metabolism of endogenous heparin have been also reported with bovine adrenal capillary endothelial cells (33).

C. Consequences of Endothelial Cell Binding for Heparins

1. Anticoagulant Activities of Bound Heparin

To determine whether heparin bound to endothelium could act as a source of immobilized anticoagulant and contribute to the nonthrombogenic properties, the anticoagulant activities of bound heparins were measured after treatment by pronase of endothelial cells preincubated with ^{35}S UH or ^{35}S LMWH (enoxaparin) for 5 hr at 4°C. ^{35}S unfractionated heparin dissociated from cultured endothelium was almost twofold more active in anti-IIa and anti-Xa activity than ^{35}S UH before binding. ^{35}S low-molecular-weight fraction and fragments of heparin extracted from cells had a fourfold higher anti-Xa and eightfold higher anti-IIa activity than ^{35}S LMWH before binding (24). Selective binding of heparin chains with high anti-IIa and anti-Xa activity is in agreement with earlier observations in which fractions of heparins with high affinity for antithrombin III had greater affinity for endothelium. In fact, both the affinity of heparin for endothelium and the affinity for antithrombin III increased with the molecular weight of the polysaccharide chains. Selective binding of molecules with high anticoagulant activity therefore seems likely related to the high-molecular-weight dependency of heparin-chain binding to the endothelium.

When anticoagulant activities of bound heparin were measured in dishes containing intact endothelial cells previously incubated with UH for 5 hr at 37°C, the results were different (21). The endothelial bound heparin slightly accelerated factor IIa and factor Xa inactivation by antithrombin III. However, the bound fractions were less available to interaction with antithrombin III. Their activities represented only 5 and 7%, respectively, of anti-IIa and anti-Xa activities of an equivalent amount of heparin in solution. Furthermore, these activities were partly provided by release of a fraction of bound heparin into the incubation medium. It appears, therefore, unlikely that cell-bound heparin may express full biological activity as an immobilized anticoagulant or mimic the action of the endogenous heparin-like molecules, as previously reported (34). In fact, binding to endothelial cells is accompanied by neutralization of heparin. The fraction of heparin released into the medium exhibited lower specific activity and a higher ratio of anti-Xa/anti-IIa potency than the applied heparin. This was a further argument for an endothelial release of the lower-M_r chains. Heparin degradation following binding and endocytosis at 37°C is probably responsible for the neutralization.

2. Implications for Pharmacokinetics

All these studies on the interactions of exogenous glycosaminoglycans with cultured endothelial cells have led to a better understanding of the pharmacokinetics of UH and LMWH. Pharmacokinetics studies indicated that the rapid clearance of heparin after intravenous injection was a consequence of a combination of a saturable and nonsaturable mechanism (35). Whereas the nonsaturable mechanism might be related to renal elimination, the saturable mechanism was suggested to result from an uptake by endothelial and reticuloendothelial cells (36). The slower disappearance of anticoagulant from the circulation after administration of LMWH has been attributed to a poor efficiency of the saturable mechanism (37), which would be in accordance with the low affinity of LMWH for endothelium. Preferential uptake from the circulation of molecules more active in both factor Xa and factor IIa neutralization might also contribute to the divergence between in vitro and in vivo anticoagulant activities. Differences found between anti-factor Xa and activated partial thromboplastin time clearance curves of UH can be explained by remaining low-molecular-weight material in the circulation possessing almost exclusively anti-factor Xa activity.

The short half-life of UH after intravenous injection in humans compared to the longer half-life of LMWH seems therefore to be a consequence of the respective affinities of these compounds for vascular endothelium.

IV. ROLE OF PROTEOGLYCANS IN VASCULAR CELL BIOLOGY

Proteoglycans and glycosaminoglycans are of enormous importance in several biological processes, such as cell-cell recognition, tissue differentiation, organization of extracellular matrix, cell-matrix and cell-substrate adhesion, and cell growth.

A. Cell Adhesion

Endothelial cell adhesion to connective tissue substrates is pivotal to the maintenance of vascular integrity and normal vascular hemostasis. Vascular endothelial cells interact with their substrates in specialized areas called focal adhesion sites. These sites concentrate (1) adhesive proteins and heparan sulfate proteoglycans on the extracellular matrix side and (2) actin microfilaments on the cytoplasmic side. Cell-associated heparan sulfate proteoglycans could interact with specific binding domains in adhesive proteins such as fibronectin and subsequently stabilize binding of fibronectin to its cell surface receptor (38). The fact that removal of heparan sulfate proteoglycans from endothelial cells does not detach cells, but does prevent cells from reattaching, is in favor of multiple adhesion mechanisms, heparan sulfate proteoglycans being involved in one of them (39). Proteoglycans also influence cell-to-cell association by self-association.

B. Cell Migration

Endothelial cell migration in response to injury is critical to vascular repair. The precise mechanism of endothelial cell migration is not yet totally clarified. Proteoglycans are supposed to facilitate endothelial cell migration by interfering with the cell adhesion process. Endothelial cell migration is accompanied by an increased synthesis of proteoglycans and by a shift within the synthetized extracellular matrix from heparan sulfate proteoglycan to chondroitin sulfate/dermatan sulfate proteoglycan (40).

Heparin also stimulates the migration of capillary endothelial cells (41) but inhibits the migration of smooth muscle cells (42).

C. Cell Growth

1. Proteoglycans as Modulators of Endothelial Cell Growth

The first observation that heparin might influence the proliferation of endothelial cells came from Thorton et al. (43). This group reported that heparin plus endothelial cell growth factor supported the clonal growth of endothelial cells. Moreover, they showed that in the absence of heparin the growth was significantly less than that stimulated in the presence of heparin. Mast cell granules containing heparin can be internalized and degraded by endothelial cells and can cause migration and proliferation of microvascular endothelial cells (44). In fact, heparin seems rather to modulate endothelial cell growth according to the existing conditions—sometimes it stimulates and sometimes it inhibits proliferation. Our group contributed to the demonstration of this modulator effect of heparin (22, 25, 26). When added alone to cultured human macrovascular endothelial cells in the presence of low concentrations of human serum, heparin inhibited ^{3}H-thymidine uptake and growth in a dose-dependent maner. This inhibition started 6–9 hr after heparin addition and was reversible. The inhibitory effect was required to cause binding and internalization of glycosaminoglycans by the endothelial cells. Pentosan polysulfate was effective as well, whereas chondroitin sulfate was ineffective. LMWH fractions and fragments induced a significant growth inhibition, although their affinity for endothelial cells is about 100 times lower than that of unfractionated heparin. The inhibitory effect of heparin was more potent when measured in the presence of human serum deprived of antithrombin III.

The effect of heparin has also been shown to be variable according to the cellular density and the cell cycle of the cultured endothelial cells. In log-phase growing human omental microvascular endothelial cells or human umbilical vein endothelial cells, heparin inhibited cell proliferation, whereas in serum-deprived endothelial cells, it stimulated cell proliferation. Heparan sulfate proteoglycan derived from postconfluent endothelial cells and smooth muscle cells also inhibited proliferation of arterial smooth muscle cells (45). Heparin and heparan sulfate have been shown to exhibite opposite activities on the growth of human umbilical vein endothelial cells in the presence of acidic and basic fibroblast growth factor (46). Confirming the observation of Thornton et al. (43), we also reported that heparin added at the same time as endothelial cell growth factor stimulated endothelial cell growth (26). However, preincubation of the cells with heparin 6–24 hr before the addition of the growth factor still exhibited an inhibitory effect. Similar inhibition was found when heparin was added 24 hr after endothelial cell growth factor. Heparin added 6–24 hr before or up to 24 hr after endothelial cell growth factor might have exerted its inhibitory effect via an intracellular action on protein kinase C (47). Heparin plus corticosteroïds has been reported to inhibit angiogenesis by an unknown mechanism, although a capillary membrane dissolution has been postulated (48). A combination of heparin (or LMWH) and steroids (devoid of any mineralo-or glucocorticoid activity) caused a strong inhibition of endothelial cell proliferation (26).

2. *Proteoglycans as Modulators of Growth Factor Activities*

Sulfated glycosaminoglycans have a strong negative charge. This allows glycosaminoglycans to bind some growth factors. The role of heparan sulfate proteoglycans as binders of fibroblast growth factors (FGFs) in protecting FGFs from degradation has been demonstrated during the last 8 years. Proteoglycan binding provides a matrix-bound or cell-surface-bound reservoir of FGFs. Vlodavsky et al. showed that FGFs are sequestered in the extracellular matrix because of their binding to heparan sulfate proteoglycan (49). Basic FGF remains biologically active when immobilized to matrix via the heparan sulfate chains of syndecan (50). Cell surface proteoglycan likely to interact with basic FGF is also syndecan. Active FGF-glycosaminoglycan complex can be generated by proteolysis of core proteins or partial degradation of heparan sulfate component.

The binding of basic FGF to its cell surface receptor protein requires prior binding either to the heparan sulfate side chains of a membrane heparan sulfate proteoglycan or to free heparin chain. FGF receptor in heparan sulfate–deficient CHO mutant does not bind basic FGF. The binding ability is restored when basic

FGF is added to the mutant cells in the form of a heparin–basic FGF complex (51). Treatment of heparin with heparinase completely abolishes its capacity to restore high-affinity basic FGF receptor binding to heparan sulfate–deficient CHO mutant cells. A heparin-derived oligosaccharide containing at least eight sugar units is needed for restoration of FGF receptor binding in heparan sulfate–deficient mutant cells (52). Basic FGF-glycosaminoglycan interactions may change the conformation of basic FGF to make possible basic FGF binding to its receptor protein. Another mechanism might favor an oligomerization of basic FGF resulting in dimerization of receptors needed for signal transduction. Whatever the mechanism, it is clear that basic FGF bound to low-affinity heparan sulfate–binding sites is not active unless it is properly presented to high-affinity basic FGF receptors, and high-affinity receptors are not accessible for basic FGF binding and signal transduction in the absence of the low-affinity heparan sulfate–binding sites. Recent work (53) on kinetics of basic FGF binding to its receptor and heparan sulfate proteoglycan suggested a mechanism of protein-glycosaminoglycan cooperativity that involves the formation of a more stable ternary complex of basic FGF–cell surface receptor–protein heparan sulfate proteoglycan. The difference in K_d for cell surface receptor binding and heparan sulfate proteoglycan binding appears to result from the faster rate at which basic FGF is released from heparan sulfate proteoglycan sites compared to the cell surface receptor. The high-affinity binding of basic FGF to intact cells therefore seems to result from the formation of a complex of basic FGF with both cell surface receptor and heparan sulfate proteoglycan, not from the interaction of basic FGF with the cell surface receptor alone. A portion of cell surface heparan sulfate proteoglycan is anchored via a covalently linked glycosyl-phosphatidyl inositol residue, which can be released by treatment with a glycosyl-phosphatidyl inositol–specific phospholipase (52). Addition of this phospholipase to sparsely seeded vascular endothelial cells stimulates cell proliferation. Three to 8% of total cellular content of basic FGF is associated with glycosyl phosphatidylinositol–anchored cell surface heparan sulfate proteoglycan. This FGF might have autocrine and paracrine effects when released by specific phospholipase and properly presented to cell surface receptor protein. Basic FGF bound to extracellular matrix is not released by phosphatidylinositol lipase, indicating that anchorage through glycosyl-phosphatidyl-inositol is unique to the cell surface. In contrast, heparinase and heparinitase release basic FGF from both cell surface and extracellular matrix. Basic FGF released by heparinitase is biologically active whereas the material released by heparinase loses its mitogenic effect. This may be due to a difference in the small size of the released fragments degraded by heparinase.

Basic FGF lacks a classic hydrophobic signal peptide and is therefore mostly an intracellular protein. How basic FGF is exported to the cell membrane or to the extracellular matrix remains unknown. Basic FGF may follow a novel route of membrane insertion and secretion involving phosphatidyl-inositol phospholipase. Transforming growth factor β, a multifunctional factor, binds to proteoglycan through the core protein of betaglycan. Glycosaminoglycan of betaglycan is not needed for the binding of transforming growth β whereas it is required for the binding of basic FGF. Thus, these two growth factors can bind to the same cell membrane proteoglycan through separate domains (54). Moreover, transforming growth factor β binds to proteoglycan decorin in the extracellular matrix. This binding also occurs to the core protein of decorin. When bound to decorin, transforming growth factor β is neutralized.

Thrombospondin, an inhibitor of angiogenesis, endothelial cell growth, and migration, binds to the surface of vascular endothelial cells. Heparin may form a complex with thrombospondin and consequently inhibit thrombospondin binding to endothelial cell surface (55).

Platelet factor 4 binds heparin and chondroitin sulfate. It is stored in the platelet α-granules in the form of a complex with chondroitin sulfate proteoglycan serglycin (56). Platelet factor 4 inhibits angiogenesis and endothelial cell proliferation. The active part of platelet factor 4 is the heparin-binding domain of the molecule (57). The potential role of platelet factor 4 alone or complexed to proteoglycan in vascular cell biology remains unclear; additional studies are needed.

REFERENCES

1. Wight TN. Arteriosclerosis 1989; 9:1.
2. Ruoslahti E, Yamagushi Y. Cell 1991; 64:867.
3. Marcum JA, Reilly CF, Rosenberg RD. In: Wight TN, Macham RP, eds. Biology of Extracellular Matrix: Biology of Proteoglycans. Orlando, FL: Academic Press, 1987:301.
4. Staprans I, Felto JM. J Clin Invest 1985; 76:1984.
5. Kojima T, Leone CW, Marchildon GA, Marcum JA, Rosenberg RD. J Biol Chem 1992; 267:4859.
6. Vannuchi S, Pasquali F, Chiarugi V, Ruggiero M. Biochem Biophys Res Commun 1986; 140:294.
7. Horne MDK, Stein CA, La Rocca RV, Myers CE. Blood 1988; 76:273.
8. Palmer RN, Rick ME, Rick PD, Zeller JA, Gradnick JR. N Engl J Med 1984; 310:1696.
9. Busch C, Owen WG. J Clin Invest 1982; 69:726.
10. Marcum JA, McKenney JB, Galli SJ, Jackman RW, Rosenberg RD. Am J Physiol 1986; 250:H879.
11. Marcum JA, Rosenberg RD. Biochem Biophys Res Commun 1985; 126:365.
12. Marcum JA, Atha DH, Fritze LMS, Nawroth P, Stern D, Rosenberg RD. J Biol Chem 1986; 261:7507.
13. Nader HB, Dietrich CP, Buonassi V, Colburn P. Proc Natl Acad Sci USA 1987; 84:3565.

14. Shimada K, Ozawa T. J Clin Invest 1985; 75:1308.
15. Kajima T, Shworak NW, Rosenberg RD. J Biol Chem 1992; 267:4870.
16. Hiebert LM. Thromb Res 1981; 21:383.
17. Mahadoo J, Hiebert LM, Jacques LB. Thromb Res 1977; 12:79.
18. Glimelius B, Busch C, Höök M. Thromb Res 1978; 13:773.
19. Jacques LB. Trends Pharmacol Sci 1982; 3:289.
20. Bârzu T, Molho P, Tobelem G, Petitou M, Caen J. Biochim Biophys Acta 1985; 845:196.
21. Bârzu T, Van Rijn JLML, Petitou M, Molho P, Tobelem G, Caen J. Biochem J 1986; 238:847.
22. Rosenbaum J, Tobelem G, Molho P, Bârzu T, Caen J. Cell Biol Int Rep 1986; 10:437.
23. Bârzu T, Van Rijn JLML, Petitou M, Tobelem G, Caen J. Thromb Res 1987; 47:601.
24. Van Rijn JLML, Trillou M, Mardiguian J, Tobelem G, Caen J. Thromb Res 1987; 45:211.
25. Bikfalvi A, Dupuy E, Ruan C, Tobelem G, Lesèche G, Caen J. Cell Biol Int Rep 1988; 12:931.
26. Cariou R, Harousseau JL, Tobelem G. Cell Biol Int Rep 1988; 12:1037.
27. Lesèche G, Bikfalvi A, Dupuy E, Tobelem G, Andreassian B, Caen J. Surgery 1989; 105:36.
28. Bleiberg I, MacGregor I, Aronson M. Thromb Res 1983; 29:53.
29. Reyser HJP, Morad N, Shen WD. Cell Biol Int Rep 1984; 7:923.
30. Castellot JI, Wong K, Herman B, Hoover RI, Albertini DE, Wright TC, Caleb BJ, Karnovski MJ. J Cell Physiol 1985; 124:13.
31. Dawes J, Pepper DS. Thromb Haemost 1992; 67:468.
32. Dawes J, Pepper DS. Thromb Res 1979; 14:845.
33. Vannucchi S, Pasquali F, Porciatti F, Chiarugi V, Magnelli L, Bianchini P. Thromb Res 1988; 49:373.
34. Rosenberg RD, Rosenberg JS. J Clin Invest 1984; 74:1.
35. De Swart CAM, Nijmejer B, Roelofs JMM, Sixma JJ. Blood 1982; 60:1251.
36. Caranobe C, Barret A, Gabarg AM, Duponu D, Sie P, Boneu B. Thromb Haemost 1985; 54:196.
37. Caranobe C, Dupuy D, Gabaig AM, Boneu B. Thromb Haemost 1985; 54:196.
38. Ruoslahti E, Hayman EG, Pierschbacher MD. Arteriosclerosis 1985; 5:581.
39. Hatcher VB, Fadl-Allah N, Levitt MA, Brown A, Margossian SS, Gordon PB. J Cell Physiol 1986; 128:353.
40. Kinsella MG, Wight TN. J Cell Biol 1986; 102:679.
41. Majak RA, Clowes AW. J Cell Physiol 1984; 118:253.
42. Terranova WP, Difloria R, Lyall RM, Hic S, Friesel R. J Cell Biol 1985; 101:2330.
43. Thornton SC, Meller SN, Levine EM. Science 1983; 222:623.
44. Marks RM, Roche WR, Czeniecki M, Penny R, Nelson DS. Lab Invest 1986; 55:289.
45. Castelot JJ, Favreau LV, Karnovsky MJ, Rosenberg RD. J Biol Chem 1982; 257:11256.
46. Imamura T, Mitsui Y. Exp Cell Res 1987; 172:92.
47. Bikfalvi A, Dupuy E, Tobelem G, Caen J, Castagna M. Blood 1987; 68(Suppl 1):1452 (abstract).

48. Folkman J, Langer R, Linhart RJ, Haudensheld O, Taylor S. Science 1983; 221:719.
49. Vlodavsky I, Folkman J, Sullivan R, Fridman R, Ishai-Michaeli R, Sasse J, Klagsbrun M. Proc Natl Acad Sci USA 1987; 84:2292.
50. Salmivirta M, Heino J, Jalkaren M. J Biol Chem 1992; 267:17606.
51. Yayon A, Klagsbrun M, Esko JD, Leder P, Ornitz D. Cell 1991; 64:841.
52. Bashkin P, Neufeld G, Gitay-Goren H, Vlodavsky I. J Cell Physiol 1992; 151:126.
53. Nugent MA, Edelman ER. Biochemistry 1992; 31:8876.
54. Andres JL, De Falcis D, Noda M, Massagué J. J Biol Chem 1992; 267:5927.
55. Murphy-Ullrich JE, Mosher DF. J Cell Biol 1987; 105:1603.
56. Périn JP, Bonnet F, Maillet P, Jollès P. Biochem J 1988; 255:1007.
57. Maione TE, Gray GS, Petro J, Hunt AJ, Donner AL, Bauer SI, Carson HF, Sharpe RJ. Science 1990; 247:77.

7
Interactions Between Heparin and Fibrinolysis

Henri Roger Lijnen and Désiré Collen
Center for Molecular and Vascular Biology, University of Leuven, Leuven, Belgium

I. INTRODUCTION

The blood coagulation system is responsible for the formation of fibrin, the solid noncellular component of the thrombus. Sequential activation of proteins in the clotting cascade occurs on the surface of various types of blood cells, primarily platelets and monocytes, and results in the generation of thrombin that converts fibrinogen into fibrin. This process is counterbalanced by inhibitors. Antithrombin III is a major thrombin-inactivating protein in plasma, and the rate of inhibition of thrombin by antithrombin III is greatly enhanced by the presence of heparin.

Human plasma also contains an enzymatic system for the dissolution of fibrin, known as the fibrinolytic system, which is responsible for restoring and maintaining vascular patency following fibrin formation. Fibrinolysis plays an important role in several biological processes, such as tissue repair, malignant transformation, macrophage function, and fertility, but we will focus on its role in the removal of fibrin from the blood stream.

The fibrinolytic system is schematically represented in Figure 1 and some properties of its main components are summarized in Table 1. The system contains a proenzyme, plasminogen, which by the action of plasminogen activators is converted to the active enzyme plasmin, which in turn digests fibrin to soluble degradation products. Inhibition of the fibrinolytic system occurs both at the level of the plasminogen activators, by plasminogen activator inhibitors (mainly plasminogen activator inhibitor-1, PAI-1), and at the level of plasmin, mainly by α_2-antiplasmin. The physiological plasminogen activators, tissue-type plasminogen activator (t-PA) and single-chain urokinase-type plasminogen activator (scu-PA, prourokinase), activate plasminogen preferentially at the fibrin

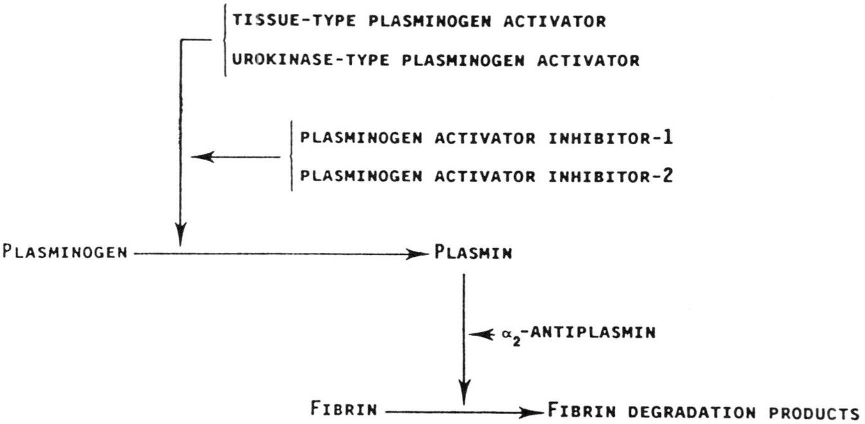

Figure 1 Schematic representation of the fibrinolytic system. The proenzyme plasminogen is activated to the active enzyme plasmin by tissue-type or urokinase-type plasminogen activator. Plasmin degrades fibrin into soluble fibrin degradation products. Inhibition of the fibrinolytic system may occur at the level of the plasminogen activators, by plasminogen activator inhibitors, or at the level of plasmin, mainly by α_2-antiplasmin.

surface. Plasmin, associated with the fibrin surface, is protected from rapid inhibition by α_2-antiplasmin and may thus efficiently degrade the fibrin of a thrombus (1).

This fibrin-specific mechanism of action of both t-PA and scu-PA has triggered great interest in the use of these agents for thrombolytic therapy. Thrombolytic therapy has become standard treatment for patients with acute myocardial infarction or some other forms of thromboembolic disease. However, successful thrombolytic therapy may be offset by reocclusion as a result of new fibrin deposition on the underlying vessel wall damage. Heparin has been used extensively as an anticoagulant agent in the early phase of thrombolysis (2–6). However, some controversy exists with respect to the efficacy of heparin in combination with different thrombolytic agents and with respect to the possible contribution of heparin to the development of bleeding complications (7). It has also been suggested that heparin may directly influence fibrinolysis via different mechanisms, including induction of t-PA release from vascular endothelial cells or binding to t-PA with enhancement of the catalytic efficiency for plasminogen activation.

In this chapter we will indicate the different levels at which heparins may affect fibrinolysis, as monitored in in vitro systems, and discuss the relevance of these effects on fibrinolysis and thrombolysis as monitored in animal models of thrombosis and in patients with thromboembolic disease.

Table 1 Some Properties of the Main Components of the Fibrinolytic System

	M_r (kDa)	Carbohydrate content (%)	Number of amino acids	Catalytic triad	Reactive site	Plasma concentration (mg/L)
Plasminogen	92	2	791	—	—	200
Plasmin	85	2	±715	His^{603},Asp^{646},Ser^{741}	—	—
t-PA	68	7	527	His^{322},Asp^{371},Ser^{478}	—	0.005
scu-PA	54	7	411	His^{204},Asp^{255},Ser^{356}	—	0.008
α_2-Antiplasmin	70	13	452	—	Arg^{364}-Met^{365}	70
PAI-1	52	ND	379	—	Arg^{346}-Met^{347}	0.05
PAI-2	47	ND	393	—	Arg^{358}-Thr^{359}	<0.005

t-PA = tissue-type plasminogen activator; scu-PA = single-chain urokinase-type plasminogen activator, prourokinase; PAI-1 = plasminogen activator inhibitor-1; PAI-2 = plasminogen activator inhibitor-2; ND = not determined.

II. MAIN COMPONENTS OF THE FIBRINOLYTIC SYSTEM

A. Plasminogen

Human plasminogen is a single-chain glycoprotein with a molecular weight of 92,000, present in plasma at a concentration of 1.5–2 μM. It consists of 791 amino acids with 24 disulfide bridges and it contains five homologous triple-loop domains, or "kringles" (8,9).

All plasminogen activators convert single-chain plasminogen to plasmin by cleavage of the Arg^{561}-Val^{562} peptide bond. The plasmin molecule is a two-chain, trypsin-like serine proteinase with an active site composed of His^{603}, Asp^{646}, and Ser^{741}. The kringle domains of plasminogen contain structures, called lysine-binding sites, that interact specifically with amino acids such as lysine and 6-aminohexanoic acid. These lysine-binding sites mediate the specific binding of plasminogen to fibrin and the interaction of plasmin with α_2-antiplasmin and play a crucial role in the regulation of fibrinolysis (1).

B. Plasminogen Activators

1. Tissue-Type Plasminogen Activator (t-PA)

Human t-PA is a serine proteinase with M_r about 70,000, composed of one polypeptide chain containing 527 amino acids (10). Limited plasmic hydrolysis of the Arg^{275}-Ile^{276} peptide bond converts the molecule to a two-chain activator held together by one interchain disulfide bond. The t-PA molecule contains four domains: (1) an aminoterminal region comprising residues 4–50 (F-domain), which is homologous with the finger domains mediating the fibrin affinity of fibronectin; (2) residues 50–87 (E-domain), which are homologous with human epidermal growth factor; (3) two regions comprising residues 87–176 and 176–262 (K_1- and K_2-domains), which share a high degree of homology with the five kringles of plasminogen; and (4) a serine proteinase domain (residues 276–527) with the active site residues His^{322}, Asp^{371}, and Ser^{478}.

t-PA is a poor enzyme in the absence of fibrin, but fibrin enhances the activation rate of plasminogen by t-PA by at least two orders of magnitude (11).

2. Urokinase-Type Plasminogen Activator (u-PA)

Single-chain urokinase-type plasminogen activator (scu-PA, prourokinase) is a glycoprotein with M_r 54,000 containing 411 amino acids (12). Upon limited hydrolysis by plasmin or kallikrein of the Lys^{158}-Ile^{159} peptide bond, the molecule is converted to a two-chain derivative (tcu-PA, urokinase) (13). The aminoterminal chain contains a region homologous to human epidermal growth factor (E-domain; residues 9–45) and one kringle region (K-domain; residues 45–134). The catalytic center is located in the proteinase domain (residues 159–411) and is composed of His^{204}, Asp^{255}, and Ser^{356}.

scu-PA has a very low reactivity toward low-molecular-weight synthetic substrates or active site inhibitors that are very reactive toward tcu-PA. In mixtures of purified scu-PA and plasminogen, both tcu-PA and plasmin are quickly generated, suggesting that scu-PA has some intrinsic plasminogen-activating activity. The magnitude of this intrinsic activity is, however, still controversial (14–16).

3. *Streptokinase and Anisoylated Plasminogen-Streptokinase Activator Complex (APSAC)*

Streptokinase is produced by several strains of hemolytic streptococci; it consists of a single polypeptide chain with M_r 47,000–50,000 and contains 414 amino acids (17). Streptokinase cannot directly cleave peptide bonds, but it activates plasminogen to plasmin indirectly, following formation of an equimolar complex with plasmin(ogen) (18).

Anisoylated plasminogen-streptokinase activator complex (APSAC) was constructed to control the enzymatic activity of the plasmin(ogen)-streptokinase complex by a specific reversible chemical protection of its catalytic center (i.e., by titration with a *p*-anisoyl group) (19). APSAC is an equimolar, noncovalent complex between human Lys-plasminogen and streptokinase, containing the titrated catalytic center and the lysine-binding sites of plasminogen. Reversible acylation of the catalytic center would thus not affect the weak fibrin-binding capacity of Lys-plasminogen in the complex. Deacylation of APSAC, which regenerates the catalytic center, occurs both in the circulation and at the fibrin surface. A plasma half-life of 70 min was found for APSAC, compared to 25 min for the plasminogen-streptokinase complex formed in vivo after administration of streptokinase (20).

C. Inhibitors of the Fibrinolytic System

Inhibition of the fibrinolytic system may occur at the level of plasmin or at the level of the plasminogen activators. Alpha$_2$-antiplasmin is the main physiological plasmin inhibitor in human plasma, whereas inhibition of the physiological plasminogen activators t-PA and u-PA occurs primarily by plasminogen activator inhibitor-1 (PAI-1) and plasminogen activator inhibitor-2 (PAI-2).

1. *Alpha$_2$-Antiplasmin*

Alpha$_2$-antiplasmin is a single-chain glycoprotein with a M_r of 70,000, consisting of 452 amino acids (21). It belongs to the *ser*ine *p*roteinase *in*hibitor protein family (serpins). Its P_1-P_1' reactive site peptide bond consists of Arg^{364}-Met^{365}. The concentration of the inhibitor in plasma is about 1 μM. In the presence of calcium ions and activated coagulation factor XIII, α_2-antiplasmin is cross-linked to the fibrin α-chain (22).

Alpha$_2$-antiplasmin forms a 1:1 stoichiometric complex with plasmin that is devoid of protease or esterase activity. The inhibition of plasmin (P) by α_2-antiplasmin (A) can be represented by two consecutive reactions: a fast, second-order reaction producing a reversible inactive complex (PA), which is followed by a slower, first-order transition resulting in an irreversible complex (PA′). This model can be represented by:

$$\mathrm{P} + \mathrm{A} \underset{k_{-1}}{\overset{k_1}{\rightleftharpoons}} \mathrm{PA} \overset{k_2}{\rightarrow} \mathrm{PA'}$$

The second-order rate constant of the inhibition of plasmin by α_2-antiplasmin ($k_1 = 2\text{–}4 \times 10^7\ \mathrm{M}^{-1}\ \mathrm{sec}^{-1}$) is among the fastest protein-protein reactions described (23). This high inhibition rate is dependent on the presence of a free lysine-binding site and active site in the plasmin molecule and of a plasminogen-binding site (in the carboxyterminal portion) and the reactive site in the inhibitor.

2. *Plasminogen Activator Inhibitor-1 (PAI-1)*

PAI-1 was first identified in conditioned media of cultured human endothelial cells and rat hepatoma cells, and subsequently in plasma, platelets, placenta, and conditioned media of fibrosarcoma cells and hepatocytes (for references cf. 24). It is a single-chain glycoprotein with M_r about 52,000, consisting of 379 amino acids. The cDNA has been sequenced, revealing that PAI-1 is a member of the serine proteinase inhibitor (serpin) family. Its reactive site consists of Arg^{346}-Met^{347} (25,26).

PAI-1 is the primary inhibitor of both t-PA and u-PA in human plasma (27, 28). Like other serpins, PAI-1 inhibits its target proteinases by formation of a 1:1 stoichiometric reversible complex, followed by formation of a convalent binding. PAI-1 is stabilized by binding to a plasminogen activator inhibitor–binding protein identified as S-protein or vitronectin (29).

The synthesis and/or release of PAI-1 from various cell types is regulated by several stimuli, including thrombin, dexamethasone, endotoxin, interleukin-1, transforming growth factor β, and tumor necrosis factor (for references cf. 24). PAI-1 levels are elevated in several disease states, including venous thromboembolism, obesity, sepsis, and coronary artery disease (30).

III. REGULATION OF THE FIBRINOLYTIC SYSTEM

The fibrinolytic system is regulated by controlled activation and inhibition of its components. Activation of plasminogen by t-PA is enhanced in the presence of fibrin or at the endothelial cell surface. Inhibition of fibrinolysis may occur at the level of plasminogen activation or at the level of plasmin. Fibrinolysis may also be regulated as a result of increased or decreased synthesis and/or secretion of t-PA and of PAI-1 from the vessel wall.

The physiological importance of the fibrinolytic system is demonstrated by the association between abnormal fibrinolysis and a tendency toward bleeding or thrombosis. Impairment of fibrinolysis is a commonly observed hemostatic abnormality associated with thrombosis. It may be due to a defective synthesis and/or release of t-PA from the vessel wall, to a deficiency or functional abnormality in the molecular interactions regulating plasminogen activation, or to increased levels of inhibitors of t-PA or of plasmin. On the other hand, excessive fibrinolysis due to increased levels of t-PA or to α_2-antiplasmin or PAI-1 deficiency may result in bleeding tendency (30, 31).

A. Plasminogen Activation by t-PA

1. At the Fibrin Surface

Although different kinetic constants have been reported for the activation of plasminogen by t-PA (11, 32–34), most authors agree that t-PA is a poor enzyme in the absence of fibrin, but that fibrin stimulates plasminogen activation by t-PA by at least two orders of magnitude. The kinetic data of Hoylaerts et al. (11) support a mechanism in which fibrin provides a surface to which t-PA and plasminogen adsorb in a sequential and ordered way yielding a cyclical ternary complex. Fibrin essentially increases the local plasminogen concentration by creating an additional interaction between t-PA and its substrate. The high affinity of t-PA for plasminogen in the presence of fibrin thus allows efficient activation on the fibrin clot, whereas plasminogen activation by t-PA in plasma is a comparatively inefficient process. Plasmin formed on the fibrin surface has both its lysine-binding sites and active site occupied and is thus only slowly inactivated by α_2-antiplasmin (half-life of about 10–100 sec); in contrast, free plasmin, when formed, is rapidly inhibited by α_2-antiplasmin (half-life of about 0.1 sec) (23).

Initial binding of t-PA to fibrin appears to be governed by the finger domain, and partial degradation of fibrin results in enhanced binding of t-PA via kringle 2 to newly exposed COOH-terminal lysine residues (35). Thus, early fibrin digestion by plasmin may accelerate fibrinolysis by increasing the binding of both t-PA (35) and plasminogen (36).

Binding studies (37, 38) as well as kinetic studies (39) have revealed that Lp(a) competes with plasminogen for binding to fibrin, as a result of binding of Lp(a) to fibrin via its lysine-binding domains. As for plasminogen, binding of Lp(a) to fibrin is enhanced by partial proteolytic degradation of the fibrin surface (37). As a functional consequence of the competition between Lp(a) and plasminogen for binding to fibrin, the fibrin-dependent enhancement of plasminogen activation by t-PA is inhibited (38, 39). Elevated levels of Lp(a), such as those seen in patients with atherosclerosis, might therefore impair physiological fibrinolysis (40).

2. *At the Endothelial Cell Surface*

Over the last years, a striking analogy between the role of fibrin and of cell surfaces in plasminogen activation has been recognized (41). Many cell types bind plasminogen activators and plasminogen, resulting in enhanced plasminogen activation (42–45) and protection of bound plasmin from inhibition by α_2-antiplasmin (46, 47). Gangliosides (48), as well as a class of membrane proteins with carboxyterminal lysine residues such as α-enolase (49), play an important role in binding of plasminogen to cells.

Several authors have demonstrated specific, saturable, reversible binding of t-PA to human umbilical vein endothelial cells (HUVEC) (42, 50). With ligand blot techniques a M_r 40,000 membrane protein has been identified that may represent the functional t-PA receptor (51). Cell-surface-bound t-PA retains it enzymatic activity and is protected from inhibition by PAI-1 (51). Assembly of plasminogen and t-PA at the endothelial cell surface thus provides a focal point for plasmin generation and may play an important role in maintaining blood fluidity and nonthrombogenicity.

Lipoprotein (a) binds to HUVEC with an affinity and binding capacity similar to those of plasminogen. Competition of Lp(a) with plasminogen for binding to endothelial cells results in strongly down-regulated activation of cell-surface-bound plasminogen by t-PA, suggesting that Lp(a) may play a role in the regulation of fibrinolysis at the endothelial cell surface (52).

B. Plasminogen Activation by u-PA

tcu-PA has no fibrin specificity and activates fibrin-bound and circulating plasminogen relatively indiscriminately. Extensive plasminogen activation and depletion of α_2-antiplasmin may occur following treatment of patients with thromboembolic disease with tcu-PA, leading to degradation of several plasma proteins, including fibrinogen, factor V, and factor VIII.

scu-PA, in contrast to tcu-PA, has a significant fibrin specificity. Several hypotheses for the mechanism of plasminogen activation and fibrin specificity of clot lysis with scu-PA in a plasma milieu have been proposed (14, 15, 53). Studies in human plasma in vitro have suggested that conversion of scu-PA to tcu-PA during clot lysis constitutes a primary positive feedback system, whereas binding of plasminogen to fibrin or predigestion of fibrin by plasmin was found to result in relatively minor additional acceleration of fibrinolysis (14). rscu-PA and tcu-PA also bind to cells (54), and conversion of single-chain to two-chain u-PA may occur at the cell surface (55). The main role of u-PA, however, is probably in proteolytic events in the basal membrane of cells, not in fibrinolysis in the circulation (56).

IV. EFFECTS OF HEPARIN ON FIBRINOLYSIS

An association between heparin and fibrinolysis was suggested for the first time in 1948 (57). Some investigators claimed that heparin had a direct effect on fibrinolysis, whereas others believed that it prevented thrombus growth through its anticoagulant properties and thereby facilitated clot lysis initiated by the endogenous fibrinolytic system. Later, it was reported by some investigators that administration of glycosaminoglycans, such as unfractionated heparin, low-molecular-weight heparin (LMWH), and pentosan polysulfate, to humans resulted in shortening of the euglobulin clot lysis time (58, 59), whereas other reports did not find a consistent effect of heparin on fibrinolysis (60, 61). More recently, the extensive use of heparin as an anticoagulant agent in the early phase of thrombolysis (2–6) has triggered renewed interest in its potential profibrinolytic properties. We will review the presently available information on the interaction(s) of heparin with the fibrinolytic system, as monitored in vitro, in animal models of thrombosis, and in patients with thromboembolic disease.

A. In Vitro

In vitro effects of heparin on the fibrinolytic system include direct effects on the efficiency of plasminogen activation by plasminogen activators as well as indirect effects, such as binding of heparin to components of the fibrinolytic system or effects of heparin on the synthesis and/or release of plasminogen activators and plasminogen activator inhibitors from endothelial cells.

1. Effect of Heparin on t-PA-Mediated Plasminogen Activation

In a buffer milieu, heparin binds stoichiometrically to t-PA, resulting in an enhancement of the catalytic efficiency of t-PA for plasminogen activation, mainly as a result of an enhanced affinity (62–68). This phenomenon may be explained by formation of a ternary complex between heparin, t-PA, and plasminogen. Binding of heparin to t-PA is mediated predominantly via the finger domain, although some binding of heparin to the second kringle domain of t-PA has been reported (68). Competition experiments have suggested that the binding sites for heparin on the t-PA A-chain are not identical to the fibrin-binding sites (65), although the enhancing effect of heparin on the catalytic efficiency of t-PA is not additive to that of fibrin or fibrin fragments (62–65). In addition, the t-PA-binding site on heparin appears to be different from the antithrombin III–binding site (67, 68).

There is apparently no consensus on whether this effect of heparin on the enzymatic activity of t-PA is also observed in blood or in plasma. Interaction of heparin with t-PA may indeed, on the one hand, enhance systemic activation of the fibrinolytic system in the absence of fibrin, as a result of enhanced plasminogen activation, and may, on the other hand, impair its fibrinolytic potency by decreasing the amount of t-PA available for binding to fibrin. Klauser (69) has reported that heparin at concentrations within the therapeutic range indeed enhances t-PA activity in plasma, whereas other in vitro studies, using whole blood, suggested that heparin either delayed the lysis of blood clots induced by recombinant t-PA (rt-PA) (70) or did not affect clot lysis (71). Furthermore, no effect of high concentrations of heparin was observed on fibrinogenolysis by high-dose rt-PA in the absence of fibrin (72). Fry and Sobel (71) showed that heparin, at therapeutic concentration, does not interfere with binding of t-PA to thrombi formed in whole blood, that it does not enhance plasminogen activation by t-PA in plasma, and that it does not affect clot lysis induced by t-PA in a plasma milieu. It has, however, been reported that therapeutic concentrations of heparin in plasma may modify fibrin polymerization, leading to the formation of clots that are more sensitive to lysis by t-PA (73). These contradictory results obtained with heparin in plasma may be explained to some extent by the presence and concentration of other heparin-binding proteins (see below).

Andrade-Gordon and Strickland (67) have reported that LMW heparin preparations, obtained by nitrous acid depolymerization or by heparinase treatment of standard heparin, do not stimulate plasminogen activation by t-PA but still efficiently enhance thrombin inhibition by antithrombin III. This was explained by the absence of binding of t-PA or native plasminogen to these heparin preparations. Furthermore, by affinity chromatography on insolubilized t-PA, a heparin fraction was isolated with low affinity for t-PA but efficient binding to antithrombin III (68). These findings suggest that it is possible to obtain heparin preparations with intact anticoagulant properties, but without profibrinolytic properties. On the other hand, following periodic oxidation of heparin, fractions have been isolated with greatly reduced anticoagulant activities, but unaffected or only slightly reduced profibrinolytic activities in vitro and ex vivo (74).

2. *Effect of Heparin on Other Fibrinolytic Components*

Several authors have reported that urokinase (62, 63, 75) also binds to heparin, resulting in an enhanced plasminogen-activating potential. The binding sites for urokinase and t-PA on heparin are probably different (67). In a buffer milieu, both unfractionated heparin and a LMWH fragment enhanced the plasminogen-activating potential of scu-PA in the absence of fibrin(ogen) fragments (75). However, neither heparin preparation strongly potentiated clot lysis induced by scu-PA in a plasma milieu in vitro, but apparently reduced fibrinogenolysis somewhat, as a result of a reduced generation of tcu-PA activity in the surrounding plasma (76). This is in apparent contradiction with the enhancing effect of heparin on the plasmin-mediated conversion of scu-PA to tcu-PA in a buffer milieu (77) and suggests a modulating role of heparin-binding proteins in plasma. The existence of a plasma factor with M_r approximately 80,000 that converts the single-chain forms of both t-PA and u-PA to their two-chain derivatives and enhances their amidolytic activities in the presence of LMW heparin has been suggested (78). The enzymatic activity of the plasminogen-streptokinase complex is not affected by heparin (62, 65).

Potential interactions of heparin with the fibrinolytic process have been suggested at several other levels. Thus, heparin enhances the inhibition rate of rt-PA by PAI-1 in a buffer milieu approximately fourfold, with a dissociation constant of 20 nM (79). Furthermore, Lp(a) competes with plasminogen for access to heparin-bound t-PA (80, 81) and prevents inhibition of t-PA by PAI-1 in the presence of heparin, without affecting the reaction in the absence of heparin (79). Heparin also strongly enhances the inhibition rate of plasmin and of the plasmin-streptokinase complex by antithrombin III (82).

The bioavailability of heparin in a human plasma milieu may be modulated by its binding to other plasma proteins. Heparin-binding proteins include antithrombin III (AT III), histidine-rich glycoprotein (HRG), heparin cofactor II, fibrinogen, albumin, fibronectin, lipoprotein lipase, α_1-acid glycoprotein, and platelet factor 4. HRG was shown to be an efficient competitor of AT III for the binding to heparin (83), and the affinity of heparin for HRG is higher than that for the other binding proteins, indicating that HRG may play a significant role in the modulation of both its anticoagulant and profibrinolytic properties in plasma (84). Vitronectin binds to complexes of thrombin with protease inhibitors, i.e., thrombin-AT III, thrombin-heparin cofactor II, and thrombin-protease nexin I, and these ternary complexes bind heparin via the vitronectin component, thus acting as heparin scavengers (85,86). In purified systems, vitronectin is an effective noncompetitive inhibitor of the inhibition of thrombin by AT III-heparin (87), but in a plasma milieu it has only a weak effect on heparin activity, possibly owing to a different (folded) conformation of vitronectin in plasma (88).

3. *Effect of Heparin on t-PA and PAI-1 Secretion from Endothelial Cells*

Several studies suggest that heparin may affect the synthesis and/or release of fibrinolytic components from endothelial cells. Thus, as early as 1977, Markwardt and Klocking (89) showed that perfusion of heparin in the isolated pig ear model increased plasminogen activator activity in a dose-dependent way, and this effect was later confirmed with LMWH fractions (59). This activity could also be demonstrated in animals (90) and in healthy volunteers (59), but conflicting results have been obtained in patients with thrombotic disease (91–93). More recently, it was reported that the t-PA-like activity induced by heparin and LMWH in rats binds to a thrombus, resulting in an enhanced fibrinolytic potential (94, 95). Also, dermatan sulfate was shown to induce release of t-PA activity in the perfused rat hindquarters (96).

The availability of specific methods for determination of t-PA and PAI-1 antigen, activity, and mRNA levels has allowed more detailed study of the effects of heparin on the fibrinolytic system, mainly using cultured endothelial cells (EC) in vitro. Thus, several authors have reported enhanced intracellular t-PA levels following addition of heparin or pentosan polysulfate to cell cultures such as rat epididymal fatpad capillary EC (97), bovine arterial EC (98), diploid human lung fibroblasts (99), and HUVEC (100, 101). In addition, several authors have reported a decreased secretion of PAI-1 upon addition of heparin to HUVEC (100, 102). Konkle and Ginsburg (100) showed that addition of endothelial cell growth factor (HBGF-1) and heparin to HUVEC induced a three-to 10-fold decrease of PAI-1 mRNA levels and of secreted PAI-1 activity. Studies in other cell types, such as human mesothelial cells derived from omentum, confirmed the stimulating effect of heparin and pentosan polysulphate on t-PA production, which was impaired in the presence of cycloheximide, but failed to demonstrate an effect on PAI-1 synthesis (103).

B. In Animal Models of Thrombosis

Over the last years, the effect of different heparin preparations on thrombolysis induced with plasminogen activators has been investigated in animal models (Table 2). Most studies report a stimulatory effect of unfractionated heparin on thrombolysis induced with the non-fibrin-specific agents streptokinase (104, 105) and tcu-PA (107), as well as with the more fibrin-specific agents t-PA (72, 106, 107, 111–113) and scu-PA (110). Other studies, however, have failed to demonstrate an enhancing effect of unfractionated heparin on thrombolysis induced with either t-PA (108, 109), scu-PA (108), or APSAC (72). LMW heparin fragments did potentiate the thrombolytic potency of t-PA and scu-PA in the rabbit jugular vein thrombosis model (108) and that of t-PA in the dog left anterior descending (LAD) coronary artery thrombosis model (111). In a randomized prospective study in a combined femoral arterial and venous thrombosis model in the dog, the concomitant use of intravenous heparin with rt-PA was found to accelerate arterial reperfusion and to enhance venous thrombolysis (114). Thus, a growing body of experimental evidence indicates that thrombolytic therapy with rt-PA requires concomitant adjunctive IV heparin for optimal efficacy.

Besides enhancing the efficacy of plasminogen activators, heparin may reduce the occurrence of reocclusion as a result of its anticoagulant properties. Agnelli et al. (115), however, reported that heparin was not efficient in preventing accretion of new fibrin on thrombi in the rabbit jugular vein thrombosis model, during and after treatment with t-PA. Several other studies have shown that conjunctive therapy with heparin or LMW heparin and t-PA results in sustained reflow and delayed reocclusion in a canine thrombosis model (113, 116), whereas in a rabbit arteriovenous shunt model heparin prevented platelet activation associ-

Table 2 Overview of Studies on the Effect of Heparin on Thrombolysis in Animal Models

Model	Thrombolytic agent	Heparin type	Observations	Ref.
Dog pulmonary embolism	Streptokinase	Unfractionated	Enhanced thrombolysis	104
Dog left circumflex coronary artery	Streptokinase	Unfractionated	Enhanced thrombolysis	105
Dog femoral artery	t-PA	Unfractionated	Enhanced thrombolysis	106
Dog LAD coronary artery	t-PA, tcu-PA	Unspecified	Enhanced thrombolysis	107
Rabbit jugular vein	t-PA, scu-PA	LMW heparin	Enhanced thrombolysis	108
		Unfractionated	No effect	108
Rabbit jugular vein	t-PA	Unfractionated	No effect	109
Guinea pig pulmonary embolism	t-PA	Unfractionated	Enhanced thrombolysis	72
	APSAC	Unfractionated	No effect	72
Rabbit femoral artery	scu-PA	Unfractionated	Enhanced thrombolysis	110
Dog LAD coronary artery	t-PA	Unfractionated	Enhanced thrombolysis	111
		LMW heparin	Enhanced thrombolysis	111
Rabbit arteriovenous shunt	t-PA	Unfractionated	Enhanced thrombolysis	112
Dog LAD coronary artery	t-PA	Unfractionated	Enhanced thrombolysis	113
Dog femoral vein and artery	t-PA	Unfractionated	Enhanced thrombolysis	114

LAD = left anterior descending.

ated with t-PA therapy (112). Also, with bolus injection of scu-PA in rabbits with femoral artery thrombosis, more persistent reperfusion was obtained with simultaneous anticoagulation with either heparin or with the thrombin inhibitor Argatroban (110).

In the canine LAD coronary artery thrombosis model (117), full heparinization did not completely prevent reocclusion after thrombolysis with t-PA, suggesting that the efficiency of heparin in this respect may be limited. In rabbits with arterial erythrocyte-rich thrombosis with superimposed endothelial damage and distal high-grade stenosis (118), with bolus administration of t-PA reflow was obtained more slowly with heparin than with Argatroban, and reocclusion after reflow was less frequent with Argatroban. This is consistent with the hypothesis that thrombin-mediated pathways of platelet activation play a significant role in the pathogenesis of arterial thrombosis (119). Also, in the prevention of occlusion in the rabbit femoral eversion graft model, heparin was inefficient compared to Argatroban (120). It is possible that in these models, heparin at much higher doses may also yield comparable results to Argatroban. It has indeed been found, in a rabbit jugular vein thrombosis model, that the efficacy of heparin as an adjunct to bolus t-PA is dose-dependent (121). In humans, such doses would, however, be outside the accepted therapeutic range, especially in association with thrombolytic therapy.

Other studies in animal models have suggested that heparin may enhance plasminogen activation or may increase release of t-PA from the vessel wall. Thus, in a rat inferior vena cava thrombosis model, administration of LMW heparin was found to reduce thrombus weight via a mechanism that was blocked by coadministration of ϵ-aminocaproic acid (122). Also, in the rabbit jugular vein thrombosis model, both ϵ-aminocaproic acid and aprotinin reversed the enhancement of thrombolysis induced by LMW heparin (59). Fareed et al. have reported that LWMH enhances endogenous fibrinolysis in a primate model by stimulating t-PA release (123).

Although somewhat conflicting and variable results have been obtained in different animal models, heparin is now used extensively in combination with thrombolytic therapy in patients with thromboembolic disease (see below).

C. Patients with Thromboembolic Disease

1. Without Thrombolytic Therapy

Several early studies have evaluated the effect of unfractionated heparin or LMWH on the components of the fibrinolytic system, both in healthy volunteers and in patients with thromboembolic disease (124–130). Variable, even contradictory, results reported in these studies may have been due to the use of heparin preparations of different origin and composition, administered via differing routes and with varying regimens with respect to both dose and duration of treatment.

Furthermore, in the earlier studies no specific assays for t-PA or PAI-1 antigen and/or activity were available, and the significant diurnal fluctuations of t-PA and PAI-1 levels, which go in opposite directions (131), had not yet been recognized. It has indeed been suggested that the increased fibrinolytic activity (measured by euglobulin clot lysis time) during the day, following a subcutaneous injection of unfractionated heparin or LMWH in healthy volunteers, may reflect only the circadian physiological fluctuation of fibrinolysis (132, 133). Therefore, it is difficult to compare results obtained in different studies in a valid way.

The results of more recent studies are summarized in Table 3 (134–142). Most studies agree that no significant effects on fibrinolysis are observed with either unfractionated or LMWH when the normal diurnal fluctuations of both t-PA and PAI-1 are accounted for. After total or elective hip replacement or surgery, elevated PAI-1 levels have been observed in patients receiving heparin (138–140), but this may be due to an acute-phase reaction (143). Increased t-PA activity after heparin administration in volunteers (135) and increased t-PA antigen in unstable angina (142) or in a general patient population (144) treated with heparin have also been reported. In none of these studies with administration of unfractionated or LMWH for up to 7 days have changes in fibrinogen, plasminogen, or α_2-antiplasmin levels been reported (135,142).

In an elderly population, a marked increase in t-PA antigen and in t-PA/PAI-1 complex was found after 30–60 days of treatment with standard heparin, but not with LMWH. This difference remained unexplained, but was observed both before and after venous occlusion (145). An enhanced response of t-PA antigen and activity to venous occlusion under heparin treatment was reported previously, for unfractionated (146) but also for LMWH (147). Agnelli et al. (148) reported an additive effect of DDAVP and standard heparin on the increase in circulating t-PA, the effect of DDAVP being potentiated and prolonged by heparin.

In conclusion, few conclusive data are available on the direct effects of heparin on fibrinolysis in patients. Small changes in t-PA or PAI-1 levels may be obscured by their large diurnal variations, but clearly no other fibrinolytic parameters are affected by heparin. Therefore, the beneficial effect of heparin, in the absence of thrombolytic therapy, appears to result mainly from its anticoagulant properties. This is probably also true for other glycosaminoglycans such as dermatan sulfate, which was found to have only a negligible effect on fibrinolysis in volunteers (149). In contrast, two studies have reported enhanced fibrinolysis after administration of pentosan polysulfate, measured either by euglobulin clot lysis time or by t-PA activity determination (150, 151).

2. *With Thrombolytic Therapy*

In the prethrombolytic era, numerous studies showed that subcutaneous administration of heparin to patients with acute myocardial infarction (AMI) reduces

Table 3 Overview of Some Studies on the Effect of Heparin on Fibrinolysis in Humans in the Absence of Thrombolytic Therapy

Condition	Heparin: Origin	Administration	Dose	Duration	Observations	Ref.
Volunteers	UH, porcine mucosa	s.c. bolus	5000 IU	1 bolus at 9 A.M.	Changes in t-PA and PAI-1 activity within diurnal range	134
	LMWH (Fragmin)	s.c. bolus	5000 anti-Xa U	1 bolus at 9 A.M.		
Volunteers	UH, porcine mucosa	i.v. bolus	5000 IU	1 bolus at 8 A.M.	Increased t-PA activity 1 hr after injection with UH and 10,000 anti-Xa U LMW; no effect on PAI-1 activity	135
	LMWH (Fragmin)	i.v. bolus	5000 or 10,000	1 bolus at 8 A.M.		
DVT	LMWH (CY222)	3 injections daily	2–4 mg/kg daily	7 days	No changes in t-PA or PAI-1 antigen	136
DVT	LMWH (CY222)	2 s.c. injections daily	750 U/kg daily	10 days	No fibrinolytic activity as monitored by measurement of FDP levels	137
	UH	2 s.c. injections daily	500 IU/kg daily	10 days		
Hip replacement	LMWH (Logiparin)	s.c. bolus	50 anti-Xa U per kg	7 days at 8 A.M.	No change in t-PA antigen or activity	138
Hip replacement	LMWH (Fragmin)	1 s.c. bolus	5000 U daily	10 days	No difference in t-PA or PAI-1 antigen or activity between LMWH and UH	139
	UH	3 s.c. injections	5000 U daily	10 days		
Hysterectomy	LMWH	s.c. injection	1500 APTT U daily	8 days, A.M.	No effect on fibrinolytic activity	140
	UH	s.c. injection	5000 IU per 12 hr	8 days, A.M.		
Hip arthroplasty	LMWH (Enoxaparin)	s.c. bolus	±4000 anti-Xa U daily	8 days	No correlation between t-PA antigen levels and development of DVT	141
Unstable angina	UH	3 s.c. injections daily	30,000 U daily	3 days	Increased t-PA antigen levels; no effect on PAI-1 activity	142

UH = unfractionated heparin; s.c. = subcutaneous; i.v. = intravenous; IU = international units; DVT = deep vein thrombosis; FDP = fibrin degradation products.

mortality. MacMahon et al. (152) have reviewed 20 of these clinical trials and concluded that patients allocated to heparin (5700 patients analyzed) had a 17% lower odds of death versus control, a 22% lower odds of reinfarction, and a 50% lower odds of stroke. In these studies 20,000 U or more of heparin was administered daily in 90% of the patients, with subcutaneous administration in about half of them. The route of administration, subcutaneous versus intravenous, therefore probably has no effect on the outcome. It is well established that heparin therapy alone is associated with a significant reduction of left ventricular thrombosis, stroke, deep vein thrombosis, pulmonary embolism, reinfarction, and death in patients with AMI (153-155).

During recent years, thrombolytic therapy has become the treatment of choice for patients with AMI. Although the clinical benefit of thrombolytic therapy is well established, the optimal thrombolytic regimen, in terms both of thrombolytic agent and of conjunctive anticoagulant and/or antiplatelet agents, has not yet been determined. The effect of the conjunctive use of heparin in combination with rt-PA on coronary artery recanalization has been intensively investigated. The rationale for this approach is the assumption that, because of the short plasma half-life and the fibrinogen-sparing properties of rt-PA, patients may be very susceptible to reocclusion if adequate anticoagulation is not maintained.

The potential role of intravenous heparin given concomitantly with streptokinase or alteplase (recombinant t-PA, rt-PA) therapy had earlier been suggested with the demonstration of fibrinopeptide A (FPA) generation during infusion of thrombolytic agents (156–158) and its rapid decrease following anticoagulation (158, 159). Persistently high or reincreasing FPA plasma levels despite anticoagulation might correlate with coronary artery reocclusion after administration of alteplase (158) or streptokinase (156). Eisenberg et al. (160) have shown that the increase in thrombin activity in patients with AMI treated with alteplase is at least in part due to enhanced activation of prothrombin by factor Xa.

Table 4 summarizes the results obtained in some recent studies on the influence of heparin on coronary patency after treatment of patients with AMI with alteplase. Whereas Topol et al. (2) found no effect of heparin on patency at 90 min, other studies showed that omission of heparin markedly reduced patency rates measured at 7–24 hr (3), 48–72 hr (4), or 48–120 hr (5). Taken together, these studies suggest that concomitant intravenous heparin improves coronary patency in patients with AMI treated with alteplase. Rapold et al. (161) recently confirmed that enhanced fibrin generation during and after thrombolytic therapy with alteplase in patients with AMI is suppressed by sustained concomitant anticoagulation with intravenous heparin. High plasma FPA levels 24 hr after alteplase therapy were shown to be specific, but insensitive, markers of vessel occlusion in anticoagulated patients, but did not correlate with clinical outcome, i.e., recurrent ischemia or left ventricular thrombosis. These authors

Table 4 Influence of Heparin on Coronary Patency in Patients with Acute Myocardial Infarction Treated with Alteplase

End-point	Without heparin	With heparin	p	Ref.
90 min	79 (54/68)	79 (50/63)	0.83	2
7–14 hr	62 (48/93)	82 (82/100)	<0.001	3
48–72 hr	43 (18/42)	71 (30/42)	0.015	4
48–120 hr	74 (181/244)	83 (214/258)	0.022	5

The data represent percentage values, with absolute numbers given in parentheses.

suggested that adequate anticoagulation warrants individual titration of the heparin dose. In two other studies, a correlation was found between the efficiency of heparinization and patency of the infarct-related coronary artery after treatment of AMI with alteplase (162, 163). Importantly, excessive anticoagulation did not appear to increase the hemorrhagic risk, except that access site-related hemorrhage was more frequent in well-anticoagulated patients (163). These studies thus confirm that patients treated with alteplase require concomitant adequate anticoagulation with heparin to sustain coronary patency. Whether this early, sustained patency will translate into a reduced mortality remains to be confirmed by large prospective studies. For streptokinase, unfortunately, very few data are available on the effect of heparin anticoagulation in patients with AMI (164). The Global Utilization of Streptokianse and t-PA for Occluded Coronary Arteries (GUSTO) trial may help to clarify this issue (165).

Of particular concern with the conjunctive use of heparin and thrombolytic agents is the occurrence of stroke (7, 166). A consistent finding of the GISSI-2 (167) and ISIS-3 (168) studies has been a significantly greater risk of stroke in patients with AMI treated with alteplase, compared to streptokinase. A meta-analysis of the combined data of both studies (169) suggested that this excess of stroke incidence was primarily due to an increased incidence of intracranial hemorrhage associated with the use of fibrin-selective thrombolytic agents. Sobel and Collen (166), however, questioned the value of this meta-analysis because the nature of stroke was qualitatively different in both megatrials and because the confidence intervals surrounding the means of the incidence of hemorrhagic stroke did not overlap. These authors suggest that the increased incidence of ischemic stroke seen with t-PA in GISSI-2 may be explained by the unopposed procoagulant effect (absence of i.v. heparin), which is more pronounced for the fibrin-selective agent (alteplase) than for streptokinase. The increased incidence of hemorrhagic stroke seen with t-PA in the ISIS-3 study, on the other hand, may have been due to the administration of large amounts of plasminogen activator activity with the t-PA (duteplase) regimen used (166). It was suggested that in the t-PA-treated patients, procoagulant effects would be less prominent under conditions in which subcutaneous heparin would be used, rather than excluded.

Interestingly, in a recent study (170), it was shown that 100 mg alteplase can be given within the first 6 hr of acute cerebral artery stroke together with heparin, with acceptable safety (<10% deleterious hemorrhage).

V. CONCLUSIONS AND PERSPECTIVES

Heparin may directly influence fibrinolysis via different mechanisms, including induction of t-PA release from vascular endothelial cells or binding to t-PA with enhancement of its catalytic efficiency for plasminogen activation. In patients, however, the beneficial effect of heparin appears to be mediated primarily via its anticoagulant properties, preventing accretion of new febrin on a thrombus and thus facilitating fibrinolysis. Data from several large clinical trials in patients with AMI suggest that optimal thrombolytic therapy with alteplase (recombinant t-PA) requires concomitant adequate anticoagulation with heparin. Less data are available for streptokinase.

However, the efficacy of heparin, and aspirin, to accelerate coronary thrombolysis, to overcome resistance to lysis, and to prevent reocclusion seems to be limited. Even with the concomitant administration of heparin and aspirin, thrombolytic therapy does not produce maximal stable coronary artery recanalization in patients with evolving myocardial infarction. Improved thrombolytic strategies may require the conjunctive use of more potent and more selective antiplatelet and anticoagulant agents with plasminogen activators (171). Such approaches include the use of thromboxane synthase inhibitors, antagonists of the serotonin or endoperoxide receptors, platelet glycoprotein IIb/IIIa receptor blocking agents, and selective thrombin inhibitors. The bleeding risk associated with such combinations will, however, need to be explored in more detail.

REFERENCES

1. Collen D. Thromb Haemost 1980; 43:77.
2. Topol EJ, George BS, Kereiakes DJ, Stump DC, Candela RJ, Abbottsmith CW, Aronson L, Pickel A, Boswick JM, Lee KL, Ellis SG, Califf RM, and TAMI Study Group. Circulation 1989; 79:281.
3. Hsia J, Hamilton WP, Kleiman N, Roberts R, Chaitman BR, Ross AM, for the Heparin-Aspirin Reperfusion Trial (HART) Investigators. N Engl J Med 1990; 323:1433.
4. Bleich SD, Nichols TC, Schumacher RR, Cooke DH, Tate DA, Teichman SL. Am J Cardiol 1990; 66:1412.
5. de Bono DP, Simoons ML, Tijssen J, Arnold AER, Betriu A, Burgersdijk C, Lopez Bescos L, Mueller E, Pfisterer M, Van de Werf F, Zijlstra F, Verstraete M, for the European Cooperative Study Group. Br Heart J 1992; 67:122.

6. The SCATI (Studio sulla Calciparina nell'Angina e nella Trombosi Ventricolare nell'Infarcto) Group. Lancet 1989; 2:182.
7. Sobel BE, Collen D. Am J Cardiol 1992; 70:385.
8. Sottrup-Jensen L, Petersen TE, Magnusson S. In: Dayhoff MO, ed. Atlas of Protein Sequence and Structure, Vol 5, Suppl 3. Washington, DC: National Biomedical Research Foundation, 1978:91.
9. Forsgren M, Raden B, Israelsson M, Larsson K, Heden LO. FEBS Lett 1987; 213:254.
10. Pennica D, Holmes WE, Kohr WJ, Harkins RN, Vehar GA, Ward CA, Bennett WF, Yelverton E, Seeburg PH, Heyneker HL, Goeddel DV, Collen D. Nature 1983; 301:214.
11. Hoylaerts M, Rijken DC, Lijnen HR, Collen D. J Biol Chem 1982; 257:2912.
12. Holmes WE, Pennica D, Blaber M, Rey MW, Guenzler WA, Steffens GJ, Heyneker HL. Biotechnology 1985; 3:923.
13. Günzler WA, Steffens GJ, Ötting F, Buse CT, Flohé L. Hoppe-Seyler's Z Physiol Chem 1982; 363:133.
14. Lijnen HR, Van Hoef B, De Cock F, Collen D. Blood 1989; 73:1864.
15. Husain SS. Biochemistry 1991; 30:5797.
16. Manchanda N, Schwartz BS. J Biol Chem 1991; 266:14580.
17. Jackson KW, Tang J. Biochemistry 1982; 21:6620.
18. Reddy KNN, Kline DL, Reddy KNN, eds. In: Fibrinolysis CRC Press, Boca Raton, FL: 1980:71.
19. Smith RAG, Dupe DJ, English PD, Green J. Nature 1981; 290:505.
20. Staniforth DH, Smith RAG, Hibbs M. Eur J Clin Pharmacol 1983; 24:751.
21. Holmes WE, Nelles L, Lijnen HR, Collen D. J Biol Chem 1987; 262:1659.
22. Ichinose A, Tamaki T, Aoki N. FEBS Lett 1983; 153:369.
23. Wiman B, Collen D. Eur J Biochem 1978; 84:573.
24. Kruithof EKO. Enzyme 1988; 40:113.
25. Ny T, Sawdey M, Lawrence D, Millan JL, Loskutoff DJ. Proc Natl Acad Sci USA 1986; 83:6776.
26. Pannekoek H, Veerman H, Lambers H, Diergaarde P, Verweij CL, van Zonneveld AJ, van Mourik JA. EMBO J 1986; 5:2539.
27. Kruithof EKO, Tran-Thang C, Ransijn A, Bachmann F. Blood 1984; 64:907.
28. Juhan-Vague I, Moerman B, De Cock F, Aillaud MF, Collen D. Thromb Res 1984; 33:523.
29. Declerck PJ, De Mol M, Alessi MC, Baudner S, Pâques EP, Preissner KT, Müller-Berghaus G, Collen D. J Biol Chem 1988; 263:15454.
30. Wiman B, Hamsten A. Semin Thromb Haemost 1990; 16:207.
31. Lijnen HR, Collen D. Fibrinolysis 1989; 3:67.
32. Takada A, Sugawara Y. Takada Y. Haemostasis 1988; 18:117.
33. Nieuwenhuizen W, Voskuilen M, Vermond A, Hoegee-de Nobel B, Traas DW, Eur J Biochem 1988; 174:163.
34. Ranby M. Biochim Biophys Acta 1982; 704:461.
35. van Zonneveld AJ, Veerman H, Pannekoek H. J Biol Chem 1986; 261:14214.
36. Suenson E, Lützen O, Thorsen S. Eur J Biochem 1984; 140:513.
37. Harpel PC, Gordon BR, Parker TS. Proc Natl Acad Sci USA 1989; 86:3847.
38. Loscalzo J, Weinfeld M Fless GM, Sxanu AM. Atherosclerosis 1990; 10:240.

39. Edelberg JM, Gonzales-Gronow M, Pizzo SV. Thromb Res 1990; 57:155.
40. Edelberg JM, Pizzo SV. Fibrinolysis 1991; 5:135.
41. Plow EF, Felez J, Miles LA. Thromb Haemost 1991; 66:32.
42. Hajjar KA, Hamel NM, Harpel PC, Nachman RL. J Clin Invest 1987; 80:1712.
43. Hajjar KA, Harpel PC, Jaffe EA, Nachman RL. J Biol Chem 1986; 261:11656.
44. Miles LA, Plow EF. J Biol Chem 1985; 260:4303.
45. Stephens RW, Pöllänen J, Tapiovaara H, Leung KC, Sim PS, Salonen EM, Ronne E, Behrendt N, Danø K, Vaheri A. J Cell Biol 1989; 108:1987.
46. Miles LA, Plow EF. Fibrinolysis 1988; 2:61.
47. Plow EF, Freaney DE, Plescia J, Miles LA. J Cell Biol 1986; 103:2411.
48. Miles LA, Dahlberg CM, Levin EG, Plow EF. Biochemistry 1989; 28:9337.
49. Miles LA, Dahlberg CM, Plescia J, Felez J, Kato K, Plow EF. Biochemistry 1991; 30:1682.
50. Barnathan ES, Kuo A, Van der Keyl H, McCrae KR, Larsen GR, Cines DB. J Biol Chem 1988; 263:7792.
51. Hajjar KA, Hamel NM. J Biol Chem 1990; 265:2908.
52. Nachman RL. Hajjar KA. Ann NY Acad Sci 1991; 614:240.
53. Pannell R, Gurewich V. Blood 1986; 67:1215.
54. Blasi F. Fibrinolysis 1988; 2:73.
55. Ellis V, Scully MF, Kakkar VV. J Biol Chem 1989; 264:2185.
56. Van Hinsbergh VWM, Kooistra T, Emeis JJ, Koolwijk P. Int J Radiat Biol 1991; 60:261.
57. Halse T. Fibrinolyse. Eine experimentelle und klinische Studie uber die 4. Phase der Blutgerinnung. Hamburg: Editio Cantor GmbH, 1948.
58. Fischer A-M, Merton RE, Marsh NA, Williams S, Gaffney PJ, Barrowcliffe TW, Thomas DP. Thromb Haemost 1982; 47:109.
59. Vairel EG, Brouty-Boye H, Toulemonde F, Doutremepuich C, Marsh NA, Gaffney PJ. Thromb Res 1983; 30:219.
60. Bergqvist D, Nilsson IM. Thromb Res 1981; 23:309.
61. Greaves M, Preston FE, Kluft C, Bertina RM, Malia RG, Simms M. In: Davidson JF, Donati MB, Coccheri S, eds. Progress in Fibrinolysis, Vol 7. Edinburgh: Churchill Livingstone, 1985:105.
62. Andrade-Gordon P, Strickland S. Biochemistry 1986; 25:4033.
63. Pâques E-P, Stöhr H-A, Heimburger N. Thromb Res 1986; 42:797.
64. Soeda S, Kakiki M, Shimeno H, Nagamatsu A. Biochim Biophys Acta 1987; 916:279.
65. Fears R. Biochem J 1988; 249:77.
66. Stein PL, van Zonneveld A-J, Pannekoek H, Strickland S. J Biol Chem 1989; 264:15441.
67. Andrade-Gordon P, Strickland S. J Biol Chem 1989; 264:15177.
68. Andrade-Gordon P, Strickland S. Proc Natl Acad Sci USA 1990; 87:1865.
69. Klauser RJ. Thromb Haemost 1988; 60:324.
70. Görög P, Ridler CD, Kovacs IB. J Intern Med 1990; 227:125.
71. Fry ETA, Sobel BE. Blood 1988; 71:1347.
72. Fears R, Esmail AF, Greenwood HC. Semin Thromb Hemost 1991; 17:389.
73. Nenci GG, Parise P, Morini M, Rossini A, Agnelli G. Blood Coag Fibrinol 1992; 3:279.

74. Porta R, Pescador R, Niada R, Diamantini G, Fedeli GF, Mantovani M, Prino G. Thromb Res 1989; 53:435.
75. Dosne AM, Bendetowicz AV, Kher A, Samama M. Thromb Res 1988; 51:627.
76. Lourenço DM, Dosne AM, Kher A, Samama M. Thromb Haemost 1989; 62:923.
77. Lijnen HR, Collen D. Thromb Res 1986; 43:687.
78. Okada K, Fukao H, Tanaka H, Ueshima S, Matsuo O. Thromb Res 1990; (Suppl X):27.
79. Edelberg JM, Reilly CF, Pizzo SV. J Biol Chem 1991; 266:7488.
80. Edelberg JM, Pizzo SV. Biochemistry 1990; 29:5906.
81. Loscalzo J, Weinfeld M, Fless GM, Scanu AM. Arteriosclerosis 1990; 10:240.
82. Anonick PK, Wolf BB, Gonias SL. Thromb Res 1990; 59:449.
83. Lijnen HR, Hoylaerts M, Collen D. J Biol Chem 1983; 258:3803.
84. Lijnen HR, Collen D. Ann NY Acad Sci 1989; 556:181.
85. Tomasini B, Mosher DF. Blood 1988; 72:903.
86. Preissner KT, Zwicker L, Müller-Berghaus G. Biochem J 1987; 243:105.
87. Preissner KT, Müller-Berghaus G. J Biol Chem 1987; 262:12247.
88. Preissner KT, Jenne D. Thromb Haemost 1991; 66:189.
89. Markwardt F, Klocking HP. Haemostasis 1977; 6:370.
90. Vairel EG, Brouty-Boye H, Toulemonde F, Doutremepuich C. Ann Pharmaceut Fses 1983; 41:339.
91. Tobelem G, Molho P, Dunn P, Barzu T, Soria C, Soria J, Dupuy E, Toulemonde F. Haemostasis 1984; 14 (abstract 220).
92. Melissari E, Scully M, Paes T, Kakkar VV. In: Davidson JF, Donati MB, Coccheri S. eds. Progress in Fibrinolysis, Vol 7. Edinburgh: Churchill Livingstone, 1985:310.
93. Faivre R, Fareed J, Neuhart E, Kieffer Y, Petiteau P, Toulemonde F, Bassand JP, Maurat JP. Fibrinolysis 1986; 1:352 (abstract).
94. Doutremepuich C, Toulemonde F, Doutremepuich F, de Sèze O, Bayrou B, Pereira F. Thromb Res 1988; 50:335.
95. Doutremepuich C, Deharo E, Doutremepuich F, Lalanne MC, Toulemonde F. Thromb Res 1989; 53:615.
96. Abbadini M, Zhu GJ, Maggi A, Pangrazzi J, Donati MB, Mussoni L. Blood 1987; 70:1858.
97. Castellot JJ, Kambe AM, Dobson DE, Spiegelman BM. J Cell Physiol 1986; 127:323.
98. Delvos U, Paul JE, Müller-Berghaus G. Blut 1985; 51:127.
99. Rappaport RS, Ronchetti-Blume M, Vogel RL, Hung PP. Thromb Haemost 1988; 59:514.
100. Konkle BA, Ginsburg D. J Clin Invest 1988; 82:579.
101. Chanquia CJ, Fontcuberta J, Fabra A, Ruttlant M. Fibrinolysis 1988; 2(Suppl 1):59 (abstract 134).
102. Chesterman CN, Marsh NA, Minter AJ. J Physiol 1990; 423:84P.
103. Grulich-Henn J, Preissner KT, Müller-Berghaus G. Thromb Haemost 1990; 64:420.
104. Cade JF, Hirsh J, Regoeczi E, Gent M, Buchanan MR, Hynes DM. J Clin Invest 1974; 54:782.
105. Schumacher WA, Lee EC, Lucchesi BR. J Cardiovasc Pharmacol 1985; 7:739.
106. Cercek B, Lew AS, Hod H, Yano J, Reddy KNN, Ganz W. Circulation 1986; 74:583.

107. Susawa T, Yui Y, Hattori R, Takahashi M, Aoyama T, Takatsu Y, Sakaguchi K, Yui N, Kawai C. Jpn Circ J, 1987; 51:431.
108. Stassen JM, Juhan-Vague I, Alessi MC, De Cock F, Collen D. Thromb Haemost 1987; 58:947.
109. Agnelli G, Pascucci C, Cosmi B, Nenci GG. Blood 1990; 76:2030.
110. Schneider J. Thromb Res 1991; 64:677.
111. Mestre M, Uzan A, Sedivy P, Cavero I. Thromb Res 1992; 66:191.
112. Rudd MA, George D, Johnstone MT, Moore RT, Collins L, Rabbani LE, Loscalzo J. Circ Res 1992; 70:829.
113. Yao SK, McNatt J, Anderson HV, Eidt J, Cui K, Golino P, Glas-Greenwalt P, Maraganore J, Buja LM, Willerson JT. Am J Physiol 1992; 262:H374.
114. Rapold H-J, Lu HR, Wu Z, Nijs H, Collen D. Blood 1991; 77:1020.
115. Agnelli G, Pascucci C, Cosmi B, Nenci GG. Thromb Haemost 1991; 66:592.
116. Nicolini FA, Nichols WW, Saldeen TGP, Khan S, Mehta JL. Am Heart J 1992; 124:280.
117. Yasuda T, Gold HK, Fallon JT, Leinbach RC, Guerrero L, Scudder LS, Kanke M, Shealy D, Ross MJ, Collen D, Coller BS. J Clin Invest 1988; 81:1284.
118. Jang IK, Gold HK, Leinbach RC, Fallon JT, Collen D. Circ Res 1990; 67: 1552.
119. Fuster V, Badimon L, Cohen M, Ambrose JA, Badimon JJ, Chesebro J. Circulation 1988; 77:1213.
120. Jang IK, Gold HK, Ziskind AA, Leinbach RC, Fallon JT, Collen D. Circulation 1990; 81:219.
121. Agnelli G, Parise P. Chest 1992; 101:172S.
122. Doutremepuich C, Gestreau JL, Kuttler MC, Masse A, Bousquet F, Toulemonde F, Vairel EG, Guilichini R. In: Davidson JF, Donati MB, Coccheri S, eds. Progress in Fibrinolysis, Vol 7. Edinburgh: Churchill Livingstone, 1985:303.
123. Fareed J, Walenga JM, Hoppensteadt DA, Messmore HL. Semin Thromb Hemost 1985; 11:199.
124. Fischer A-M, Merton RE, Marsh NA, Williams S, Gaffney PJ, Barrowcliffe TW, Thomas DP. Thromb Haemost 1982; 47:109.
125. Vinazzer H, Woler M. Thromb Res 1985; 40:135.
126. Fareed J, Walenga M, Hoppensteadt A, Messore L. In: Davidson JF, Donati MB, Coccheri S, eds. Progress in Fibrinolysis, Vol 7. Edinburgh: Churchill Livingstone, 1985:356.
127. Schulman S, Granqvist S, Wiman B, Lockner D. Thromb Res 1985; 39:607.
128. Melissari E, Scully MF, Paes T, Kakkar VV. Thromb Res 1985; 37:115.
129. Fareed J, Walenga JM, Hoppensteadt DA, Emanuele RM. Haemostasis 1986; 16:123.
130. Arnesen H, Engebretsen LF, Ugland OM, Seljeflot I, Kierulf P. Thromb Res 1987; 45:553.
131. Kluft C, Jie AFH, Rijken DC, Verheijen JH. Thromb Haemost 1988; 59:329.
132. Neerstrand H, Østergaard P, Bergqvist D, Mätzsch T, Hedner U. Fibrinolysis 1987; 1:39.
133. Grimaudo V, Omri A, Kruithof EKO, Hauert J, Bachmann F. Thromb Haemost 1988; 59:388.

134. Eriksson E, Wollter IM, Christenson B, Stigendal L, Risberg B. Thromb Haemost 1988; 59:284.
135. Agnelli G, Borm J, Cosmi B, Levi M, ten Cate JW. Thromb Haemost, 1988; 60:311.
136. Juhan-Vague I, Stassen JM, Alessi MC, Elias A, Aillaud MF, Serradimigni A, Collen D. Semin Thromb Hemost 1989; 15:390.
137. Faivre R, Neuhart E, Mirshahi M, Mirshahi M, Soria C, Soria J, Bassand JP, Caen JP, Maurat JP. Semin Thromb Hemost 1989; 15:435.
138. Sørensen JV, Borris LC, Lassen MR, Christiansen HM, Schøtt P, Olsen AD, Neerstrand HS. Thromb Res 1990; 59:131.
139. Eriksson BI, Eriksson E, Risberg B. Thromb Res 1991; 62:55.
140. Bounameaux H, Lijnen HR, Hellemans H, Verstraete M. Thromb Haemost 1986; 55:298.
141. Borris LC, Sørensen JV, Lassen MR, Walenga JM, Fareed J, Jørgensen LN, Hauch O, Wille-Jørgensen P. Thromb Res 1991; 63:21.
142. Huber K, Resch I, Rosc D, Probst P, Kaindl F, Binder BR. Thromb Res 1989; 55:779.
143. Kluft C, Verheijen JH, Jie AF, Rijken DC, Preston FE, Sue-Ling HM, Jespersen J, Aasen AO. Scand J Clin Lab Invest 1985; 45:605.
144. Klein P. Thromb Res 1989; 56:649.
145. Vergnes C, Manciet G, Bourdenx V, Roudaut MF, Lacombe F, Boisseau MR. Thromb Res 1991; 63:521.
146. Arnesen H, Engebretsen LF, Ugland OM, Seljeflot I, Kierulf P. Thromb Res 1987; 45:553.
147. Molho PM, Dunn FW, Barzu TL, Soria C, Soria J, Dupuy E, Tobelem GM. In: Davidson JF, Donati MB, Coccheri S, eds. Progress in Fibrinolysis, Vol 7. Edinburgh: Churchill Livingstone, 1985:307.
148. Agnelli G, Levi M, Cosmi B, ten Cate JW, Nenci GG. Thromb Haemost 1989; 61:507.
149. Tripodi A, Moia M, Bottasso B, Tenconi PM, Gianese F, Mannucci PM. Thromb Res 1991; 62:663.
150. Vinazzer H. Semin Thromb Hemost 1991; 17:375.
151. Losonczy H, David M, Nagy I. Semin Thromb Hemost 1991; 17:394.
152. MacMahon S, Collins R, Knight C, Yusuf S, Peto R. Circulation 1988; 78:II-98 (abstract).
153. Neri Serneri GG, Gensini GF, Carnovali M, Rovelli F, Pirelli S, Fortini A. Lancet 1987; 1:937.
154. Turpie AGG, Robinson JG, Doyle DJ, Mulji AS, Mishkel GJ, Sealey BJ, Cairius JA, Skingley L, Hirsh J, Gent M. N Engl J Med 1989; 320:352.
155. The SCATI Group. Lancet 1989; 2:182.
156. Eisenberg PR, Sherman LA, Jaffe AS. J Am Coll Cardiol 1987; 10:527.
157. Owen J, Friedman KD, Grossman BA, Wilkins C, Berke AD, Powers ER. Blood 1988; 72:616.
158. Rapold HJ, Kuemmerli H, Weiss M, Baur H, Haeberli A. Circulation 1989; 79:980.
159. Rapold HJ. Lancet 1990; 1:481.
160. Eisenberg PR, Sobel BE, Jaffe AS. J Am Coll Cardiol 1992; 19:1065.

161. Rapold HJ, de Bono D, Arnold AER, Arnout J, De Cock F, Collen D, Verstraete M, for the European Cooperative Study Group. Circulation 1992; 85:928.
162. Arnout J, Simoons M, de Bono D, Rapold HJ, Collen D, Verstraete M. J Am Coll Cardiol 1992; 20:513.
163. Hsia J, Kleiman N, Aguirre F, Chaitman BR, Roberts R, Ross AM, for the HART Investigators. J Am Coll Cardiol 1992; 20:31.
164. Col JJ, Col-De Beys CM, Renkin JP, Lavenne-Pardonge EM, Bachy JL, Moriau MH. Am J Cardiol 1989; 63:1185.
165. Global Utilization of Streptokinase and t-PA for Occluded Coronary Arteries (GUSTO) Study Protocol, March 21, 1991.
166. Sobel BE, Collen D. Am J Cardiol 1993; 71:424.
167. The International Study Group. Lancet 1990; 336:71.
168. ISIS-3 (Third International Study Group of Infarct Survival) Collaborative Group. Lancet 1992; 339:753.
169. Collins R, Peto R, Parish S, Sleight P. Lancet 1992; 339:1226.
170. von Kümmer R, Hacke W. Stroke 1992; 23:646.
171. Gold HK. N Engl J Med 1990; 323:1483.

8

Low-Molecular-Weight Heparins for Prevention of Venous Thromboembolism Following General Surgery

David Bergqvist
University Hospital, Uppsala, Sweden

I. INTRODUCTION

Prevention of postoperative venous thromboembolism is now well established although the principles and methods vary considerably (1). Use of low-dose standard unfractionated heparin (UFH) has been predominant worldwide since the mid-1970s, and it is indeed effective (2). In many hospitals this prophylactic modality is now replaced by low-molecular-weight heparins (LMWH) (3), and the number of publications analyzing their effects in various situations is rapidly increasing. In the early studies based on in vitro data and animal experiments, it was hoped that thromboprophylaxis might be possible without influencing hemostasis with increased bleeding risk. This hope was not totally realized, and the remaining clinical advantages with LMWHs are better bioavailability and longer biological half-life after subcutaneous injection, less interaction with platelets, and less influence on lipolysis. The immediate clinical application of this would be the need for less frequent injections than with UFH, which is given 2–3 times daily. Thromboprophylaxis with LMWHs has already been reviewed many times (4–16), and there is also a recent meta-analysis (17). Conclusions from the many studies on LMWH have led to more general recommendations on their use in various risk situations (18,19).

The first clinical study on LMWH was uncontrolled, but it was shown that the principle of one daily injection did work with a low frequency of postoperative deep vein thrombosis (DVT) as a result, a Choay LMW fraction being used (20). Although no untreated group was included, there was no apparant increase in intra- or postoperative bleeding.

The aim of this chapter is to discuss the use of LMWH for thromboprophylaxis in patients undergoing nonorthopedic surgery, which mainly means elective general abdominal surgery. Only studies with proper methodology have been used in the analysis, that is, prospective comparative studies with a randomized design and where some objective tests have been used for diagnosis of DVT and pulmonary embolism (PE). As far as DVT is concerned, the predominant method has been the ^{125}I-fibrinogen uptake test (FUT). Only full publications from peer-reviewed journals have been analyzed. Also, with these restrictions there are great differences between studies, making it difficult to make comparisons. Hopefully, however, the groups within a randomized study should be comparable. One further concern is the sample size of the various investigations. Only rarely this has been estimated on the basis of a biostatistical analysis before the start of the study. Moreover, the analysis in this chapter is restricted to LMWH and does not deal with low-molecular-weight heparin analogs.

II. PREVENTION OF THROMBOEMBOLISM

A. Prevention of DVT

1. Comparison with Untreated Controls

At present, most surgeons believe it is unethical not to give prophylaxis, and the inclusion of untreated control or placebo groups in thromboprophylactic studies is only rarely possible. There is one placebo-controlled study from one center in New Zealand, where routine prevention was not used in general surgical patients when the investigation started (21). Of 88 placebo patients, 14 developed DVT (FUT diagnosis) compared to four of 95 in the dalteparin group, a reduction in frequency from 15.9% to 4.2%, which is statistically significant ($p < 0.008$). On subgroup analysis, the effect was seen only in patients operated on for malignant diseases, the frequency of DVT being very low in those with benign disorders. In another placebo-controlled study by Valle et al. (22) from Geneva, Italy, 50 patients were included in each group. The study is mentioned because of the design with placebo, but unfortunately the diagnostic surveillance was suboptimal, using Doppler sonography, which so far has not been sufficiently evaluated in this setting. Although the authors stated that they studied patients who had major surgery, the majority of patients underwent minor procedures and three thrombi were found in the placebo group.

2. Comparison with Low-Dose Unfractionated Heparin

The vast majority of studies have used unfractioned low-dose heparin for comparison. The studies are summarized in Table 1. In some, either dihydroergotamine or graded elastic compression stockings have been used as a routine in all patients in addition to heparin and LMWH. Whether such a combination adds any prophylactic benefit has not been properly evaluated, but this would probably be difficult to show, bearing in mind the very low frequencies of DVT. In fact, there is no convincing evidence that addition of dihydroergotamine to LMWH has a prophylactic benefit.

The ^{125}I-fibrinogen uptake test was used for diagnosis in all studies, venographic verification being added only occasionally. In the study by Speziale et al. (41), patients undergoing aortofemoral reconstructions were investigated, and in this group the test may be less reliable in the proximal thigh because of the surgical wound. Baumgartner et al. (24) could confirm only half the FUT-detected DVT with phlebography, but there was still no difference between the two groups. Many of the studies were fairly small and thus the confidence intervals are wide. The prophylactic protocols varied considerably. Except for differences in the method of production of the LMWH, the doses varied from 1500 to 7500 anti-factor Xa units; in most of the studies LMWH were given once daily, whereas UFH was given 2 or 3 times daily in the conventional way. In the study by Leizorovicz et al. (35), two groups receiving LMWH were included; one received 2500, and the other 3500, anti-factor Xa units of tinzaparin daily. The lower dose resulted in a significantly higher incidence of DVT than the higher, the results of which did not differ from those after a UFH regimen. The reasonable conclusion from the studies reported in Table 1 is that LMWH seems to be at least as effective as low-dose unfractionated heparin in preventing postoperative DVT as diagnosed by the ^{125}I-fibrinogen test. Analyzing the open studies shows a relative risk reduction of DVT of 44% in favor of LMWH. The corresponding reduction is only 8% when the double-blind studies are compared.

One randomized study compared UFH dihydroergotamine with dalteparin in patients undergoing hysterectomy and found no difference in the incidence of thrombosis detected by thermography (leg temperature profile) with phlebographic verification (45). In a similar study of patients undergoing gynecological surgery, Heilmann et al. (46) used impedance plethysmography to diagnose DVT and found no significant difference between UFH and LMWH (Sandoz). These methods of diagnosis are inadequate for surveillance, but likely faults should be equally distributed among the groups.

In the meta-analysis by Nurmohamed et al. (17), a classification of study methodology was made. The studies were scored according to eight predefined criteria that were considered to reflect the methodological strength of the study. In investigations classified as strong, the relative risk was 0.91 (95% confidence interval 0.68–1.23) in favor of LMWH in contrast to those with weaker methodology, where it was 0.67 (0.54–0.85).

In a recent preliminary analysis, the use of LMWH was more cost-effective than UFH in prophylaxis in both elective general and hip surgery (47).

Table 1 Incidence of Deep Vein Thrombosis in Nonorthopedic Studies of Low-Molecular-Weight Heparin Compared with Low-Dose Unfractionated Heparin

		LMWH			Low-dose UFH		
	Type of study	Type	No. of patients	No. (%) of DVT	No. of patients	No. (%) of DVT	Comments
Adolf et al., 1989 (23)	Double blind	Sandoz	202	25 (12)	202	24 (12)	Abdominal surgery
Baumgartner et al., 1989 (24)	Double blind	Sandoz	99	14 (14)	102	14 (14)	Dihydroergotamine also given to both groups; abdominal surgery
Bergqvist et al., 1986 (25)	Double blind	Kabi	215	13 (6)	217	9 (4)	Abdominal surgery
Bergqvist et al., 1988 (26)	Double blind	Kabi	505	28 (6)	497	41 (8)	Abdominal surgery; LMWH started 12 hr before operation
Caen, 1988 (27)	Double blind	Kabi	195	6 (3)	190	7 (4)	General surgery
Corrado et al., 1989 (28)	Open	Fluxum	29	3 (10)	29	3 (10)	Urological surgery
European Fraxiparin Study, 1988 (29)	Open	CY 216	960	27 (3)	936	42 (5)	Elastic stockings also used in both groups; abdominal surgery
Fricker et al., 1988 (30)	Open	Kabi	40	2 (5)	40	0	Abdominal surgery
Hartl et al., 1990 (31)	Double blind	Kabi	126	9 (7)	124	9 (7)	Abdominal surgery
Kakkar and Murray, 1985 (32)	Double blind	CY 216	196	5 (3)	199	14 (7)	Abdominal surgery
Kakkar et al., 1989 (33)	Double blind	Sandoz	88	10 (11)	91	10 (11)	Dihydroergotamine also given to both groups; general surgery

Koller et al., 1986 (34)	Double blind	Kabi	97	2	(2)	92	2	(2)	Abdominal surgery
Leizorovicz et al., 1991 (35)	Double blind	Novo	861	50	(6)	429	18	(4)	General surgery[a]
Onarheim et al., 1986 (36)	Double blind	Kabi	25	2	(8)	27	2	(7)	Abdominal surgery
Roder et al., 1988 (37)	Open	Kabi	102	5	(5)	104	18	(17)	Abdominal surgery
Samama et al., 1988 (38)	Open	Enoxaparin	448	13	(3)	437	20	(5)	General surgery[a]
Sasahara et al., 1986 (39)	Double blind	Sandoz	137	14	(10)	132	13	(10)	Dihydroergotamine also given to both groups; abdominal surgery
Schmitz-Hübner et al., 1984 (40)	Open	Sandoz	81	3	(4)	39	0		Abdominal surgery
Speziale et al., 1988 (41)	Open	Fluxum	46	3	(7)	46	4	(9)	Vascular surgery
Verardi et al., 1989 (42)	Open	Fluxum	44	1	(2)	44	3	(7)	General surgery
Verardi et al., 1989 (43)	Open	Fluxum	308	10	(3)	302	19	(6)	General surgery
Welzel et al., 1988 (44)	Open	Sandoz	115	4	(4)	116	14	(12)	Dihydroergotamine also given to both groups; abdominal surgery
Total			4919	249	(5)	4395	286	(7)	
Open studies			2173	71	(3.3)	2093	123	(5.9)	
Double blind studies			2746	178	(6.5)	2302	163	(7.1)	

[a]Including abdominal, gynecological, urological, and thoracic surgery.

Table 2 Total Number of Deaths and Number Caused by Pulmonary Embolism or Bleeding in Comparative Nonorthopedic Studies on Low-Molecular-Weight Heparin and Low-Dose Heparin

	LMWH				Low-dose heparin			
		No. of deaths				No. of deaths		
	No. of patients	Total	Pulmonary embolism	Bleeding	No. of patients	Total	Pulmonary embolism	Bleeding
Adolf et al., 1989 (23)	202	1	0	0	202	1	0	0
Baumgartner et al., 1989 (24)	99	1	0	1	102	2	1	0
Bergqvist et al., 1986 (25)	215	3	0	0	217	6	0	0
Bergqvist et al., 1988 (26)	505	10	0	0	497	10	1	0
Borstad et al., 1988 (50)	105	0	0	0	110	0	0	0
Borstad et al., 1992 (51)	71	1	0	0	70	0	0	0
Caen, 1988 (27)	195	2	0	0	190	3	0	0
Catania and Salanitri, 1988 (52)	88	2	0	0	85	3	0	0
Corrado et al., 1989 (28)	29	0	0	0	29	0	0	0
European Fraxiparin Study, 1988 (29)	960	11	0	0	936	12	1	0

Fricker et al., 1988 (30)	40	2	0	0	40	2	1	0
Haas et al., 1987 (53)	55	0	0	0	55	0	0	0
Hartl et al., 1990 (31)	126	6	1	0	124	4	1	0
Heilmann et al., 1989 (46)	150	0	0	0	150	0	0	0
Kakkar and Murray, 1985 (32)	196	5	0	0	199	5	1	0
Koller et al., 1986 (34)	97	0	0	0	92	0	0	0
Liezorovicz et al., 1991 (35)	861	20	0	0	429	9	0	0
Onarheim et al., 1986 (36)	25	0	0	0	25	0	0	0
Salcuni et al., 1988 (54)	73	0	0	1	68	0	0	0
Samama et al., 1988 (38)	448	4	0	0	437	0	0	0
Sasahara et al., 1986 (39)	137	2	0	0	132	5	1	0
Schmitz-Hübner et al., 1984 (40)	81	1	0	0	39	0	0	0
Steiner et al., 1989 (55)	92	0	0	0	99	0	0	0
Valle et al., 1988 (22)	50	0	0	0	50	0	0	0
Verardi et al., 1989 (42)	44	0	0	0	44	0	0	0
Verardi et al., 1989 (43)	308	0	0	0	302	0	0	0
Voigt et al., 1986 (56)	107	4	0	0	103	6	0	0
Total (%)	5359	75	1	2	4826	68	7	0

B. Prevention of Pulmonary Embolism

There are no LMWH studies where scintigraphic or angiographic techniques have been used for surveillance of postoperative PE in patients undergoing general surgery. In one study on elective hip replacement, dalteparin significantly reduced the frequency of scintigraphic perfusion defects compared with UFH (48). It should be stressed, however, that the clinical relevance of scintigraphic defects detected during surveillance is completely unknown. Only one placebo-controlled study has been large enough for evaluation of the effect of LMWH on the incidence of fatal PE (49). This was a multicenter (18 centers), double-blind Italian study with a total of 4498 patients undergoing general surgical operations, who were randomized to receive one daily injection of 7500 anti-Xa units of LMWH (CY 216) or placebo. There were eight deaths in the LMWH group (0.3%) compared with 18 in the placebo group (0.8%), a significant difference ($p < 0.05$). Twenty-three of the 26 patients who died (89%) underwent necropsy, and pulmonary embolism was confirmed as the cause of death in two patients in the LMWH group (0.09%) and four in the placebo group (0.2%); this difference is, however, not significant.

The extent of the problem of fatal PE is further analyzed in Table 2, where all randomized studies from which it is possible to collect data on mortality, fatal PE, and fatal bleeding are summarized. The overall incidence of fatal PE was 0.02% in the LMWH groups compared with 0.15% in the UFH groups. Total mortality was 1.4% in both groups. Similar results were reported in the meta-analysis by Nurmohamed et al. (17): two fatal PE in LMWH patients and nine in patients receiving UFH.

When all data available on fatal PE in patients having received LMWH prophylaxis, including those who had orthopedic surgery, are compiled, this low frequency is still present (11). Thus, among 55,545 patients, 20 were reported having died from PE (0.04%).

C. Prevention of Late Sequelae

This problem has not been analyzed, but the extent of it is probably small (57).

III. SIDE EFFECTS

A. Hemorrhagic Complications

The greatest problem when dealing with bleeding complications is the variability in reporting routines and criteria for hemorrhage and what is considered "abnormal" bleeding. Thus it is important that the studies be blinded, when bleeding complications are analyzed. As there are great differences between centers concerning indications and routines for blood replacement, the transfusion amount is a suboptimal parameter of bleeding potential. The studies in which exact measurements of blood loss were made are shown in Table 3. There were no differences in perioperative blood loss or loss from drains between LMWH and UFH groups. In some of the earlier studies, however, a higher incidence of bleeding complications occurred with LMWH (25, 34, 40, 50), but in retrospect it is clear that the dose was too high, as indicated by high plasma concentrations of anti-factor Xa activity (5). With today's knowledge these studies should be looked upon as dose-finding studies. Data from the hip arthroplasty studies by Levine et al. showed a relationship between anti-factor Xa concentration during the first 3 postoperative days and the risk of bleeding (58). From this study and from those summarized by Levine and Hirsh (5), it seems reasonable to conclude that the anti-factor Xa concentration should be kept between 0.1 and 0.2 units/ml. This provides good prophylaxis as well as a good margin of safety as far as hemorrhage is concerned.

In the dose comparison study by Bansillon et al. (59), 200 anti-factor Xa units/kg body weight was clearly too high in patients undergoing total hip replacement, as shown by the high incidence of wound hematoma. In a study of 1290 patients undergoing general surgery, there was no correlation between anti-factor Xa activity and the occurrence of bleeding postoperatively, tinzaparin being used (60). Planes et al. (61) found more hematomas when they gave 60 mg enoxaparin daily in elective hip surgery than when they gave 40 mg. In all recent studies, bleeding complications have been no more common in the LMWH groups than in the UFH groups. In the study by Ockelford et al. (21), there was no difference in hemorrhagic variables between dalteparin and placebo. The LMWH dose was 2500 anti-factor Xa units once daily. In the large Italian multicenter study previously mentioned, 7500 anti-Xa units daily of CY 216 resulted in significantly more wound hematomas, injection site hematomas, and transfusions than did placebo (49). The incidence of severe bleeds, however, did not differ. In the meta-analysis by Nurmohamed et al. (17), there was no difference in incidence of major bleeding, and this was true for studies with both strong and weak methodology.

One important aspect of safety and potential hemorrhagic complications is whether it is safe to combine epidural/spinal anesthesia with LMWH. This problem is analyzed in another chapter in this volume.

B. Thrombocytopenia

One great concern with UFH is its potential to induce thrombocytopenia (62–64). Initially LMWHs were considered safe from this point of view, and it was also recommended that patients with heparin-induced thrombocytopenia be switched to LMWH (65). It is now clear, though, that LMWH preparations can induce platelet aggregation and thrombocytopenia (66–69). The frequency is, however,

Table 3 Blood Loss (ml) Measured During Operation and from Drains in Comparative Nonorthopedic Studies in Which Low-Molecular-Weight Heparin and Low-Dose Heparin Were Compared

	Type of study	LMWH	Low-dose heparin	Site of blood loss
Bergqvist et al., 1986 (25)	DB	300 (0–4000)	300 (0–2500)	Perioperative
Bergqvist et al., 1988 (26)	DB	300 (0–3500)	300 (0–10000)	Perioperative
Briel et al., 1988		45 (3–695)	26 (5 150)	Drain
Borstad et al., 1988 (50)		262 ± 151	286 ± 215	Perioperative
Caen, 1988 (27)	DB	405 ± 378	421 ± 427	Perioperative
		209 ± 252	226 ± 237	Drain
European Fraxiparin Study, 1988 (29)	O	315 ± 437	321 ± 414	Total blood loss
Fricker et al., 1988 (30)	O	922	992	Drain
Haas et al., 1987 (53)		304 ± 146	368 ± 218	Drain and perioperative
Heilmann et al., 1989 (46)		86 (2–1630)	150 (2–1170)	Drain
Kakkar and Murray, 1985 (32)	DB	270.2	213.3	Drain
Kakkar et al., 1989 (33)	DB	745 ± 666	738 ± 875	Perioperative
Samama et al., 1988 (38)	O	308 ± 486	294 ± 364	Drain (after 20 mg enoxaparin)
		247 ± 466	278 ± 559	Drain (after 40 mg enoxaparin)
		230 ± 35	253 ± 53	Drain (after 60 mg enoxaparin)
Sasahara et al., 1986 (39)	DB	49 ± 71	69 ± 145	Drain
Schmitz-Hübner et al., (40)	O	568.8, 703.7[a]	659	Perioperative
Steiner et al., 1989 (55)		124 ± 130	118 ± 125	Drain

[a] Two different LMWHs.

Units are ml of blood in mean ± SD or median and range.

DB = double blind; O = open.

not known, and the relative risk compared with UFH has not been analyzed in properly designed studies. In several small studies there has been no influence on platelet count (30, 36, 41, 50). In the 4498-patient study by Pezzuoli et al. (49), the frequency of postoperative platelet count lower than 100,000/ml was 0.6% in the CY 216 group and 0.4% in the placebo group. This indicates a very low frequency of drop in platelet count with LMWH prophylaxis, and in this situation a true immunologically induced thrombocytopenia is certainly a rarity.

C. Influence on Liver Enzymes

ASAT and ALAT were uninfluenced in a study using 5000 anti-factor Xa units daily of dalteparin in general surgery (25) or 15,000 units of fluxum (41). In a similar analysis of patients undergoing gynecological surgery, there was a postoperative increase, which, however, was significantly higher for patients receiving UFH than LMWH (50).

D. Other Complications

Local pain at the injection site may occur but was actually significantly less common in an LMWH group (dalteparin) than in the group receiving standard low-dose heparin (26). This corresponds to less injection site hematoma (23, 52), but this is probably dose dependent, as shown in a study on tinzaparin (35).

IV. DOSE AND TIMING

A. Dose

As the optimal concentration of anti-factor Xa activity is between 0.1 and 0.2 unit/ml, the reasonable dose seems to be 2500 units once daily subcutaneously in low-risk patients and 5000 units in high-risk patients undergoing operations for malignant disease (70).

One daily dose is adequate, and the subcutaneous injection should be made in the abdominal wall or the thigh. In patients with transverse lower abdominal surgical incisions and transection of the lymph vessels, the injection should not be given near the incision because it may increase the risk of hematoma formation, as it does with UFH (71).

B. Start of Prophylaxis

In the large International Multicentre Trial on low-dose heparin (72), the first heparin injection was given subcutaneously 2 hr preoperatively.

When, some 10 years later, LMWHs were developed, the time for the first injection was adopted from the low-dose heparin routines, the first of which was published by Kakkar et al. (20). A fixed 2-hr interval before surgery can be rather

Table 4 Time of First LMWH Injection in Relation to Surgery

Time of first injection	No. of studies
Day before surgery	1
At 10 P.M. evening before	3
Evening before	1
12 hr preoperatively	2
8 hr preoperatively	1
At 5 A.M. morning before surgery	1
At 7 A.M. morning before surgery	1
2 hr preoperatively	42
1 hr preoperatively	3
12–24 hr postoperatively	2
Postoperative day 3	1
Not stated	3
Total	61

The individual studies are analyzed in Bergqvist (79).

impractical, and some patients get their initial dose too close to the time of operation to be totally safe. In a study in which we measured the exact time lapse between the first injection and surgery, the median was 2.3 hr before operation, with a range of 0.2–9.3 hr (26). In two studies the first LMWH injection was instead given the evening before operation, and the effect was at least as good (26, 73). In our study on elective abdominal surgery, this injection was given a median of 12.7 hr before operation (range 9.4–18.4 hr), and there was no correlation between the time interval and effect. The registered elapsed time between first dose and the operation did not differ between patients with hemorrhagic complications and patients who developed DVT, in neither the UFH nor the LMWH groups. This means that it is reasonable to give the first injection the evening before operation. Pharmacodynamic investigations indicate that this may also be beneficial from the point of view of the circadian rhythm (74).

One reason for the limited use of thromboprophylaxis in North America has been the fear of postoperative bleeding complications. A pragmatic attitude to this problem was taken by the McMaster group when starting prophylaxis 12–24 hr postoperatively; they were able to show a good prophylactic effect compared with placebo in elective hip surgery (75). This was further verified in comparisons of LMWH and UFH (76). In their study, Planes et al. (77) found that preoperative start of prophylaxis was more effective than postoperative start, but the sample size was too small to make a firm conclusion. In another study on hip replacement, different prophylactic doses of enoxaparin were compared; in all groups prophylaxis was started postoperatively (no later than 1 day postoperatively) (78). By increasing the dose from 10 to 40 mg, it was possible to significantly reduce the frequency of DVT, as well as proximal vein thromboses. However, the only scientific way to show if a postoperative start of prophylaxis is sufficiently effective would be a randomized comparison between pre-and postoperative injection of the first dose, other factors being kept constant. This is considered one of the key questions, needing an urgent answer, that were defined in the recent European Consensus Statement (18). Probably, to be equally effective, the postoperative start requires at least a higher dose of LMWH than a preoperative start. It may also be preferable to give twice-daily injections when postoperative start is used. One of the potential advantages with LMWH would then be missed.

Published articles on LMWHs show that in most studies the first injection was given 2 hr preoperatively, but there is a wide time range when the first injection was given in relation to surgery (Table 4). In the majority of studies, a preoperative dose was given, but in as many as eight (13%), it was given several hours before surgery.

C. Duration of Prophylaxis

In the vast majority of studies, the duration of prophylaxis has been around 1 week, but the optimal duration has not been investigated. There has been some concern about delayed development of DVT, even after discharge from hospital (80). This may partly explain late postoperative occurrence of fatal pulmonary embolism in some patients (81, 82). This is not, however, motivation enough to prolong prophylaxis after discharge until adequately performed studies have shown that it really is beneficial. The present duration of 5–7 days is effective in keeping the frequency of fatal PE at a very low level (see above).

D. Neutralization of LMWH

One disadvantage of LMWH is neutralization of the anticoagulant effect with protamine. When LMWH is administered intravenously as well as subcutaneously, anti-factor Xa is not fully reversed by equimoler concentrations of protamine sulfate, although the anti-factor IIa activity is reversed (83–89). There is a gradual return of anti-factor Xa activity as well as anti-factor IIa activity when LMWH is given subcutaneously, indicating a continuing absorption (88). Despite the partial neutralization of anti-factor Xa activity, prolonged experimental bleeding time is neutralized by protamine sulfate (87, 90, 91).

V. CONCLUSION

The main advantage of LMWH in general surgery seems to be practical, i.e., the need for only one injection daily. The effect may be slightly improved compared with UFH. The prophylaxis in recommended doses is safe.

REFERENCES

1. Bergqvist D. Thromb Haemorrh Disord 1990; 2:69.
2. Collins R, Scrimgeour A, Yusuf S, Phil D, Peto R. N Engl J Med 1988; 318:1162.
3. Mätzsch T, Bergqvist D, Johansson A. Regional lumbar anaesthesia and thromboprophylaxis—attitudes of Swedish anaesthetists. Läkartida 1992; 89:4028.
4. Levine M, Hirsh J. Semin Thromb Hemost 1988; 14:116.
5. Levine MN, Hirsh J. Acta Chir Scand 1988; 543(suppl):73.
6. Samama M, Boissel JP, Combe-Tamzali S, Leizorovicz A. Ann NY Acad Sci 1989; 506:386.
7. Daures JP, Schved JF, Momas I, Gril JC, Azoulay P, Gremy F. Rev Epidémiol Santé Publ 1989; 37:363.
8. Nenci GG, Agnelli G. Thromb Res 1990; (Suppl XI):69.
9. Hirsh J. Am J Surg 1991; 161:512.
10. Lassen MR, Borris LC, Christiansen HM, Schøtt P, Olsen AD, Sørensen, JV, Rahr H, Jensen HP. Semin Thromb Hemost 1991; 17:284.
11. Bergqvist D. Eur J Surg 1992; 158:67.
12. Bergqvist D, Lindblad B, Mätzsch T. In: Lane D, Björk I, Lindahl U, eds. Heparin and Related Polysaccharides. Advances in Experimental Medicine and Biology. New York: Plenum Press, 1992.
13. Breddin HK, Haas S, Encke A. Heparin and low molecular weight heparins in the prevention of venous thrombosis. An overview of clinical trials. In: Florence Proceedings, Florence: Scientific Press, 1992.
14. Hirsh J, Levine MN. 1992; Blood 79:1.
15. Barrowcliffe TW, Johnson EA, Thomas DP. Low Molecular Weight Heparin. Chichester: Wiley, 1992.
16. Boisseau M. In: Doutremepuich C, ed. Low Molecular Weight Heparins in Clinical Practice. New York: Marcel Dekker, 1992.
17. Nurmohamed M, Rosendaal F, Büller H, Dekker E, Hommers D, Vandenbroucke J, Briët E. Lancet 1992; 340:152.
18. European Consensus Statement. Int Angiol, 1992; 11:151.
19. Thromboembolic Risk Factors (THRIFT) Consensus Group. Br Med J 1992; 305:567.
20. Kakkar VV, Djazaeri B, Fok J, Fletcher M, Scully MF, Westwick J. Br Med J 1982; 284:375.
21. Ockelford PA, Patterson J, Johns AS. Thromb Haemost 1989; 62:1046.
22. Valle I, Sola G, Origone A. Curr Med Res Opin 1988; 11:80.
23. Adolf J, Knee H, Roder JD, van de Flierdt E, Siewert JR. Dtsch Med Wochenschr 1989; 114:48.
24. Baumgartner A, Jacot N, Moser G, Krähenbühl B. VASA 1989; 18:152.
25. Bergqvist D, Burmark US, Frisell J, Hallböök T, Lindblad B, Risberg B, Törngren S, Wallin G. Br J Surg 1986; 73:204.
26. Bergqvist D, Mätzsch T, Burmark US, Frisell J, Guilbaud O, Hallböök T, Horn A, Lindhagen A, Ljungnér H, Ljungström KG, Onarheim H, Risberg B, Törngren S, Örtenwall P, Br J Surg 1988; 75:888.
27. Caen JP. Thromb Haemost 1988; 59:216.

28. Corrado F, Fini M, Severini G, Benati A, Monetti N, Levorato M, Fusconi E, Mazzucca A. Clin Trials J 1989; 26:138.
29. European Fraxiparin Study (EFS) Group. Br J Surg 1988; 75:1058.
30. Fricker J-P, Vergnes Y, Schach R, Heitz A, Eber M, Grunebaum L, Wiesel M-L, Kher A, Barbier P, Cazenave J-P. Eur J Clin Invest 1988; 18:561.
31. Hartl P, Brücke P, Dienstl E, Vinazzer H. Thromb Res 1990; 57:577.
32. Kakkar VV, Murray WGJ. Br J Surg 1985; 72:786.
33. Kakkar VV Stringer MD, Hedges AR, Parker CJ, Welzel D, Ward VP, Sanderson RM, Cooper D, Kakkar S. Am J Surg 1989; 157:413.
34. Koller M, Schoch U, Buchmann P, Largiadèr F, von Felten A, Frick PG. Thromb Haemost 1986; 56:243.
35. Leizorovicz A, Picolet H, Peyrieux JC, Boissel JP, and the HBPM Research Group. Br J Surg 1991; 78:412.
36. Onarheim H, Lund T, Heimdal A, Arnesjøo B. Acta Chir Scand 1986; 152:593.
37. Roder JD, Weber R, Adolf J, van de Flierdt E. Intensivbehandlung 1988; 13:149.
38. Samama M, Bernard P, Bonnardot JP, Combe-Tamzali S, Lanson Y, Tissot E, on behalf of the participants of the Group d'Etude de l'Enoxaparine (GENOX) multicenter trial. Br J Surg 1988; 75:128.
39. Sasahara AA, Koppenhagen K, Häring R, Weizel D, Wolf H. Br J Surg 1986; 73:697.
40. Schmitz-Hübner U, Bünte H, Freise G, Reers B, Rüschemeyer C, Scherer R, Schulte H, van de Loo J. Klin Wochenschr 1984; 62:349.
41. Speziale F, Verardi S, Taurino M, Nicolini G, Rizzo L, Fiorani P, Palazzini E. Pharmatherapeutica 1988; 5:261.
42. Verardi S, Cortese F, Boffo V, Baroni B, Verardi V, Casciani CU. Chirurgia 1989; 2:349.
43. Verardi S, Cortese F, Baroni B, Boffo V, Casciani CU, Palazzini E. Curr Ther Res 1989; 96:366.
44. Welzel D, Wolf H, Koppenhagen K. Arzneim-Forsch/Drug Res 1988; 38:120.
45. Briel RC, Doller P, Hermann CU. Geburtsh Frauenheilk 1988; 48:160.
46. Heilmann L, Kruck M, Schindler AE. Geburtsh Frauenheilk 1989; 49:803.
47. Bergqvist D, Mätzsch T. Hemostasis 1993; 23 (Suppl 1):15–19.
48. Eriksson B, Kälebo P, Anthmyr B, Wadenvik H, Tengborn L, Risberg B. J Bone Joint Surg 1991; 73-A:484.
49. Pezzuoli G, Neri Serneri GG, Settembrini P, Coggi G, Olivari N, Buzzetti G, Chierichetti S, Scotti A, Scatigna M, Carnovali M, and the STEP-Study Group. Int Surg 1989; 74:205.
50. Borstad E, Urdal K, Handeland G, Abildgaard U. Acta Obstet Gynecol Scand 1988; 67:99.
51. Borstad E, Urdal K, Handeland G, Abildgaard U. Acta Obstet Gynecol Scand 1992; 71:471.
52. Catania G, Salanitri G. Int J Clin Pharmacol Ther Toxicol 1988; 26:304.
53. Haas S, Zielke E. Medwelt 1987; 38:1658.
54. Salcuni PF, Azzarone M, Palazzini E. Curr Ther Res 1988; 43:824.
55. Steiner RA, Keller K, Lüscher T, Schreiner WE. Arch Gynecol Obstet 1989; 244:141.

56. von Voigt J, Hamelmann H, Hedderich J, Seifert J, Buchhammer T, Köhler A. Zentralbl Chir 1986; 11:1295.
57. Lindhagen A, Bergqvist D, Hallböök T. Br J Surg 1984; 71:511.
58. Levine MN, Planes A, Hirsh J, Goodyear M, Vochelle N, Gent M. Thromb Haemost 1989; 62:940.
59. Bansillon V, Dejour H, Besson L, Davidas JL, Rondelet B, Azzar D, Massignon D. Ann Chir 1987; 41:377.
60. Bara L, Leizorovicz A, Picolet H, Samama M. Thromb Res 1992; 65:641.
61. Planes A, Vochelle N, Ferru J, Przyrowski D, Clerc J, Fagola M, Planes M. Hemostasis 1986; 16:152.
62. Warkentin T, Kelton J. Ann U Rev Med 1989; 40:31.
63. Bell W. J Lab Clin Med 1989; 11:600.
64. Becker S, Miller V. Stroke 1989; 20:1449.
65. Gouault-Heilmann M, Huet Y, Adnot S, Contant G, Bonnet F, Intrator R, Payen D, Levent M. Hemostasis 1987; 17:134.
66. Vitoux JF, Mathieu JF, Roncato M, Fiessinger JN, Aiach M. Thromb Haemost 1986; 55:37.
67. Blockmans D, Bounameaux H, Vermylen J, Verstraete M. Thromb Haemost 1986; 55:90.
68. Horellou MH, Conard J, Lecrubier C, Samama M, Roque-D'Orbcastel O, de Fenoyl O, Di Maria G, Bernadou A. Thromb Haemost 1984; 51:124.
69. Leroy J, Leclerc MH, Delahousse B, Guerois C, Foloppe P, Gruel Y, Toulemonde F. Semin Thromb Haemost 1985; 11:326.
70. Bergqvist D, Burmark US, Frisell J, Guilbaud O, Hallböök T, Horn A, Lindhagen A, Ljungnér H, Ljungström K-G, Mätzsch T, Onarheim H, Risberg B, Törngren S, Örtenwall P. Semin Thromb Hemost 1990; 16:19.
71. Briel RC. Int Surg 1983; 68:241.
72. International Multicentre Trial. Lancet 1975; 2:45.
73. Planes A, Vochelle N, Mazas F, Mansat C, Zucman J, Landais A, Pascariello JC, Weill D, Butel J. Thromb Haemost 1988; 60:407.
74. Mätzsch T, Bergqvist D, Burmark U-S, Holmer E, Söderberg K. Thromb Haemost 1989; 62:525.
75. Turpie AGG, Levine MN, Hirsh J, Carter CJ, Jay RM, Powers PG, Andrew M, Hull RD, Gent M. N Engl J Med 1986; 315:925.
76. Levine MN, Hirsh J, Gent M, Turpie AG, Leclerc J, Powers PJ, Jay RM, Neemeh J. Ann Intern Med 1991; 114:545.
77. Planes A, Vochelle N, Fagola M, Feret J, Bellaud M. J Bone Joint Surg 1991; 73-B:418.
78. Spiro T. Thromb Haemost 1991; 65:927 (abstract).
79. Bergqvist D, In: Neri Serneri GG, Gensini GF, Abbate R, Prisco D, eds. Thrombosis. An Update. Florence: Scientific Press, 1982: 509.
80. Scurr JH, Coleridge-Smith PD, Hasty JH. Br Med J 1988; 297:28.
81. Lindblad B, Eriksson A, Bergqvist D. Br J Surg 1991; 78:849.
82. Huber O, Bounameaux H, Borst F, Rohner A. Arch Surg 1992; 127:310.
83. Massonet-Castel S, Pelissier E, Bara L, Terrier E, Abry B, Guibourt P, Swanson J, Jaulmes B, Carpentier A, Samama M. Hemostasis 1986; 16:139.

84. Harenberg J, Gnasso A, de Vries JX, Zimmermann R, Augustin J. Thromb Res 1985; 38:11.
85. Harenberg J, Wurzner B, Zimmermann R, Schettler G. Thromb Res 1986; 44:549.
86. Racanelli A, Fareed J, Walenga JM, Coyne E. Semin Thromb Haemost 1985; 11:176.
87. van Ryn-McKenna J, Cai L, Ofusu FA, Hirsh J, Buchanan MR. Thromb Haemost 1990; 63:271.
88. Holst J, Lindblad B, Mätzsch T, Bergqvist D. Thromb Res 1992; 65:651.
89. Gram J, Mercker S, Bruhn HD. Thromb Res 1988; 52:353.
90. Diness V, Østergaard P. Thromb Haemost 1986; 56:318.
91. Doutremepuich C, Bonini F, Toulemonde F, Bertrand H, Bayrou B, Quilichini R. Semin Thromb Haemost 1985; 11:318.

9

Low-Molecular-Weight Heparins for Prevention of Venous Thromboembolism Following Orthopedic Surgery

Fedor Bachmann
University of Lausanne Medical School, Lausanne, Switzerland

Pierre-François Leyvraz
Hôpital Orthopédique de la Suisse Romande, Lausanne, Switzerland

I. INTRODUCTION

The incidence of postoperative deep vein thrombosis (DVT) after total hip replacement without thromboprophylaxis is about 50% and that of fatal pulmonary embolism (PE) is about 2%, but in some studies up to 6% of fatal PE has been observed. The mortality of hip fractures without antithrombotic prophylaxis varies from 3 to 12% and is mainly due to thromboembolic complications (1, 2). After knee arthroplasty the incidence of DVT is still higher (50–80%), but principally located in the calf veins (3–5). In the seventies, only a minority of orthopedic surgeons routinely used pharmacological prophylaxis with antithrombotic drugs (6), in part because of the fear of inducing excessive bleeding (which is considered to be an iatrogenic complication, whereas a thromboembolic event is a fatality). During the last decade many surgeons have become increasingly aware of the benefits of regimens preventing postoperative DVT and PE. In a recent survey of over 600 orthopedic surgeons in the United Kingdom, 90% used some form of prophylaxis, with 83% using drugs. The subcutaneous injection of low doses of unfractionated heparin was, by far, the preferred antithrombotic regimen, followed by oral anticoagulation and intravenous infusion of dextran (7).

II. PATHOGENIC FACTORS CONTRIBUTING TO THE HIGH INCIDENCE OF DVT IN ORTHOPEDIC SURGERY

Hypercoagulability, due to tissue damage and perioperative stasis during general anesthesia, is a common pathogenic factor for the development of DVT in all types of surgery. Fixed doses of low-dose heparin appear to be an effective means to correct the hypercoagulable state and reduce the incidence of postoperative DVT. In a widely quoted meta-analysis of prophylactic trials, Collins et al. calculated that the administration of two to three subcutaneous injections of 5000 IU of unfractionated heparin (UH) reduced the DVT incidence by about 65% after general and orthopedic surgery (8). The American College of Chest Physicians Third Consensus Conference on antithrombotic therapy considered only trials with strong methodology and arrived at very different conclusions. After elective hip replacement, the administration of fixed doses of UH reduced the relative risk to develop DVT by 32% and by only 9% after hip fracture (2).

In prosthetic hip surgery, some intraoperative manipulations of the lower limb are pathogenic factors that do not exist in abdominal surgery. The distortion and kinking of the femoral vein during hip dislocation temporarily produces almost complete occlusion and probably causes damage to portions of the proximal third of the femoral vein (9). The stasis in and trauma of this portion of the femoral vein has been shown to produce a local increase in the concentration of tissue-type plasminogen activator (t-PA), as measured in blood samples taken from a femoral vein catheter (10), and could lead to local exhaustion of t-PA stores in the endothelial cells. Failure to release appropriate amounts of t-PA in response to forming fibrin may then result in uncontrolled local accumulation of fibrin. During reaming of the acetabulum and of the femur shaft, very high concentrations of tissue factor are released into the circulation (11), accompanied by a 20-to 30-fold increase of circulating fibrinopeptide A and thrombin–antithrombin III complexes (12), both markers of thrombin generation. The latter are still elevated three-to fourfold 1 day after surgery (13). Crushed adipose tissue derived from fractured bone has abundant tissue factor activity (14) and was shown to cause shortening of the plasma recalcification time and to produce microemboli in the lungs after its release into the circulation (15). It has been demonstrated that the generation of heat during polymerization of methacrylate used for cemented prostheses and the pressure effect produced by introduction of the prosthesis stem into the femur shaft also release some fat particles into the circulation.

Most patients having undergone hip or knee surgery develop some degree of swelling in the operated region, in part due to inflammatory reactions, in part due to the formation of wound hematomas. Both may result in compression of leg veins and stasis of blood flow. Early mobilization is often difficult for many older patients undergoing hip surgery. Hip fracture patients are frequently immobilized for a few days before operation, and it has been shown that the length of time until operation is correlated with an increased incidence of (preoperative?) DVT (16). During total knee replacement, a tourniquet is usually applied to reduce blood losses. The resulting anoxia may produce complete exhaustion of t-PA stores in the distal portion of the leg and may in part explain the extremely high incidence of DVT in this type of surgery.

It has been argued that two different kinds of DVT are seen after hip surgery. The first, probably due to hypercoagulability and stasis, is also encountered in general surgery, concerns mainly the calf veins, and also occurs in the nonoperated limb. The second kind observed typically after hip surgery is located in the femoral vein of the operated limb (9). The latter type is particularly worrisome because of its high frequency (about 50% of all DVTs observed after hip surgery) and because release of thrombi from larger veins is more likely to cause fatal PE.

The advanced age of the majority of patients and the concerted action of several of the above-mentioned factors may well explain why patients undergoing orthopedic surgery are at a higher risk to develop thromboembolic complication than general surgery patients.

III. DIAGNOSIS OF DVT IN ORTHOPEDIC SURGERY

There is general agreement that the "gold standard" for the diagnosis of asymptomatic DVT after orthopedic surgery of the lower extremities is phlebography (reviewed in 17, 18). Nevertheless, more than half of all studies evaluating the incidence of DVT after total hip replacement, hip fractures, and knee arthroplasty have used the ^{125}I-fibrinogen uptake test (FUT). This test has been extremely useful in general surgery to collect data on the epidemiology of DVT. It is not sensitive enough, however, to detect the important proximal DVT, which is so frequent after hip surgery, because of the high background radioactivity stemming from large vessels in the upper thigh, from the wound itself, and from ^{125}I accumulation in the bladder (19). Because phlebography may be painful, is invasive and expensive, and may cause hypotension and allergic reactions, clinicians have sought to develop other, noninvasive tests for the diagnosis of DVT. Impedance plethysmography has been widely used since the seventies and is a useful test for the detection of proximal DVT in symptomatic patients. Its sensitivity for the detection of clinically suspected DVT is around 66% (20) but unacceptably low (19%) in hip surgery patients (19). The same can be said for computerized impedance plethysmography (21). The diagnosis of proximal DVT, by Doppler ultrasonography, in patients with an important edema of the thigh is very difficult. In our own experience it was not sufficiently sensitive to detect four out of five femoral vein thrombi verified by phlebography. Newer methods have yielded disappointing results for the detection of proximal DVT in asymptomatic high-risk patients. Compared to phlebography, real-time B-mode ultrasonography exhibited a sensitivity of 57% (22) in a recent study of 60 patients with hip fracture and 40 patients with elective hip replacement. Color Doppler ultrasound had a sensitivity of only 38% in a series of 319 patients undergoing unilateral hip or knee arthroplasty (23).

Phlebography, the so-called gold standard, also has some shortcomings. Some patients refuse to submit to phlebography, and in others it is not possible to find a suitable foot vein for injection of the contrast medium. With the classic Rabinov-Paulin technique, the interobserver disagreement for the presence or absence of DVT or inadequacy of the film was reported to be 21%. The inadequacy rate was found to be only 2% for long-leg films taken after the injection of 150 ml of contrast medium, and interobserver disagreement was 4% (24). Interobserver disagreement was much more pronounced for radiographs suggesting DVT than for those thought to be negative (25).

IV. PROPHYLACTIC REGIMENS FOR THE PREVENTION OF DVT IN ORTHOPEDIC SURGERY

The expert committee of the third ACCP Consensus Conference on antithrombotic therapy has evaluated 14 different prophylactic regimens used in orthopedic surgery (2). Some of these regimens have been used in small series of patients only, and the incidence figures given for DVT may not be representative for a larger group. Pooled data were derived from studies using phlebography to screen for DVT. Table 1 demonstrates that after elective hip replacement, the use of aspirin, elastic stockings, and fixed low doses of subcutaneous UH with or without dihydroergotamine was not very effective in reducing the relative risk of DVT in these patients. The most effective thromboprophylaxes were: adjusted (low)-dose heparin, low-molecular-weight heparins (LMWHs), oral anticoagulants, and intermittent pneumatic compression of the legs. Dextran 70 had an intermediate position.

Fewer trials have been conducted in hip fracture surgery, and several of the incidence figures are derived from very small series of patients. This is particularly the case for studies where a combination of drugs was evaluated, such as low-dose heparin plus oral anticoagulants, and dextran plus dihydroergotamine or oral anticoagulants or aspirin. It appears that in hip fractures also, LMWHs are the most effective regimen for the prophylaxis of DVT.

V. CLINICAL TRIALS WITH LMWHs IN ORTHOPEDIC SURGERY

We have analyzed 25 prospective, randomized clinical trials using LMWHs or a heparinoid for the prevention of postoperative DVT after elective hip surgery, hip fracture, or knee arthroplasty. Many more studies have been conducted over

Table 1 Prevention of DVT After Hip Surgery

Regimen	Elective hip replacement				Hip fracture			
	No. of trials	No. of patients	DVT incidence (%)	Reduction of rel. risk (%)	No. of trials	No. of patients	DVT incidence (%)	Reduction of rel. risk (%)
Untreated control subjects	10	459	50		8	297	43	
Fixed LDUH	6	257	34	32	2	43	39	9
LDUH + oral anticoagulation					1	75	61	0
Adjusted LDUH	2	78	11	77				
LDUH/DHE	3	223	37	26	2	116	36	17
LMWH	6	581	16	68	2	254	11	74
Oral anticoagulation	3	162	18	63	6	301	25	43
Dextran 70	5	229	30	41	8	486	30	32
Dextran/DHE					1	28	36	17
Dextran/oral anticoagulation					1	39	10	76
Dextran/aspirin					1	42	33	23
Aspirin	6	418	45	11	1	66	41	6
IPC	3	261	21	60				
Elastic stockings	2	137	38	25				

Pooled data from trials based on routine phlebography.
LDUH = low-dose heparin; LMWH = low-molecular-weight heparin; DHE = dihydroergotamin; IPC = intermittent pneumatic compression of the legs.
Source: From Clagett et al. (2).

the last 7 years, but we excluded dose-ranging studies and trials using dosage regimens no longer in use (too high or too low). We have not found a randomized prospective study using LMWH for multiple-trauma patients.

For total hip replacement, only studies in which routine phlebography was attempted in every patient were included. As a rule, phlebographies were interpreted by radiologists unaware of the patient's treatment. In hip fractures and knee surgery, few clinical trials have been conducted, and we have also included studies in which phlebography was used to confirm or invalidate a suspicion for DVT based on some other diagnostic tests. In general, we have tabulated the figures given for evaluable patients, that is, those in whom bilateral phlebography was done. In several studies an intention-to-treat analysis was also performed. This will be discussed later. All LMWH dosages indicated have been converted into international units of anti-factor Xa activity. There is no uniform definition for the term "major bleeding." Most of the investigators defined it as an episode with cerebral hemorrhage, retroperitoneal bleeding, a drop of the hemoglobin of more than 20 g/L, or any bleeding that led to interruption of the treatment. There also is no consistency for the label PE. In most studies only clinically manifest PE, verified by perfusion lung scan, angiography, or autopsy, was recorded. In a few studies, pulmonary perfusion-ventilation scans were performed in all patients, and these trials show significantly higher incidences of PE. Missing data are tabulated as NR (not reported), and statements indicating that there was no difference between two treatment groups without indication of actual figures are listed as n.s. (not significant). Many of these trials have been the object of two recent meta-analyses (26, 27). The present review contains several recent reports, which were not yet published at the time these meta-analyses were made.

A. Clinical Trials in Elective Hip Surgery

LMWHs and a heparinoid preparation have been used in thousands of patients undergoing orthopedic surgery. Their antithrombotic effect has been compared to that of UH, UH plus dihydroergotamine (DHE), dextran, and oral anticoagulants; four trials included an untreated control group. One firm has developed a combination preparation containing LMWH and DHE.

1. Trials Including a Placebo Control Group

Table 2 lists the four trials comparing a LMWH or the heparinoid Lomoparan with placebo controls. The study of Turpie et al. (28) comprised 100 patients, but mandatory phlebographies were done only during the second study period and the figures listed in Table 2 indicate only these latter patients. The specific activity of enoxaparin (Clexane, Lovenox) used in this study was 80 anti-factor Xa units/mg. (Note however, that in the majority of later studies with enoxaparin, preparations with a specific activity of 100 anti-factor Xa units were used.) The treatment group received twice-daily injections of 2400 IU of enoxaparin, and the first injection was started 12–24 hr postoperatively. Treatment was continued until day 14 or less if the patients were discharged earlier. A FUT was done daily in all patients, and impedance plethysmography was performed at entry and on alternate days after day 5. Only the intention-to-treat analysis was reported. It demonstrates a highly significant reduction of the incidence of total DVT from 51% to 11% and of proximal DVT from 23% to 5%. No case with clinically apparent PE occurred in this study. Major hemorrhagic complications occurred in one patient of the enoxaparin group and in two of the placebo group.

The study of Tørholm et al. compared the efficacy of dalteparin (Fragmin, Low Liquemin) versus placebo (29). The methodology used in this trial is weaker than that of other trials in total hip replacement because mandatory phlebography was not used in all patients. Patients were screened daily with the FUT, and 86% of those with a suspect scan had phlebography. Dalteparin was given in two doses of 2500 IU on the operative day, the first 2 hr before and the next 12 hr after surgery. On the following days one dose of 5000 IU was given daily for 7 days. If only those patients with phlebography are tabulated, 31% in the control group developed DVT (an unusually low figure, see Table 11) versus 14% in the dalteparin group. There were no significant differences in the incidence of PE, major bleeding, or deaths between the two groups. In the placebo group a higher number of DVTs occurred during the first 4 postoperative days than in the remaining study period ($p < 0.02$). Such a difference was not found in the treatment group.

The two remaining studies each comprise some 200 patients. Lassen et al. (30) were the only investigators in this series of reports to use a body-weight-adjusted dose of tilziparin (Logiparin). The first dose of 50 IU/kg was given 2 hr before surgery and then daily for 7 days. Thigh-length graded compression stockings (TED antiembolism stockings, Kendall Co.) were applied to both legs 1 hr before the operation in both groups. Bilateral ascending phlebography was carried out in all patients from days 8 to 10, or earlier if DVT was suspected. DVT occurred in 45% of the placebo patients and in 31% of the tilziparin patients, and 80% of the thrombi were proximal in both groups. The odds for contracting DVT were lower in patients who had been mobilized successfully during the first 4 days ($p = 0.02$), most of the effect being attributable to a reduction of DVT in the treated group (placebo patients 44%, tilziparin 23%). There were no significant differences in the incidence of PE, major bleeding, or deaths.

Hoek et al. examined the effect of Lomoparan, a LMWH composed mainly of heparan sulfate and dermatan sulfate, in elective hip surgery (31). Patients received twice daily a subcutaneous injection of 750 IU of Lomoparan or of saline. The first injection was given 15–45 min before the induction of anesthesia. All patients underwent mandatory phlebography. The incidence of total DVT

Table 2 Clinical Trials in Elective Hip Surgery, LMWH Versus Placebo

Author, year	Type of LMWH	Dosage regimen, LMWH: Dose (IU/day)	Dosage regimen, LMWH: First injection[a] (days)	Dosage regimen, LMWH: Duration (days)	End-point # of events/# of patients: DVT LMWH	DVT Placebo	Pulmonary embolism LMWH	Pulmonary embolism Placebo	Major bleeding LMWH	Major bleeding Placebo	Total mortality LMWH	Total mortality Placebo
Turpie, '86 (28)	Enoxaparin	2 × 2400	12–24	≤14	4/37	20/39	0/50	0/50	1/50	2/50	0/50	1/50
Tørholm, '91 (29)	Fragmin	2 × 2500 d0 1 × 5000 d1 +	−2	7	8/57	16/51	0/58	1/54	n.s.		1/58	0/54
Lassen, '91 (30)	Logiparin	1 × 50/kg	−2	7	29/93	44/97	1/105	1/104	0/105	1/104	1/105	1/104
Hoek, '92 (31)	Lomoparan	2 × 750	−1	10	15/97	56/99	0/97	0/99	0/97	0/99	0/97	0/99
Total					56/284	136/286	1/310	2/307	1/252	3/253	2/310	2/307
Percent					**19.7**	**47.6**	0.3	0.7	0.4	1.2	0.7	0.7
Rel. risk reduction					**59%**							

[a] Hours before (−) or after surgery.

was significantly lower in the Lomoparan group (15.5% vs. 56.6%), as was the frequency of proximal DVT (8.2 vs. 25.3%). There was no case of PE, major bleeding, or death in the two groups.

Taking all four studies together, the relative risk reduction of LMWH prophylaxis compared to untreated controls amounts to 59%.

2. *Comparative Trials of LMWH and UH*

Table 3 lists four trials that compared the antithrombotic effect of a fixed dose of LMWH with that of a fixed dose of 15,000 IU per day of UH, given in two or three injections, and three trials that compared LMWH with adjusted doses of UH. In several studies a LMWH preparation was given the evening before surgery, probably in an attempt to minimize intraoperative bleeding (the peak action of most LMWHs occurs some 3–5 hr after subcutaneous injection, whereas the peak action of UH occurs after 1–2 hr. Enoxaparin was used in two randomized double-blind trials and administered once daily in a dose of 4000 IU in the study conducted by Planes et al. (32) and given twice daily at a dose of 2400 IU per injection in the trial reported by Levine et al. (33). In the former study, use of enoxaparin resulted in a reduction of total DVT from 25% to 12.5% and of proximal DVT from 18.5% to 7.5%. The Levine study belongs to a small minority of trials where antithrombotic prophylaxis was started 12–24 hr after surgery. In the enoxaparin group, there were 258 patients with evaluable venograms, exhibiting an incidence of 19.4% total and 5.4% proximal DVT, whereas the UH group comprised 263 patients with evaluable films of which 23.2% were positive for total DVT and 6.5% for proximal DVT (n.s).

Fragmin, 5000 IU, given once daily, was compared to UH, 5000 IU, given once every eight hours, in a double-blind fashion by Eriksson et al. (34). This study comprised also mandatory pulmonary perfusion-ventilation scintigraphy for every patient. This explains the relatively high frequency of PE recorded in this study. Only three patients with positive lung scans had clinical signs of PE. Bilateral ascending phlebography was performed in 122 of 136 patients entering the study (27 PE/136 patients). As observed in several other studies, the total rate of thrombosis in the two groups was not statistically different. However, thrombosis of the femoral veins occurred in only 10% of patients in the Fragmin group, but in 31% in the UH group ($p = 0.01$). PE embolism occurred in 12.3% of patients in the LMWH group and in 30.6% in the UH group. Total loss of blood and the total amount of blood transfused were significantly lower in the patients who had received LMWH.

It is interesting to compare the German Hip Arthroplasty Trial (GHAT) with the multicenter trial reported by Leyvraz et al. Both compared nadroparin (Fraxiparin) with UH. In the GHAT study (35), both drugs were given at fixed doses, whereas the Leyvraz trial (36) administered the LMWH on a weight-adjusted dosage, which was probably lower in the majority of patients during

Table 3 Clinical Trials in Elective Hip Surgery, LMWH Versus UH

		Dosage regimen						End-point # of events / # of patients							
		LMWH			Unfractionated heparin			DVT		Pulmonary embolism		Major bleeding		Total mortality	
Author, year	Type of LMWH	Dose (IU/day)	First injection[a]	Duration (days)	Dose (IU/day)	First injection[a]	Duration (days)	LMWH	UH	LMWH	UH	LMWH	UH	LMWH	UH
					Fixed doses of UH										
Planes, '88 (32)	Enoxaparin	1 × 4000	−12	≤14	3 × 5000	−2	≤14	15/120	27/108	0/124	0/113	2/124	0/113	0/124	0/113
Levine, '91 (33)	Enoxaparin	2 × 2400	12–24	≤14	2 × 7500	12–24	≤14	50/258	61/263	0/333	2/332	11/333	19/332	0/333	0/332
Eriksson, '91 (34)	Fragmin	1 × 5000	−12	10	3 × 5000	−2	10	19/63	25/59	8/67	19/69	1/67	5/69	0/67	1/69
GHAT, '92 (35)	Fraxiparine	1 × 4000	−12	≤14	3 × 5000	−2	≤14	45/136	47/137	2/167	6/168	2/167	2/168	0/167	3/168
Total								129/577	160/567	10/691	27/682	16/691	30/682	0/691	4/682
Percent								**22.4**	**28.2**	**1.5**	**4**	**2.3**	**4.4**	0	0.6
Rel. risk reduction								**21%**		**63%**		**48%**			
					Adjusted doses of UH										
Barre, '87 (38)	Fragmin	2 × 2500	−2	10	3 × 3750 initial	−2	10	7/38	3/38	0/40	0/40	5/40	4/40	0/40	0/40
Dechavanne, '89 (39)	Fragmin	A: 2 × 2500 B: 2 × 2500 d 0–1 1 × 5000 d2+	−2	10–13	3 × 5000 initial	−2	10–13	5/77	4/38	NR	NR	0/82	0/40	0/82	0/40
Leyvraz, '91 (36)	Fraxiparine	41/kg d 0–3 62/kg d 4–10	−12	10	3 × 4000 initial	−16	10	22/174	28/175	1/198	4/199	1/198	3/199	1/198	2/199
Total								34/289	35/251	1/238	4/239	6/320	7/279	1/320	2/279
Percent								**11.8**	**13.9**	**0.4**	**1.7**	**1.9**	**2.5**	0.3	0.7
Rel. risk reduction								**15%**				**24%**			

[a] Hours before (–) or after surgery.
NR = not recorded in publication.

the first 3 days of treatment (41 IU/kg in a 70-kg patient amounts to only 2870 IU/day), but higher after the third postoperative day, when the dose was increased 50%. UH was given in doses adjusted according to the APTT, based on the experience of an earlier study that had given excellent results with this regimen (37). Incidences of phlebographically diagnosed total thromboses with UH were 34.4% in the GHAT and 16% in the Leyvraz trial and with Fraxiparin 33.1% and 12.6%, respectively. Neither of the differences between LMWH and UH were statistically significant. However, in both studies a significant reduction of proximal DVT was observed in the LMWH group: in the German trial from 19% to 10.3% ($p < 0.05$) and in the Leyvraz trial from 13.1% to 2.9% ($p < 0.001$). In both studies, an intention-to-treat analysis yielded results comparable to those of the efficacy analysis. Subgroup analysis in the German trial revealed a higher incidence of DVT in patients >60 years of age and in patients with a body weight >70 kg. The latter had received a daily mean dose of 53 IU/kg/day and exhibited a DVT rate of 38%, whereas those with a bodyweight of <70 kg had received a mean daily dose of 67 IU/kg of Fraxiparin, and in 25% of these DVT was diagnosed. There was no difference in the DVT incidence in patients with less than or more than 70 kg body weight in the group who had received fixed doses of UH.

The two studies of Barre et al. (38) and of Dechavanne et al. (39) both compared Fragmin with UH. In the Barre study, peridural anesthesia was used for all patients, and this might be one of the reasons why low DVT incidences with LMWH and with UH were observed. Dechavanne et al. attempted to determine whether it was preferable to give Fragmin once or twice daily. There was no significant difference between these two Fragmin groups; in Table 3 the corresponding results have been consolidated into one larger group.

The relative risk reduction for DVT when using a fixed dose of a LMWH was 21%, for PE it was 63%, and for major bleeding episodes 48%. Compared to adjusted UH, the relative risk reduction for LMWH is even smaller (15%), and there is an insufficient number of events to judge with any certainty the incidence of PE, major bleeding, or death in the two treatment groups.

3. *Comparative Trials with Dextran*

Three comparative studies have been conducted with dextran (Table 4). In the studies of Eriksson et al. (40) and of Mätsch et al. (41, 42), peridural anesthesia was used in most patients. In all three studies, dextran was given in a standardized manner after an injection of a small volume of a monovalent hapten-dextran to prevent allergic reactions from dextran. The first infusion of 500 ml of 6% Macrodex was always given during operation and was followed by a second dose several hours later, and on the first, third, and, in case the patient was not yet mobilized, on the fifth postoperative day. Fragmin and enoxaparin were given in fixed doses; Logiparin was administered on a body weight basis. Eriksson et

Table 4 Clinical Trials in Elective Hip Surgery, LMWH Versus Dextran

		Dosage regimen					End-point # of events / # of patients							
		LMWH			Dextran		DVT		Pulmonary embolism		Major bleeding		Total mortality	
Author, year	Type of LMWH	Dose (IU/day)	First injection[a]	Duration (days)	Dose ml/day	First infusion[a]	LMWH	Dextran	LMWH	Dextran	LMWH	Dextran	LMWH	Dextran
Eriksson, '88 (40)	Fragmin	2 × 2500	−2	7	2 × 500 d 0 1 × 500 d 1 + 3	Periop	10/49	22/49	2/49	2/49	0/49	2/49	0/49	0/49
Mätsch, '88 (41, 42)	Logiparin	1 × 35/kg	−2	7	2 × 500 d 0 1 × 500 d 1,3,5	Periop	13/47	19/49	NR	NR	0/49	0/49	NR	NR
DES group, '91 (43)	Enoxaparin	1 × 4000	−12	7–11	2 × 500 d 0 1 × 500 d 1,3,(5)	Periop.	7/108	24/111	NR	NR	1/120	0/126	1/126	0/126
Total							30/204	65/209	2/49	2/49	1/218	2/224	1/169	0/175
Percent							**14.7**	**31.1**	4.1	4.1	0.5	0.9	0.6	0
Rel. risk reduction							**53%**							

[a] Hours before surgery.

NR = not recorded in publication.

Table 5 Clinical Trials in Elective Hip Surgery, LMWH ± DHE Versus UH ± DHE

		Dosage regimen						End-point # of events / # of patients							
		LMWH DHE			UH DHE			DVT		Pulmonary embolism		Major bleeding		Total mortality	
Author, year	Type of LMWH	Dose (IU/d; mg/d)	First injection[a]	Duration (d)	Dose (IU/d; mg/d)	First injection[a]	Duration (d)	LMWH +DHE	UH+ DHE	LMWH +DHE	UH+ DHE	LMWH +DHE	UH+ DHE	LMWH +DHE	UH+ DHE
					Unfractionated heparin										
Weber, '91 (44)	Embolex LM	1 × 6000 plus 0.5 mg DHE	−2	14	3 × 5000	−2	14	8/35	11/36	0/35	0/36	0/35	0/36	0/35	0/36
Percent								**22.8**	**30.6**	0	0	0	0	0	0
Rel. risk reduction								**25%**							
					UH plus DHE										
Lassen, '88 (45)	Embolex LM	1 × 6000 + 0.5 mg DHE	−2	7	2 × 5000 + 0.5 mg DHE	−2	7	35/107	34/112	0/107	0/112	1/107	1/112	0/107	0/112
Freick, '91 (46)	Embolex LM	1 × 6000 + 0.5 mg DHE	−2	10	2 × 5000 + 0.5 mg DHE	−2	10	5/52	12/48	0/55	1/55	0/55	2/55	NR	NR
Total								40/159	46/160	0/162	1/167	1/162	3/167	0/107	0/112
Percent								**25.2**	**28.8**	0	0.6	0.6	1.8	0	0
Rel. risk reduction								**13%**							
Leyvraz, '92 (47)	Lomoparan	2 × 750	−2	10	2 × 5000 UH + 0.5 mg DHE	−2	10	25/145	44/139	1/153	1/150	1/153	1/150	1/153	1/150
Percent								**17.2**	**31.7**	0.6	0.6	0.6	0.6	0	0
Rel. risk reduction								**46%**							

[a] Hours before surgery.

NR = not recorded in publication.

al. confirmed an observation reported earlier; that is, the onset of DVT in patients treated with LMWH occurs later (days 5–8) than in those receiving dextran (maximum on days 1–5). The unusually low DVT incidence in the Danish Enoxaparin Study (DES) (43) is probably due to the fact that not all patients underwent mandatory phlebography.

LMWHs appear to be significantly more efficacious to prevent DVT than dextran, and the relative risk reduction was 53%.

4. *Other Randomized Trials with LMWH*

Table 5 contains the results of several other trials, in which a LMWH or Lomoparan were compared to some other prophylactic regimen. Three trials compared Embolex LM (a combination of a LMWH and of DHE) with straight UH or with the combination of UH and DHE. Weber et al. (44), in a relatively small trial, found that LMWH, given once daily at the dose of 6000 IU combined with DHE, reduced the relative risk of DVT by 25% compared to thrice-daily 5000 IU of UH. In the two other studies, Embolex LM given once daily was compared with the combination UH plus DHE, administered twice daily (45,46). The LMWH + DHE combination was slightly and insignificantly better to prevent postoperative DVT after elective hip surgery. The largest trial was our tricenter study comparing the effect of twice-daily doses of 750 IU of Lomoparan with that of the combination of UH with DHE (Sandoz), given twice daily (47). Lomoparan significantly reduced the rate of total DVT from 32% to 17% ($p = 0.007$), a relative risk reduction of 46%, but not of proximal DVT.

B. Clinical Trials in Hip Fracture Patients

We have included in this review only six trials in patients with hip fracture (Table 6). Studies in this condition are more difficult to perform, because patients are in general older than those undergoing elective hip replacement and often have other pathological conditions that have not been adequately treated prior to surgery. The mortality in most studies is much higher than that encountered in elective hip surgery. Several of the studies reported here lack rigorous methodology.

A small therapeutic trial comparing Fragmin with no treatment was conducted by Jørgensen et al. (16). All patients were screened for DVT with the FUT, but phlebographies were done in only 35% of these. Despite this deficiency, the 57% incidence of DVT in the placebo group is comparable to that encountered in other studies using mandatory phlebography in all patients. Fragmin reduced this DVT rate by 47%.

Oral anticoagulation started on admission of the patient has been fairly effective as antithrombotic prophylaxis after hip fracture (see Table 1). Gerhart et al. (48) evaluated the antithrombotic effect of 750 IU of Lomoparan given twice daily and of oral anticoagulation in a fairly large trial. All patients were screened daily by FUT, and additionally other diagnostic tests, such as impedance plethysmography and compression ultrasonography, were used, but phlebography was performed in only a minority of patients. The DVT rate in the anticoagulated patients is somewhat lower, but comparable to the mean found in six other studies listed in Table 1. In the Lomoparan group, the DVT incidence appears to be surprisingly low and represents a relative risk reduction of 68%. The difference in total mortality between the two groups is significant at the 0.04 level, but none of these deaths were considered to be related to thromboembolism.

Two smaller studies compared a LMWH preparation with UH, and in neither of these was venography systematically performed. The small study of Pini et al. (49) concerns a new LMWH preparation, Fluxum, which has not been widely tested so far. The study of Montreal et al. (50) is surprising with respect to the unusually good results obtained with thrice-daily injection of 5000 IU of UH. The DVT incidence of 19% is far below that of other studies and might be due to the fact that mandatory phlebography was performed only in the last 33 patients. In this trial all patients underwent ventilation-perfusion lung scanning on the eighth day after surgery. Again, the number of positive lung scans was significantly higher in the LMWH group than in the UH group ($p < 0.02$)

Dextran has always been one of the preferred prophylactic agents for hip fracture patients and has provided significant protection from DVT (see Table 1) and PE. Bergqvist et al. (51) have coordinated the largest multicenter trial in hip fracture and compared the effect of Lomoparan with that of Dextran. A FUT was done in all patients, and mandatory phlebography was successful in 85% of all patients. Lomoparan reduced the incidence of total DVT from 34.8% to 13.1%, the best results ever encountered in patients with hip fracture evaluated with strong methodology. The significantly better effect of Lomoparan was evident when analyzed on an intention-to-treat basis and in patients given correct prophylaxis ($p < 0.001$) and corresponds to a relative risk reduction of 62%. In the LMWH group there were three major bleedings, but the number of transfused units after surgery was significantly greater in the dextran group ($p < 0.01$).

The last trial listed in Table 6 compares the antithrombotic effect of a once-daily injection of Embolex LM with that of twice-daily injected Heparin-Dihydergot, both produced by Sandoz (52). Phlebography was performed only in patients with positive or suspect ^{99m}Tc-plasmin scans. The LMWH + DHE combination seemed to be more effective than the UH + DHE combination and resulted in a 38% reduction of the relative risk to develop DVT (n.s.).

C. Clinical Trial in Elective Knee Surgery

We found only one study conducted with adequate methodology in elective knee surgery (Table 7). Leclerc et al. (53) enrolled 131 patients undergoing knee

Table 6 Clinical Trials in Hip Fractures, LMWH Versus Various Other Regimens

Author, year	Type of LMWH	Dosage regimen: LMWH Dose (IU/day)	LMWH First injection[a]	LMWH Duration (days)	Comparative drug or placebo: Dose	Comparative First injection[a]	Comparative Duration (days)	DVT LMWH	DVT Other	Pulmonary embolism LMWH	Pulmonary embolism Other	Major bleeding LMWH	Major bleeding Other	Total mortality LMWH	Total mortality Other
					Placebo										
Jørgensen, '92 (16)	Fragmin	2 × 2500 d 0–1 1 × 5000 d 2–	−2	7				9/30	22/38	0/30	1/38	n.s.		3/30	4/38
Percent								**30**	**57**	0	2.6			10	10.5
Rel. risk reduction								**47%**							
					Oral anticoagulation										
Gerhart, '91 (48)	Lomoparan	2 × 750	Preop.	9	According to prothrombin time			9/132	28/131	0/132	1/131	8/132	5/131	1/132	7/131
Percent								**6.8**	**21.4**	0	0.8	6.1	3.8	0.8	5.3
Rel. risk reduction								**68%**							

					Unfractionated heparin										
Pini, '89 (7536)	Fluxum	2 × 7500	NR	≤14	3 × 5000 IU	NR	≤14	5/25	7/24	0/25	1/24	0/25	0/24	0/25	1/24
Montreal, '89 (50)	Fragmin	1 × 2500 d 0 1 × 5000 d 1–	−2	9	3 × 5000 IU	−2	9	14/46	6/44	6/46	0/44	2/46	1/44	2/46	3/44
Total								19/71	13/68	6/71	1/68	2/71	1/68	2/71	4/68
Percent								**27**	**19**	8.4	1.5	2.8	1.5	2.8	5.9
					Dextran										
Bergqvist, '91 (51)	Lomoparan	2 × 750	Preop.	≤12	1 × 500 ml preop. 1 × 500 ml d 0–2			14/107	40/115	1/143	5/146	3/143	0/146	9/143	8/146
Percent								**13.1**	**34.8**	0.7	3.4	2.1	0	6.3	5.5
Rel. risk reduction								**62%**							
					LMWH + DHE versus UH + DHE										
Lassen, '89 (52)	Embolex LM	1 × 6000 plus 0.5 mg DHE	Preop.	~7	2 × 5000 IU + 0.5 mg DHE	Preop.	7	14/53	23/54	1/53	0/54	1/53	0/54	4/53	2/54
Percent								**26.4**	**42.6**	1.9	0	1.9	0	7.5	3.7
Rel. risk reduction								**38%**							

[a] Hours before surgery.
NR = not recorded in publication.

Table 7 Clinical Trials in Elective Knee Surgery, LMWH Versus Placebo

		Dosage regimen, LMWH			End-point # of events / # of patients							
					DVT		Pulmonary embolism		Major bleeding		Total mortality	
Author, year	Type of LMWH	Dose (IU/day)	First injection[a]	Duration (days)	LMWH	Placebo	LMWH	Placebo	LMWH	Placebo	LMWH	Placebo
Leclerc, '91 (53)	Enoxaparin	2 × 3000	12–24	≤14	8/41	35/54	0/66	1/65	4/66	5/65	0/66	0/65
Percent					**19.5**	**64.8**	0	1.5	6.1	7.7	0	0
Rel. risk reduction					**70%**							

[a] Hours after surgery.

arthroplasty in a trial comparing twice-daily administration of 3000 IU of enoxaparin to no treatment. All patients underwent daily FUT screening and impedance plethysmography on every second day from the 5th to the 14th postoperative day. Ninety-five patients had an adequate bilateral venography. Enoxaparin reduced the DVT incidence significantly in an intention-to-treat analysis ($p < 0.0001$) as well as in the analysis of those patients in whom an adequate venography could be performed ($p < 0.0001$). The relative risk reduction was 70% for total thrombosis and 100% for proximal thrombosis.

D. Overall Comparison Between Various Regimens Used for DVT Prophylaxis in Orthopedic Surgery

Table 8 tabulates the number of events observed in the 25 reviewed studies for patients with no treatment and for six different forms of DVT prophylaxis. The number of events for PE, major bleeding, and total mortality is too small for an adequate evaluation of the usefulness of a particular type of prophylaxis, except for UH and LMWH. Clearly, LMWH appears to be the most efficacious form of thrombosis prevention, and the incidence rates for PE and major bleeding also appear to be lower than with UH.

E. Total Versus Proximal DVT

We have been particularly interested in evaluating whether UH or LMWH reduces the incidence of proximal DVT to a larger extent than that of total DVT, because fatal PE is much more common in patients with thrombosis of larger veins. If one considers the phlebographic findings in untreated patients of the three studies undertaken with strong methodology (every patient had mandatory bilateral ascending phlebography), the following incidences of total and proximal thromboses, respectively, were found: 51.3% and 23.1% (28), 45.4%and 36.1% (54), and 56.6% and 25.3% (31), resulting in a mean incidence of 51.1% total and 29.4% proximal DVT. The proportion of proximal/total DVT is thus a very high 57.4%. We were also struck by the finding that in several of the studies comparing LMWH or a heparinoid with UH, the total DVT rate observed was not significantly lower with LMWH than with UH (Table 9), but that of proximal DVT was. This applies to the studies of Eriksson et al. (34), Leyvraz et al. (36), and to the GHAT trial (35). The average relative risk reduction using LMWH was only 21% for total, but 54.9% for proximal DVT in the studies listed in Table 9. It can thus be legitimately argued whether one should not include, as the primary end-point, *proximal* DVT in all further medium-sized studies on the prophylaxis of postoperative DVT, since thrombi in the femoral, the iliac, and to a lesser extent the popliteal veins are of much greater concern to the orthopedic surgeons than calf vein thrombi. Table 10 summarizes the mean incidences of proximal/total DVT in untreated controls (from Table 2) and in patients in

Table 8 Number of Events in Orthopedic Surgery in Response to the Administration of Various Prophylactic Regimens

Regimen	# and % of DVT	# and % PE	Major bleeding	Total mortality
Placebo				
# events	193	4	8	6
# patients	378	410	318	410
% of events	**51.1**	i.n.	i.n.	i.n.
Dextran				
# events	105	7	2	8
# patients	324	195	370	321
% of events	**32.4**	i.n.	i.n.	i.n.
Rel. risk reduction	**37%**			
UH + DHE				
# events	113	2	4	2
# patients	353	371	371	316
% of events	**32.0**	i.n.	i.n.	i.n.
Rel. risk reduction	**37%**			
LMWH + DHE				
# events	62	1	2	4
# patients	247	250	250	195
% of events	**25.1**	i.n.	i.n.	i.n.
Rel. risk reduction	**51%**			
UH				
# events	219	32	38	10
# patients	922	1025	1065	1065
% of events	**23.8**	**3.0**	**3.6**	**0.9**
Rel. risk reduction	**53%**			
Oral anticoagulation				
# events	28	1	5	7
# patients	131	131	131	131
% of events	**21.4**	i.n.	i.n.	i.n.
Rel. risk reduction	**58%**			
LMWH				
# events	333	22	42	19
# patients	1880	1883	2046	2085
% of events	**17.7**	**1.2**	**2.1**	**0.9**
Rel. risk reduction	**65%**			

i.n. = insufficient number of events to calculate percentages.

Table 9 Total Versus Proximal DVT in Patients Treated with LMWH or UH: Phlebographic Studies in Elective Hip Surgery

	# of patients		# and (%) of total DVT			# and (%) of proximal DVT		
Author, year	LMWH	UH	LMWH	UH	P	LMWH	UH	P
Planes, '88 (32)	120	108	15 (12.5)	27 (25)	0.03	9 (7.5)	20 (18.5)	0.01
Levine, '91 (33)	258	263	50 (19.5)	61 (23.2)	n.s.	14 (5.4)	17 (6.5)	n.s.
Eriksson, '91 (34)	63	59	19 (30.2)	25 (42.4)	0.19	6 (9.5)	18 (31.5)	0.01
GHAT, '92 (35)	136	137	45 (33.1)	47 (34.3)	0.46	14 (10.3)	27 (19.7)	0.04
Barre, '87 (38)	38	38	7 (18.4)	3 (7.9)	0.17	2 (5.3)	1 (2.6)	0.5
Dechavanne, '89 (39)	77	38	5 (6.5)	4 (10.5)	n.s.	2 (2.6)	3 (7.9)	n.s.
Leyvraz, '91 (36)	174	175	22 (12.6)	28 (16)	0.45	5 (2.9)	23 (13.1)	<0.001
Total	866	818	163	195		52	109	
Percent			18.8	23.8		6.0	13.3	

The first four studies used fixed doses of UH; the last three studies used dose-adjusted UH.

Table 10 Percentage of Proximal DVT in Elective Hip Surgery in Untreated Controls and After UH and LMWH Prophylaxis

	Number of cases with DVT		
Patient group	Total	Proximal	% proximal
Untreated controls	120	69	57.5
Unfractionated heparin	195	109	54.4
Low-molecular-weight heparins and heparinoids	163	52	31.9

Figures were derived from studies listed in Tables 2 and 9.

whom UH was compared with LMWH (from Table 9). It is noteworthy that the administration of UH reduced the proportion of proximal DVT from 57.5% to only 54.4%, but that treatment with LMWH lowered this ratio to 31.9%. We also calculated the proximal/total DVT ratio in all trials reported in this review using LMWH as one of the comparative treatments and arrived at the slightly higher figure of 38% (Table 11). We believe that this important aspect of thromboembolic prophylaxis has so far not received the attention it merits.

F. Clinical Trial in Ambulatory Patients

The convenience of having to inject LMWH only once a day makes these preparations suitable for thromboprophylaxis in outpatients. We found only one randomized study that compared the efficacy of LMWH to no treatment (55). A total of 204 patients who required immobilization with a plaster cast because of injury to the lower extremity were included. The treatment group received one daily injection of 3075 IU of Fraxiparine. Real-time ultrasonography was performed when the cast was removed. Patients with positive scans underwent phlebography. The incidence of DVT was 6% in the Fraxiparin group and 17% in the control group ($p < 0.05$). Excluding those patients with fractures of the leg, the difference was still significant: 2 of 72 patients (2.8%) treated with Fraxiparine but 8 of 70 controls (11.4%) developed DVT ($r < 0.05$).

VI. SHOULD LMWH DOSES BE ADJUSTED ACCORDING TO THE PATIENT'S WEIGHT?

Vitoux et al. have clearly established a highly significant ($r = -68; p < 0.001$) negative relationship between ex vivo anti-factor Xa activity and the patient's body weight after the injection of a fixed dose of 3075 IU of Fraxiparine (56). In the GHAT study, the DVT incidence in patients >70 kg, receiving a mean daily

Table 11 Total Versus Proximal DVT in Patients Undergoing Elective Hip Surgery Who Were Treated with LMWH: Phlebographic Studies

Author, year	# of patients	# and (%) of DVT Total	Proximal	% proximal/total
Turpie, '86 (28)	37	4 (10.8)	2 (5.4)	50
Barre, '87 (38)	38	7 (18.4)	3 (7.9)	43
Planes, '88 (32)	120	15 (12.5)	9 (7.5)	60
Eriksson, '88 (40)	49	10 (20.4)	0 (0)	0
Mätsch, '88 (41)	47	13 (27.7)	6 (12.8)	46
Dechavanne, '89 (39)	77	5 (6.5)	2 (2.6)	40
Lassen, '91 (30)	93	29 (31.2)	24 (25.8)	83
Levine, '91 (33)	258	50 (19.4)	14 (5.4)	28
Eriksson, '91 (34)	63	19 (30.2)	6 (9.5)	32
Leyvraz, '91 (36)	174	22 (12.6)	5 (2.9)	23
DES group, '91 (43)	108	7 (6.5)	2 (1.8)	29
Hoek, '92 (31)	97	15 (15.5)	8 (8.2)	53
GHAT group, '92 (35)	136	45 (33.1)	14 (10.3)	31
Leyvraz, '92 (47)	145	25 (17.2)	7 (4.8)	28
Total	1442	266 (18.5)	102 (7.1)	38

dose of 53 IU/kg of Fraxiparine, was 38%, whereas only 25% of those with a weight <70 kg (mean daily dose 67 IU/kg) developed DVT. Adapting the dose of a LMWH renders thromboprophylaxis somewhat more complicated and is probably not necessary in general surgery. In orthopedic surgery, one might argue that an additional effort is warranted to optimize DVT prevention. The studies reviewed here do not provide sufficient information to answer the question whether weight adjustment of LMWH will improve the benefit/side effect ratio. We tabulated the three studies using weight-adjusted LMWH in one treatment arm (30,36,41) and arrived at a DVT incidence of 20.4% (64/314 patients), a figure that is quite similar to the mean DVT rate of 17.7% shown in Table 8. Only 1 of 352 patients in these three studies, an incidence of 0.3%, had major bleeding, which compares favorably with the figure of 2.1% recorded in Table 8. More clinical studies are definitely needed before any clear conclusion can be drawn concerning this question.

VII. ARE LABORATORY TESTS NECESSARY TO MONITOR THE IN VIVO ACTIVITY OF LMWHs?

This question relates in some way to that dealing with dosage adjustments according to the weight of the patient. The most widely used laboratory test for assessing LMWH concentrations in vivo is a chromogenic assay measuring the plasma's ability, in the presence of UH, LMWH, or heparinoids, to neutralize the activity of exogenously added activated factor Xa. In animal experiments, a clear dose-response relationship was observed between plasma anti-factor Xa activity and antithrombotic effect of LMWHs, on the one hand, and bleeding, on the other hand (reviewed in 57). These studies do not prove that anti-factor Xa activities are causally related to the antithrombotic or hemorrhage-producing effect in humans; they may just be a marker of some other biological activity. In several early studies, using very high doses of LMWH, a high number of peri- and postoperative bleeding in association with high anti-factor Xa levels has been reported. Levine et al. determined the anti-factor Xa levels in 163 patients undergoing elective hip surgery who were treated with 3200 IU, respectively 4800 IU of enoxaparin, given once daily (57). Blood was taken 12 hr after the evening injection on days 0, 1, 3, and 6. When the mean anti-factor Xa activity was ≤0.05 unit/ml, no postoperative wound hematomas were observed, but the risk of developing DVT was 23%. Conversely, when the mean anti-factor Xa activity exceeded 0.2 unit/ml, the risk of thrombosis was decreased to 3.3%, but the risk of hematomas increased to 30%. This carefully conducted study, which seems to suggest that anti-factor Xa levels should be measured 12 hr after injection of enoxaparin to adjust the dose to obtain plasma anti-Xa concentrations between 0.05 and 0.2 unit/ml, unfortunately has not attempted to correlate anti-Xa levels with body weight. We do not know, therefore, if high levels of anti-Xa occurred mainly in patients with low body weight, and vice versa.

LMWHs are excreted into the urine and consequently clearance is reduced in patients with renal failure. We believe that in certain, selected patients monitoring of anti-Xa activity might be warranted, such as in patients with renal failure, in those with a history of bleeding diathesis, and in those who have had recurrent episodes of thromboembolic complications. In the large majority of patients, monitoring of LWWH plasma activity is not necessary in our opinion.

VIII. CONCLUSION

In orthopedic surgery of the hip, the most efficacious, presently available thromboprophylaxis is obtained with LMWHs or the heparinoid Lomoparan. The incidence of total thrombosis is only slightly lower compared to other efficacious regimens, such as thrice-daily injections of UH with or without DHE and oral anticoagulation. However, the incidences of proximal thrombosis and of PE appear to be lower and that of major bleeding complications comparable to the treatment with low-dose UH.

In orthopedic surgery of the knee, LMWH provided effective prophylaxis in one study. More data are needed to determine whether LMWHs can be recommended as a treatment of choice in this condition.

REFERENCES

1. Haake DA, Berkman SA. Clin Orthop 1989; 242:212.
2. Clagett GP, Jr, Anderson FA, Levine MN, Salzman EW, Wheeler HB. Chest 1992; 102 (Suppl):391S.
3. Hull R, Delmore TJ, Hirsh J, et al. Thromb Res 1979; 16:37.
4. McKenna R, Galante J, Bachmann F, Wallace DL, Kaushal SP. Br Med J 1980; 1:514.
5. Lynch AF, Bourne RB, Rorabeck CH. J Bone Joint Surg 1988; 70:11.
6. Morris GK. Lancet 1980; 2:572.
7. Laverick MD, Croal SA, Mollan RAB. Br Med J 1991; 303:549.
8. Collins R, Scrimgeour A, Yusuf S, Peto R. N Engl J Med 1988; 318:1162.
9. Planès A, Vochelle N, Fagola M. J Bone Joint Surg 1990; 72-B:9.
10. Eriksson BI, Hultman E, Martinell S, Eriksson E, Tengborn L, Risberg B. Thromb Res 1991; 62:441.
11. Giercksky KE, Bjørklid E, Prydz H, Renck H. Eur Surg Res 1979; 11:296.
12. Mammen EF. Diagnose & Labor 1988; 38:93.
13. Hoek JA, Nurmohamed MT, ten Cate JW, et al. Thromb Haemost 1989; 62:1050.
14. Giercksky KE. Scand J Haematol 1977; 19:385.
15. Modig J, Busch C, Olerud S, Saldeen T. Acta Anaesthesiol Scand 1975; 18:133.
16. Jørgensen PS, Knudsen JB, Broeng L, et al. Clin Orthop 1992; 278:95.
17. Heijboer H, ten Cate JW, Büller HR. Semin Thromb Hemost 1991; 17(Suppl 3):259.
18. Büller HR, Lensing AWA, Hirsh J, ten Cate JW. Thromb Haemost 1991; 66:133.
19. Cruickshank MK, Levine MN, Hirsh J. Thromb Haemost 1989; 62:830.
20. Anderson DR, Lensing WA, Wells PS, Levine MN, Weitz JI, Hirsh J. Ann Intern Med 1993; 118:25.
21. Prandoni P, Lensing AWA, Huisman MV, et al. Thromb Haemost 1991; 65:229.
22. Agnelli G, Volpato R, Radicchia S, et al. Thromb Haemost 1992; 68:257.

23. Davidson BL, Elliott CG, Lensing AWA. Ann Intern Med 1992; 117:735.
24. Lensing AWA, Büller HR, Prandoni P, et al. Thromb Haemost 1992; 67:8.
25. Wille-Jørgensen P, Borris L, Jørgensen LN, et al. Acta Radiol 1992; 33:24.
26. Nurmohamed MT, Rosendaal FR, Büller HR, et al. Lancet 1992; 340:152.
27. Leizorovicz A, Haugh MC, Chapuis F-R, Samama MM, Boissel J-P. Br Med J 1992; 305:913.
28. Turpie AGG, Levine MN, Hirsh J, et al. N Engl J Med 1986; 315:925.
29. Tørholm C, Broeng L, Jørgensen PS, et al. J Bone Joint Surg 1991; 73-B:434.
30. Lassen MR, Borris LC, Christiansen HM, et al. Acta Orthop Scand 1991; 62:33.
31. Hoek JA, Nurmohamed MT, Hamelynck KJ, et al. Thromb Haemost 1992; 67:28.
32. Planes A, Vochelle N, Mazas F, et al. Thromb Haemost 1988; 60:407.
33. Levine MN, Hirsh J, Gent M, et al. Ann Intern Med 1991; 114:545.
34. Eriksson BI, Kälebo P, Anthmyr BA, Wadenvik H, Tengborn L, Risberg B. J Bone Joint Surg 1991; 73-A:484.
35. van de Loo J, for the German Hip Arthroplasty Trial (GHAT) group. Arch Orthop Trauma Surg 1992; 111:110.
36. Leyvraz PF, Bachmann F, Hoek J, et al. Br Med J 1991; 303:543.
37. Leyvraz PF, Richard J, Bachmann F, et al. N Engl J Med 1983; 309:954.
38. Barre J, Pfister G, Potron G, et al. J Mal Vasc 1987; 12:90.
39. Dechavanne M, Ville D, Berruyer M, et al. Haemostasis 1989; 1:5.
40. Eriksson BI, Zachrisson BE, Teger-Nilsson A-C, Risberg B. Br J Surg 1988; 76:1053.
41. Mätzsch T, Bergqvist D, Fredin H, Hedner U. Acta Chir Scand 1988; (Suppl 543):80.
42. Mätzsch T, Bergqvist D, Fredin H, Hedner U. Acta Chir Scand 1990; 156:445.
43. Danish Enoxaparin Study Group. Arch Intern Med 1991; 151:1621.
44. Weber U, Koppenhagen K, Mälzer H, Matthes M. Langenbecks Arch Chir 1991; 376:147.
45. Lassen MR, Borris LC, Christiansen HM, et al. Br J Surg 1988; 75:686.
46. Freick H, Haas S. Thromb Res 1991; 63:133.
47. Leyvraz P-F, Bachmann F, Bohnet J, et al. Br J Surg 1992; 79:911.
48. Gerhart TN, Yett HS, Robertson LK, Lee MA, Smith M, Salzman EW. J Bone Joint Surg 1991; 73-A:494.
49. Pini M, Tagliaferri A, Manotti C, Lasagni F, Rinaldi E, Dettori AG. Int Angiol 1989; 8:134.
50. Monreal M, Lafoz E, Navarro A, et al. J Trauma 1989; 29:873.
51. Bergqvist D, Kettunen K, Fredin H, et al. Surgery 1991; 109:617.
52. Lassen MR, Borris LC, Christiansen HM, et al. Arch Orthop Trauma Surg 1989; 108:10.
53. Leclerc JR, Geerts WH, Desjardins L, et al. Thromb Haemost 1992; 67:417.
54. Saksela O, Hovi T, Vaheri A. J Cell Physiol 1985; 122:125.
55. Kujath P, Spannagel U, Habscheid W, Schindler G, Weckbach A. Dtsch Med Wochenschr 1992; 117:6.
56. Vitoux JF, Aiach M, Roncato M, Fiessinger JN. Thromb Haemost 1988; 59:120.
57. Levine MN, Planes A, Hirsh J, Goodyear M, Vochelle N, Gent M. Thromb Haemost 1989; 62:940.

10

Low-Molecular-Weight Heparins and Heparinoids for Prevention of Venous Thromboembolism in Stroke and Neurosurgical Patients

Alexander G. G. Turpie
McMaster University and Hamilton General Hospital, Hamilton, Ontario, Canada

I. INTRODUCTION

Venous thromboembolism (VTE) is a common and serious complication in patients following neurosurgical procedures, after spinal cord trauma, and following stroke that results in lower limb paralysis. The rates of VTE in neurosurgical and stroke patients are summarized in Table 1. These patients fall into the moderate- to high-risk category for deep vein thrombosis (DVT) and pulmonary embolism (PE) as defined by the Consensus Development Conference of the National Heart Lung and Blood Institute (1), the Thromboembolic Risk Factors (THRIFT) Consensus Group (2), and the European Consensus Statement (3). The risk of VTE is increased by a number of clinical factors, including increasing age, obesity, malignant disease, heart disease, prolonged immobility or lower limb paralysis, use of oral contraceptives, and a history of prior VTE. In addition, a number of the risk factors for DVT may coexist and multiply the risk (4, 5).

II. NEUROSURGERY

DVT and PE are common causes of morbidity and mortality in neurosurgical patients. The incidence of DVT detected by ^{125}I-labeled fibrinogen leg scanning and impedance plethysmography (IPG) in neurosurgical patients has been reported in a number of carefully performed studies to be between 20% and 30% (6–9). In the absence of prophylaxis, fatal PE occurs in approximately 1% of neurosurgical patients (10, 11). Because of the high frequency of VTE in neurosurgery, several methods for preventing DVT following neurosurgery have

Table 1 Venous Thromboembolism in Stroke and Neurosurgery

	DVT (%)	Prox. DVT (%)	Fatal PE (%)
Stroke	30–75	10–20	1.2
Neurosurgery	20–30	5–10	0.5–1
CNS trauma	20–30	7–10	0.1–1
Spinal cord trauma	80–100	15–20	0.5–1

Prox. = proximal; CNS = central nervous system.

been evaluated and shown to be effective. The most widely accepted methods in neurosurgery are the physical methods, including graduated compression stockings or intermittent pneumatic compression devices (IPC) because they are not associated with any bleeding risk (12). Anticoagulant prophylaxis with low-dose heparin is highly effective in general surgical patients, but the use of anticoagulants in neurosurgical patients is problematic because of the potential for serious bleeding, and although there are a number of reports demonstrating the efficacy of low-dose heparin in this patient group, its use is not widely accepted. The evaluation of low-molecular-weight heparins (LMWH) for thromboprophylaxis in neurosurgery has been limited to descriptive studies involving only small numbers of patients. To date, there have been no well-designed, randomized trials of LMWH prophylaxis in neurosurgery involving the brain. An additional unresolved problem regarding thrombosis prophylaxis in neurosurgery is the duration of treatment since many patients are immobilized for prolonged periods and remain at risk.

A. Physical Methods

The main attraction of physical methods of prophylaxis in neurosurgical patients is that they are free of the potential for hemorrhagic side effects.

Intermittent pneumatic compression is an effective method of prophylaxis in both general surgical patients and neurosurgical patients (6, 7, 8, 12). Despite its demonstrated efficacy, IPC is not widely used for the prevention of DVT in neurosurgical patients, possibly because of the perception that it is inconvenient to both patients and nursing staff. Graduated compression stockings, which are much easier to use, are also effective in the prevention of DVT in general surgical patients (13–17). In one study in neurosurgical patients, graduated compression stockings alone were as effective as graduated compression stockings plus IPC for the prevention of venous thrombosis. In this study, the frequency of DVT detected by fibrinogen leg scanning and IPG was 8.8% in the graduated compression stocking alone group, 9.0% in the stockings plus IPC group, and 19.8% in

Table 2 Prevention of Deep Vein Thrombosis in Neurosurgery

Study	Modality	Control	Treatment	p
Turpie et al., 1977 (6)	Intermittent calf compression	12/63 (19.1%)	1/65 (5%)	0.0008
Skillman et al., 1978 (7)	Intermittent calf compression	12/48 (25.0%)	4/47 (8.5%)	<0.05
Turpie et al., 1979 (8)	Sequential pneumatic compression	20/96 (20.8%)	8/103 (7.8%)	0.01
Turpie et al., 1989 (18)	Graduated compression stockings	16/81 (19.8%)	7/80 (8.8%)	0.023
	Graduated compression stockings plus intermittent pneumatic compression	16/81 (19.8%)	7/78 (9.0%)	0.27

the control group. However, the risk of DVT after IPC was discontinued appeared to be increased, suggesting that the combined treatment may be better than graduated compression stockings alone (18). The results of the four randomized trials of IPC in the prevention of DVT in neurosurgery are shown in Table 2.

In a recent nonrandomized trial (19) involving 138 consecutive patients undergoing major neurosurgical procedures, intermittent pneumatic compression followed by postoperative subcutaneous heparin was reported to be associated with very low risk of DVT without increasing the risk of bleeding. This two-step approach of perioperative prophylaxis by physical methods followed by anticoagulant prophylaxis warrants further study since it reduces the risk of bleeding at the time of greatest risk.

B. Low-Dose Heparin

There have been few reports on the use of low-dose heparin prophylaxis in neurosurgical patients. Powers and Edwards (20), in a review of the low-dose heparin studies, concluded that low-dose heparin was indicated in all patients undergoing elective neurosurgical procedures and that the regimen was efficacious and safe. However, the studies were too small to exclude the possibility that heparin might result in clinically important bleeding, including intracranial bleeding. In addition, the studies included only a small number of patients who had intracranial surgery. Thus, low-dose heparin is not widely used in neurosurgical patients because of the concern regarding the risk of bleeding, particularly in patients in whom intracranial surgery is performed.

C. Low-Molecular-Weight Heparin

Experience with LMWH in neurosurgery is limited and mainly involves patients undergoing surgery to the axial skeleton. There are no reports of randomized trials of LMWH in intracranial neurosurgery. In a recent prospective randomized trial (21), LMWH (1500 aPPT units) was compared with standard unfractionated heparin (5000 units every 8 hr) for the prevention of venous thrombosis in patients undergoing microneurosurgical lumbar disease procedures and found to be as effective and safe as the standard treatment, with very low rates of DVT or PE clinically detected in each group.

A number of large-scale randomized trials of LMWH in the prevention of venous thromboembolism in neurosurgical patients are underway but the results are not yet available.

III. SPINAL CORD TRAUMA

Venous thrombosis has been reported to occur in 15–60% of patients with spinal cord injuries, depending on the severity of the injury, the presence of lower limb paralysis, and the presence of other associated risk factors. (4, 5, 22). The reported incidence of fatal PE has ranged from 2% to 16% of patients within 2–3 months of spinal cord injury (22). The majority of the reports indicate that venous thrombosis in spinal cord injury patients occurs most commonly early after injury during the period of flaccidity, but a significant number of DVT occur late. To cover the early period of risk, mechanical methods of prophylaxis are generally recommended.

A. Physical Methods

There are few reports on the use of physical methods of DVT prophylaxis in spinal-cord-injured patients, and most have involved small numbers of patients or were not randomized. Most of the data on IPC or graduated compression stockings are derived from subgroups from randomized studies in neurosurgery, none of which involved sufficient numbers of patients with spinal cord injury to provide meaningful comparisons (6, 7, 8, 22).

B. Low-Dose Heparin

Because of the evidence for the efficacy of low-dose heparin prophylaxis in general surgical and medical patients without increased risk of significant haemorrhage, low-dose heparin has been proposed as the method of preventing DVT in spinal-cord-injured patients. There have been several reports on the use of low-dose heparin in spinal-cord-injured patients, but these studies have been nonrandomized and involved only small numbers of patients (23–25). In one study using retrospective controls, there was a highly significant reduction in the frequency of DVT in spinal-cord-injured patients, using objective tests to diagnose DVT (25). In none of the studies was a significant increase in bleeding reported. In one randomized controlled trial involving 32 patients with spinal cord injury, the frequency of venous thrombosis was unexpectedly low in both the control and heparinized groups, but in this study, only impedance plethysmography was used to detect DVT, which would be insensitive to calf vein thrombi and nonoccluding proximal thrombi (26), and thus the frequency of DVT would be underestimated. A recent study (27) compared fixed with adjusted-dose heparin in 58 patients with complete motor paralysis. One-half the patients were randomized to receive 5000 U of heparin twice daily, and the remainder received sufficient heparin (on average 14,300 U every 12 hr) to prolong their activated partial thromboplastin times to 1.5 times the normal control value. Nine patients receiving the fixed dose but only two receiving the adjusted dose developed venous thrombosis ($p < 0.05$). However, bleeding necessitating withdrawal of prophylaxis occurred in seven patients treated with the higher dose but in none receiving the low-dose regimen ($p < 0.02$). Although there are limited data on anticoagulant prophylaxis following spinal cord trauma, most authors recommend heparin or oral anticoagulant prophylaxis for 3 months started after the period of risk for bleeding (17, 23–25).

C. Low-Molecular-Weight Heparin

LMWH have great potential in the prevention of venous thromboembolism in spinal-cord-injured patients. In a recent study (28), a LMWH (Logiparin) was compared with low-dose unfractionated heparin for the prevention of DVT in spinal-cord-injured patients. Twenty-one patients were randomized to receive standard heparin and 20 patients to receive LMWH. Five patients in the standard heparin group had thrombotic events, including two patients who had fatal pulmonary embolism; two other patients had bleeding severe enough to necessitate discontinuing the heparin. The cumulative rate of adverse events (venous thromboembolism and bleeding) in the heparin group was 34.7% (95% CI, 13.7–55.2%) and none in the patients treated with LMWH (CI, 0–14%); the difference between the two groups was significant ($p = 0.006$). The results of this small study suggest that LMWH may be safe and effective in the prevention of thromboembolism in patients with spinal cord injury and is superior to standard heparin when given in doses of 5000 units three times per day. However, more extensive experience with LMWH in spinal-cord-injured patients is required before it can be recommended for routine use.

IV. STROKE

Venous thromboembolism is a common complication in patients with acute ischaemic stroke. Without prophylaxis, DVT occurs, usually in the paralyzed limb, in 60–75% of patients with dense hemiplegia (29, 30), and 1–2% suffer fatal pulmonary embolism (31).

A. Low-Dose Heparin

Several methods of preventing DVT have been shown to be safe and effective in other high-risk medical patients, and of these, low-dose subcutaneous heparin has been the most extensively evaluated (32). Three randomized trials using low-dose heparin prophylaxis in patients with acute stroke have been reported. In two studies, heparin given subcutaneously in doses of 5000 units every 8 hr reduced the frequency of DVT from 75% of 16 patients to 13% of 16 patients (30) and from 73% of 161 patients to 22% of 144 patients (33) in the placebo- and heparin-treated groups, respectively. In the third study (34), a combination of low-dose heparin, 5000 units with dihydroergotamine (DHE) subcutaneously every 12 hr reduced the frequency of DVT from 56% of 41 patients in the placebo-treated group of 28% of 40 patients in the combined heparin/DHE group. Despite the demonstration in all three studies of a significant benefit of treatment, low-dose heparin is not widely used in stroke patients because of concern about a possible increased risk of intracranial hemorrhage. In addition, the rates of venous thrombosis in patients with paralytic stroke remain high even with low-dose heparin prophylaxis.

B. Low-Molecular-Weight Heparin or Heparinoid

Experience of DVT prophylaxis with LMWH in stroke patients is limited. There have been two studies using LMWH for the prevention of DVT in patients with ischemic stroke (35, 36). The results of these studies are conflicting. The first study compared LMWH in a dose of 2500 anti-factor Xa units twice a day with placebo and demonstrated a reduction in the rate of venous thrombosis from 50% to 22% (35). In the second study (36), LMWH was given in a dose of 50–65 units/kg body weight once daily (equivalent to 3500–4550 anti-factor Xa units daily), but in contrast to the first study, there was no difference in the frequency of DVT in the LMWH-treated patients (36%) compared with the placebo-treated patients (34%).

A low-molecular-weight heparinoid (Orgaran) has been shown to be effective in preventing venous thrombosis in high-risk surgical patients without significant bleeding risk and has been evaluated for the prevention of DVT in patients with acute ischemic stroke in two studies. In a double-blind, placebo-controlled study (37), 75 patients were randomized to receive LMWH (50 patients) in a loading dose of 1000 anti-Xa units intravenously followed by 750 anti-Xa units subcutaneously every 12 hr or placebo (25 patients). Prophylaxis was commenced within 7 days of stroke onset and continued for 14 days or until discharge from hospital, if earlier. Venous thrombosis was diagnosed by ^{125}I-labeled fibrinogen leg scanning and impedance plethysmography. DVT, confirmed by venography, occurred in 2 of 50 (4%) in the LMW heparinoid group and 7 of 25 (28%) in the placebo group ($p = 0.005$). The corresponding rates for proximal DVT were 0% and 16%, respectively ($p = 0.01$). There was one major hemorrhage in the LMW heparinoid-treated group and one minor hemorrhage in the placebo group. Plasma heparin levels (anti-factor Xa units/ml: mean $\pm$ SED) gradually rose from 0.18 $\pm$ 0.001 and 0.06 $\pm$ 0.001, 6 and 12 hr after injection on the first day, to 0.24 $\pm$ 0.02 and 0.12 $\pm$ 0.01, respectively, after 11 days of treatment. The results of the placebo-controlled trial demonstrate that LMW heparinoid is highly effective in the prevention of DVT in stroke patients without causing bleeding.

In the second study (38), the safety and efficacy of LMW heparinoid was compared with unfractionated heparin in the prevention of DVT in a double-blind, randomized trial in patients with acute thrombotic stroke. Eighty-seven patients with marked lower limb paralysis secondary to stroke were randomized to receive LMW heparinoid (45 patients) in a dose of 750 anti-factor Xa units

Table 3 Rates of DVT in Prophylaxis Trials in Stroke

	Placebo (%)	Heparin (%)	LMWH (%)	LMW heparinoid (%)
Warlow et al., 1972 (29)	60	—	—	—
McCarthy et al., 1977 (30)	75	12	—	—
Czechanowski and Heinrich, 1981 (34)	56	28[a]	—	—
McCarthy and Turner, 1986 (33)	73	22	—	—
Turpie et al., 1987 (37)	28	—	—	4
Prins et al., 1989 (35)	50	—	22	—
Sandset et al., 1990 (36)	34	—	36	—
Turpie et al., 1992 (38)	—	31	—	9

[a] Plus DHE.

subcutaneously every 12 hr or unfractionated heparin (42 patients) in a dose of 5000 units subcutaneously every 12 hr. Prophylaxis was commenced within 5 days of stroke onset on average and continued for 14 days. Venous thrombosis surveillance was carried out with ^{125}I-labeled fibrinogen leg scanning and impedance plethysmography confirmed by ascending venography. Venous thrombosis occurred in 4 of 45 (8.9%) of the LMW heparinoid group and 13 of 42 (31%) in the unfractionated heparin group ($2p = 0.02$). The corresponding rates for proximal vein thrombosis were 2.2% and 11.9%, respectively ($2p = 0.17$). There were no clinically significant hemorrhagic complications in either group, and the frequency of hemorrhagic conversion of the infarct was 6.9% overall with no difference in the incidence between the two treatment groups ($p > 0.1$). The results of this study indicate that LMW heparinoid is more effective prophylaxis against DVT than conventional low-dose subcutaneous heparin in patients with acute stroke. The rates of DVT in the studies of prophylaxis in ischemic stroke patients are shown in Table 3.

V. CONCLUSION

Additional studies with LMWH in the prevention of neurosurgical and stroke patients are required to determine the efficacy and safety of this approach. The limited experience to date indicates that the LMWHs and heparinoids have great potential in these patients.

REFERENCES

1. National Institutes of Health Consensus Development Conference Statement. Prevention of venous thrombosis and pulmonary embolism. JAMA 1986; 256(6):744–749.
2. Thromboembolic Risk Factors (THRIFT) Consensus Group. Risk of and prophylaxis for venous thromboembolism in hospital patients. Br Med J 1992; 305(6853):567–574.
3. European Consensus Statement. Prevention of venous thromboembolism. Int Angiol 1992; 11(3):151–159.
4. Hull RD. Venous thromboembolism in spinal cord injury patients. Chest 1992; 102(6):658S–663S.
5. Weingarden SI. Deep venous thrombosis in spinal cord injury. Overview of the problem. Chest 1992; 102(6):636S–639S.
6. Turpie AGG, Gallus AS, Beattie WS, et al. Prevention of venous thrombosis in patients with intracranial disease by intermittent pneumatic compression of the calf. Neurology 1977; 5:435–438.
7. Skillman JJ, Collins EC, Coe NP, et al. Prevention of deep vein thrombosis in neurosurgical patients: a controlled randomized trial of external pneumatic compression boots. Surgery 1978; 83:354–358.
8. Turpie AGG, Delmore T, Hirsh J, et al. Prevention of venous thrombosis by intermittent sequential calf compression in patients with intracranial disease. Thromb Res 1979; 15:611–616.
9. Turpie AGG, Gent M, Doyle DJ, et al. An evaluation of suloctidil in the prevention of deep vein thrombosis in neurosurgical patients. Thromb Res 1985; 39:173–181.
10. Sigel B, Ipsen J, Felix WR. The epidemiology of lower extremity deep venous thrombosis in surgical patients. Ann Surg 1974; 179:278–290.
11. Watson N. Anticoagulant therapy in the treatment of venous thrombosis and pulmonary embolism in acute spinal injury. Paraplegia 1974; 12:197–201.
12. Turpie AGG, Hirsh J. Venous thromboembolism. II. Current concepts. Hosp Med November 1984; pp 13–41.
13. Holford CP. Graded compression for preventing deep venous thrombosis. Br Med J 1976; 2:969–970.
14. Scurr JH, Ibrahim SZ, Faber RG, et al. The efficacy of graduated compression stockings in the prevention of deep vein thrombosis. Br J Surg 1977; 64:371–373.
15. Allan A, Williams JT, Bolton JP, et al. The use of graduated compression stockings in the prevention of postoperative deep vein thrombosis. Br J Surg 1983; 70:172–174.
16. Bergqvist D, Lindblad B. The thromboprophylactic effect of graded elastic compression stockings in combination with dextran 70. Arch Surg 1984; 119:1329–1331.
17. Colditz GA, Tuden RL, Oster G. Rates of venous thrombosis after general surgery: combined results of randomized clinical trials. Lancet 1986; 2:143–146.
18. Turpie AGG, Hirsh J, Gent M, Julian D, Johnson J. Prevention of deep vein thrombosis in potential neurosurgical patients: a randomized trial comparing graduated compression stockings alone or graduated compression stockings plus intermittent pneumatic compression with control. Arch Intern Med 1989; 149:679–681.
19. Frim DM, Barker FG, Poletti CE, Hamilton AJ. Postoperative low-dose heparin

decreases thromboembolic complications in neurosurgical patients. Neurosurgery 1992; 30(6):830–832.
20. Powers SK, Edwards MSB. Prophylaxis of thromboembolism in the neurological patient: a review. 1982; Neurosurgery 10:509–513.
21. Prestar FJ. Prevention of thromboembolism with low-molecular weight heparin in micro-neurosurgery of lumbar disc disease. Neurochirurgia 1992; 1:35.
22. Turpie AGG. Thrombosis prevention and treatment in spinal cord injured patients. In: Bloch RF, Basbaum M, eds. Spinal Cord Rehabilitation. Baltimore: Williams & Wilkins, 1986:212–240.
23. Rocha Casas E, Sanchez MP, Arias CR, et al. Prophylaxis of venous thrombosis and pulmonary embolism in patients with acute traumatic spinal cord lesions. Paraplegia 1976; 14:178.
24. Rocha Casas E, Sanchez MP, Arias CR, et al. Prophylaxis of venous thrombosis and pulmonary embolism in patients with acute traumatic spinal cord lesions. Paraplegia 1977; 15:209.
25. Silver JR. The prophylactic use of anticoagulant therapy in the prevention of pulmonary emboli in one hundred consecutive spinal injury patients. Paraplegia 1974; 12:188.
26. Frisbie JH, Sasahara AA. Low dose heparin prophylaxis for deep venous thrombosis in acute spinal cord injury patients: a controlled study Paraplegia 1981; 19:141.
27. Green D, Lee MY, Ito VY, et al. Fixed vs adjusted-dose heparin in the prophylaxis of thromboembolism in spinal cord injury. JAMA 1988; 260:1255–1258.
28. Green D, Lee MY, Lim AC, et al. Prevention of thromboembolism after spinal cord injury using low-molecular-weight heparin. Ann Intern Med 1990; 113:571–574.
29. Warlow C, Ogston D, Douglas AS. Venous thrombosis following strokes. Lancet 1972; 1:1305–1306.
30. McCarthy ST, Robertson D, Turner JJ, Hawkey CJ. Low-dose heparin as a prophylaxis against deep vein thrombosis after acute stroke. Lancet 1977; 2:800–801.
31. Brown M, Glassenberg M. Mortality factors in patients with acute stroke. JAMA 1973; 224:1493–1495.
32. Turpie AGG, Leclerc J. Prophylaxis of venous thromboembolism. In: Leclerc J, ed. Venous Thromboembolic Disorders. 1990:303–345.
33. McCarthy ST, Turner J. Low-dose subcutaneous heparin in the prevention of deep vein thrombosis and pulmonary emboli following acute stroke. Age Ageing 1986; 15:84–88.
34. Czechanowski B, Heinrich F. Prophylaxe venoser Thrombosen bei frischem ischamischem zerebrovaskularem Indult—Doppelblind studie mit Heparin-Dihydrogot. Dtsch Med Wochenschr 1981; 106:1254–1260.
35. Prins MH, Gelsema R, Sing AK, et al. Prophylaxis of deep venous thrombosis with a low-molecular weight heparin (Kabi 2165/Fragmin) in stroke patients. Haemostas 1989; 19:245–250.
36. Sandset PM, Dahl T, Stiris M, et al. A double-blind and randomized placebo-controlled trial of low molecular weight heparin once daily to prevent deep vein thrombosis in acute ischemic stroke. Semin Thromb Hemost 1990; 16:25–33.

37. Turpie AGG, Hirsh J, Jay RM, et al. Double-blind randomized trial of ORG 10172 low-molecular weight heparinoid in prevention of deep vein thrombosis in thrombotic stroke. Lancet 1987; 1:523–526.
38. Turpie AGG, Gent M, Cote R, Levine MN, Ginsberg JS, Powers P, et al. A low-molecular-weight heparinoid compared with unfractionated heparin in the prevention of deep vein thrombosis in patients with acute ischaemic stroke. Ann Intern Med 117 1992; (5):353–357.

11

Low-Molecular-Weight Heparins for Prevention of Venous Thromboembolism in Medical Patients

Meyer M. Samama and Gregory T. Gerotziafas
Hôtel Dieu Hospital, Paris, France

I. INTRODUCTION

In daily clinical practice, medical patients frequently have one or more risk factors for thrombosis. Patients with acute myocardial infarction, heart failure, arrhythmias, thrombotic stroke, malignancy, metabolic diseases (diabetes) or peripheral vascular disease, inflammatory syndrome, autoimmune disorders associated with lupus anticoagulant and/or anticardiolipins, chronic renal or respiratory insufficiency, and patients treated with drugs such as l-asparaginase and estrogens are at risk of venous thrombosis. Moreover, age, obesity, immobilization, and paralysis all favor blood stasis and frequently lead to deep vein thrombosis (DVT) or pulmonary embolism (PE).

The prevalence of the congenital deficiency in AT III in normal persons has been estimated to be 1/5000 (0.02%) (1). The incidence in healthy individuals of congenital protein S deficiency seems of the same order of magnitude. Congenital deficiency in protein C may be slightly more frequent (2). The thromboembolic disease therefore appears to be most frequently the consequence of preexisting diseases with a heterogeneous origin. Prophylaxis of DVT and PE is crucial because thromboembolism is a frequent cause of death.

According to diverse epidemiological studies, the incidence of thromboembolic disease ranges from 18% to 23% among medical patients (3,4). The frequency of DVT or/and PE in immobilized neurological patients is even higher. DVT occurs in 60–75% of paraplegic and hemiplegic patients, usually in the paralyzed limb (5). Furthermore, 1–2% of these patients have a fatal PE (6).

During the last decades, unfractionated heparin (UFH) has been used as an effective prophylactic treatment. The introduction of low-molecular-weight heparins (LMWHs) substantially changed the prevention of thromboembolic disease. LMWHs are widely used in Europe in the prophylaxis of postoperative thromboembolism. The mean molecular weight of LMWH represents about half that of UFH—5000 daltons versus 12,000 daltons, respectively. Yet, LMWHs are still somewhat heterogeneous and seem to differ, from preparation to preparation, in some of their biological properties. Despite these differences, the existing common characteristics may represent advantages for their clinical use. Reduction of the molecular weight has the following consequences (7, 8):

An ex vivo increase of anti-Xa activity over anti-IIa activity.

A greater bioavailability due to a better absorption of LMWH fragments and a delayed clearance. According to their pharmacokinetic profile, one daily subcuteneous injection seems to be as effective as two or three daily injections of unfractionated heparin.

LMWH are more resistant to the neutralizing activity of platelet factor 4 (pf4) originating from activated platelets.

LMWH exhibit no significant proaggregating activity on platelets in the presence of ADP. Furthermore, clinical trials, mainly in surgical patients, showed that preventive antithrombotic treatment with LMWH seems to be at least as effective as that with UFH and is also better tolerated (9,10).

As LMWH has proven to be useful for prophylaxis of postoperative venous thromboembolism, a review of the trials performed in medical patients seems also of interest. Eighteen trials are analyzed in this chapter. They are quite heterogeneous as they refer to different groups of patients. We classified them, therefore, in three categories: (1) elderly patients, (2) neurological patients and (3) other medical and cardiological patients.

II. STUDIES IN ELDERLY PATIENTS

Dahan et al. (1986) (11), in a placebo-controlled, randomized, double-blind trial, studied the efficacy of a LMWH (enoxaparin) in 263 elderly patients (mean age 80 years), with diverse pathological disorders. The patients were equally divided into two groups (LMWH-treated and placebo group). According to the protocol, one subcutaneous injection of 60 mg of enoxaparin was given daily. The treatment lasted 10 days. DVT was diagnosed with ^{125}I-fibrinogen scanning. The incidence of DVT was 3% in the LMWH group versus 9.2% in the placebo group. The difference was statistically significant ($p = 0.03$). During treatment, 2.29% of patients receiving placebo died from fatal PE. Also, 0.75% of the LMWH group died from acute myocardial infarction with previous pulmonary embolism. Mortality in all patients studies was 4.5%.

In the placebo group, analysis of the risk factors for thrombosis revealed the main role of confinement to bed (19.5% of DVT occurred in this subgroup). The hemorrhagic problems in the patients treated with LMWH were limited. No severe complication was reported. Only one patient had hematoma larger than 10 cm at the site of the injection at the abdominal wall.

Àcquino et al. (1990) (12), in a prospective, comparative, randomized open trial, studied the efficacy of preventive treatment with LMWH in 99 elderly medical patients older than 70 years. The patients were equally divided into two groups. One group was treated with calcium nadroparin (3100 anti-Xa IU, one subcutaneous injection daily) and the other group was treated with UFH (subcutaneous injection twice a day of 5000 IU or 7500 IU depending on body weight). DVT was confirmed with Doppler ultrasound and phlebography. Pulmonary embolism was assessed by clinical monitoring and lung scan perfusion studies. The duration of treatment was 10 days. The incidence of DVT was similar (2%) in both groups. In contrast, the treatment with LMWH was slightly better tolerated than that with UFH. The incidence of major hemorrhagic complications was 0% and 4% in the LMWH and UFH groups, respectively. There was no mention of deaths caused by possible side effects of the drug.

Manciet et al. (1990) (13) performed a similar randomized, double-blind clinical study including 256 elderly medical patients (mean age 84 years) divided into two equivalent groups (LMWH-and UFH-treated groups). LMWH (calcium nadroparin) was given as one subcutaneous injection of 3100 anti-Xa IU daily. UFH was given subcutaneously (5000 IU), twice per day. The duration of the treatment was 3 months. Doppler ultrasound, plethysmographic tests, and phlebography were performed for the diagnosis of DVT.

The antithrombotic action of both heparins was equal. The incidence of DVT was 0% in the LMWH group versus 0.78% in the UFH group. The incidence of bleeding was 0.79% in LMWH-treated patients versus 3.14% in UFH-treated patients. Fatal hemorrhagic accidents caused possibly by side effects of the drugs occurred in one patient of each treated group. Mortality was 6.25% for the entire series of elderly medical patients.

Bergmann (1992) (14) performed a randomized, controlled, double-blind clinical trial including 442 elderly patients (mean age 83.2 years) hospitalized for an acute medical disease inducing a recent (less than 3 days) bedridden period. The patients were equally divided into two groups (LMWH-and UFH-treated groups). LMWH (enoxaparin) was given as one subcutaneous injection of 20 mg daily. UFH was given subcutaneously (5000 IU), twice daily. The treatment lasted more than 7 days. Venous thrombosis was detected by ^{125}I-fibrinogen scanning and phelbography in 12 (5.6%) of the 226 patients receiving LMWH and in 11 (4.9%) of the 226 patients receiving UFH ($p = 0.73$). Bleeding complications and deaths were similar in the two groups. Two patients in the

LMWH group and six patients in the UFH group had to stop their treatment because of intolerance.

III. STUDIES IN NEUROLOGICAL PATIENTS

Turpie et al. (1987) (15), in a randomized, double-blind clinical trial, evaluated the effectiveness of a low-molecular-weight heparinoid (ORG 10172) in 67 patients with acute thrombotic stroke. ORG 10172 is a mixture of sulfated glycosaminoglycans derived from animal intestinal mucosa, which consists mainly of heparan sulfate and dermatan sulfate. The patients were divided into two groups (LMWH-treated and placebo). The treatment was started immediately after the onset of stroke and lasted 14 days. ORG 10172 was given intravenously at a loading dose of 1000 anti-Xa IU, followed by a subcutaneous injection of 750 anti-Xa IU every 12 hr. All patients underwent surveillance with ^{125}I-fibrinogen leg scanning, impedance plethysmography, and computed-tomography (CT) scan. Phlebography was carried out if either test became positive.

The incidence of DVT and PE was 2.27% versus 30.4% in the LMWH and placebo groups, respectively. The difference was statistically significant ($p = 0.002$). After 3 months of follow-up, 2.27% of patients in the LMWH group and 8.7% of patients in the placebo group had DVT and/or PE. A serious hemorrhagic accident occurred in one patient of the LMWH group. It was a hemorrhagic extension of the original cerebral infraction. This patient received only one dose of ORG 10172. In addition, the patient's anti-Xa plasma level was <0.1 U/ml. The bleeding might have been unrelated to treatment. Some minor bleedings occurred in the placebo group. In the LMWH group, 2.27% of the patients died of thrombosis versus 4.3% in the placebo group. The mortality was 4.4% for the entire series of patients.

Prins et al. (1987) (16), in a randomized, double-blind clinical trial, evaluated the antithrombotic efficacy of treatment with LMWH (dalteparin) in 60 elderly patients with severe acute thrombotic stroke. Treatment with two daily subcutaneous injections of 2500 anti-Xa IU was compared with placebo, in two groups of 30 patients. The treatment lasted 14 days and the patients were examined with CT scan, ^{125}I-fibrinogen scanning, and phlebography. In the LMWH-treated group, 20% of the patients developed DVT whereas in the placebo group DVT occurred in 50% of the patients, the difference being statistically significant ($p = 0.05$). Cerebral bleeding occurred in 13.3% of the patients in the LMWH group versus 6.6% of the patients in the placebo group (the difference was not statistically significant). PE occurred in one patient of the LMWH group versus two patients in the placebo group. During the trial, 30% of the patients in the LMWH-treated group and 13.3% of the placebo group died. Cause of deaths was not indicated.

Green et al. (1990) (17), in a randomized, double-blind clinical trial, controlled the efficacy of a preventive antithrombotic treatment with LMWH (logiparin) versus UFH in 41 patients with complete motor paralysis after spinal cord injury. The patients were divided into two groups. The first one received LMWH subcutaneously once a day (3500 anti-Xa IU) and the other received UFH subcutaneously every 8 hr (5000 IU). Impedance plethysmography, Doppler ultrasound, and phlebography were performed. The treatment lasted 8 weeks. In the LMWH-treated group, neither DVT nor PE occurred. In the UFH-treated group, the incidence of DVT and PE was 23.8%. In addition, 9.5% of the patients in the UFH group died from PE. Mortality was 4.8% for all patients studied. The incidence of major hemorrhages was 0% versus 9.5% in the LMWH- and UFH-treated groups, respectively. The difference in event rate is statistically significant ($p = 0.006$). Examining the frequency of thrombosis alone also yielded a significant difference ($p = 0.02$).

Sandset et al. (1990) (18), in a randomized, double-blind, controlled trial, evaluated the preventive treatment with dalteparin in 103 patients who had acute thrombotic stroke. Patients were divided into two groups (LMWH-treated and placebo). The two groups were heterogeneous regarding the delay of the treatment, from the onset of stroke to the first injection. The delay was shorter (33 hr) in the LMWH group than in the placebo group (44 hr) ($p = 0.045$). In addition, the LMWH group had more severe paresis ($p = 0.009$). The prognosis index was significantly poorer in the LMWH group. The treatment lasted 14 days. One subcutaneous injection of LMWH was given. The dose was adjusted to body weight and ranged from 3000 to 5500 anti-Xa IU daily. Clinical examination, CT scan, phlebography of the paretic limb, B-mode ultrasound scanning, and plethysmography were performed for screening for DVT.

The frequency of total thromboembolism was 36% [95% confidence interval (CI) 22–52%] in the LMWH group and 34% (21–49%) in the placebo group. The relative probability ratio for DVT of the LMWH group to placebo was 1.06 (95% CI 0.60–1.85%). The incidence of proximal DVT was 12% (95% CI 4–26%) versus 16% (95% CI 7–29%) in the LMWH and placebo groups, respectively. No severe bleeding complications were mentioned, whereas hemorrhagic transformation of the infarction occurred in 8% of the LMWH patients versus 6% under placebo. In the LMWH group the mortality rate was 10% and 7.6% of deaths were due to thrombotic events. In the placebo group, the mortality rate was 2% and the deaths were due to thromboembolism. Analysis of the points of heterogeneity between the two groups showed that the degree of paresis and the delay of treatment start did not contribute to the incidence of thromboembolism. In addition, thromboembolism was more frequent in patients with large cerebral lesions. However, the two groups were similar with regard to the size of the cerebral lesion. The mortality was 5.8% in the entire series of patients.

Yelnik at al. (1991) (19) studied the prevalence of DVT and PE in 147 patients with complete motor paralysis of different etiologies except neoplasia. Paralysis occurred within 48 hr of spinal cord injury, and the average time between onset of paraplegia and inclusion in the trial was 42 days. Clinical follow-up covered the entire hospital stay (an average of 6 months for paraplegics and 13 months for tetraplegics). The evaluation of prophylactic treatment was based on systematic detection of asymptomatic DVT with phlebography, which was performed between the first and the seventh day following admission in the department. A second phlebography was performed 1 month later. Among the patients, 127 received preventive anticoagulant treatment—either low dose of UFH (89 patients, 5000 IU, three subcutaneous injections daily), LMWH nadroparin (17 patients, 3100 anti-Xa IU daily), or oral anticoagulants (21 patients). The incidence of DVT on average after 45 days of the onset of paraplegia (at the time of the first phebography) was 33.4%. DVT occurred in 29% of the patients treated with UFH, in 41% of the patients treated with LMWH, in 24% of the patients treated with oral anticoagulants, and in 55% of the untreated patients. Bleeding complications were the same regardless of treatment. The incidence of DVT on average 80 days after the onset of paraplegia in 87 patients who underwent a second phlebography was 13%. DVT occurred in 18% of the patients treated with UFH, in 11% of the patients treated with LMWH, and in 50% of the untreated patients. Only one minor clinical PE occurred during the trial. The efficacy of LMWH did not appear to be significantly different from that of UFH ($p = 0.05$). In addition, the two groups were not randomized.

Turpie et al. (1992) (20), in a more recent randomized, double-blind clinical trial, compared the efficacy of ORG 10172 versus UFH in 87 patients with acute thrombotic stroke. In 45 patients, 750 anti-Xa IU ORG 10172 was administrated subcutaneously every 12 hr. In the other 42 patients, 5000 IU UFH was administrated subcutaneously every 12 hr. The treatment lasted 14 days. Impedance plethysmography, ^{125}I-fibrinogen scanning, CT scan, and phlebography were performed. The incidence of DVT was 9% versus 31% in the ORG 10172 and UFH groups, respectively ($p = 0.014$). In 4% of the LMWH group and 12% of the UFH group proximal thrombosis occurred ($p > 0.2$). Major hemorrhagic events occurred in 2% of the LMWH-treated patients. Asymptomatic hemorrhagic transformation of the infarction occured in 9% and 5.6% of the ORG 10172 and UFH group, respectively. No death caused by hemorrhage or thrombosis was reported. After a 3-month follow-up, seven patients in the ORG-treated group and seven in the heparin-treated group died from cerebrovascular accidents or secondary complications.

IV. STUDIES IN MEDICAL AND CARDIOLOGICAL PATIENTS

Caulin (1989) (21) published the preliminary results of a European multicenter study of the influence of LMWH treatment on the mortality of hospitalized medical patients. In a randomized, double-blind clinical trial, a LMWH (calcium nadroparin, 3100 anti-Xa IU, subcutaneously once a day) was compared to placebo. The treatment lasted 21 days. The two groups were comparable (1230 and 1244 patients in each). Comparison of the mortality on the 21st day did not show a significant difference: 10.08% in the LMWH group and 10.29% in the placebo group. The incidence of PE, documented by necropsy, was 15.87% in the LMWH group, versus 28.33% in the placebo group ($p = 0.12$). The incidence of thromboembolic accidents was 2.93% in the LMWH group versus 3.94% in the placebo group ($p = 0.18$). The incidence of side effects was not significantly different between the LMWH group (5.5%) and the placebo group (3.95%).

Poniewierski et al. (1988) (22) studied 200 hospitalized medical patients in a randomized, double-blind clinical trial and compared the antithrombotic efficacy of LMWH treatment (dalteparine, 2500 anti-Xa IU subcutaneously once a day) versus UFH treatment (5000 IU subcutaneously twice a day). The two groups were equivalent (100 patients in each). The patients were divided into high- and low-risk groups according to the risk of DVT. The treatment lasted 7–10 days. Thermographic screening of the legs and phlebography were performed to control for DVT. According to the authors, neither a DVT nor a clinically apparent PE was observed. No relevant bleeding complications were observed in either group.

Harenberg et al. (1989) (23) investigated the efficacy of the LMWH treatment (dalteparin) in 66 outpatients with cardiological diseases. These patients had previous severe hemorrhages and other side effects on conventional oral anticoagulants. The patients were classified according to risk factors for thrombosis. The dose was adjusted according to the risk group and to anti-Xa activity. Fifty patients with a relatively lower risk of thromboembolism were treated on average with 7500 anti-Xa IU daily; 16 patients with artificial heart valve or severe recurrent thromboembolism received a daily dose on average of 10,000 anti-Xa IU. Duration of treatment was about 18 weeks. DVT and arterial thromboembolism occurred in 6% of the patients. The incidence of thrombosis was 4% in the low-risk group and 12.5% in the high-risk group. LMWH was well tolerated without any major hemorrhagic complications. Unfortunately, there was no control group in this study.

Harenberg et al. (1989) (24), in a randomized, double-blind clinical trial, studied the antithrombotic efficacy of LMWH treatment in 32 outpatients with atrial fibrillation. A LMWH (nadroparin) was administered in 13 patients subcutaneously (3100 anti-Xa IU) once a day. The other 19 patients constituted the placebo group. The trial lasted 6 months. The incidence of thromboembolism was 7.6% in the LMWH-treated group and 15.7% in the placebo group ($p = 0.02$). There was no mention of hemorragic incidents or accidents.

Haas and Biegholdt (1990) (25), in an open multicenter trial, studied a group of 44 patients with indications for long-term prophylaxis of thromboembolism and contraindications or intolerance to oral anticoagulants. In 80% of the patients, the treatment was prophylaxis following previous occurrences of thromboembolism. A LMWH (calcium nadroparine) was administered subcutaneously as a single daily injection of 3100 anti-Xa IU. The average duration of the treatment was 164 days. Treatment effect was studied from a clinical viewpoint. In 93.2% of the patients, no thromboembolism or relapse occurred. In 4.5% of the patients, a relapse occurred, and in 2.3% of the patients, the clinical condition did not change. There was no mention of hemorragic accidents or fatal side effects of the drug.

Harenberg et al. (1990) (26), in a third, randomized, double-blind clinical trial, compared the efficacy of the LMWH treatment (Sandoz 1500 APTT U, one subcutaneous daily injection) with UFH treatment (5000 IU subcutaneously 3 times a day). The study lasted 10 days. Two groups of 84 and 82 hospitalized medical patients were studied. Systematic scanning with Doppler ultrasound and impedance plethysmography were performed. Phlebography was performed when there were clinical symptoms of DVT. The incidence of DVT and/or arterial thrombosis was 3.4% in the LMWH group, versus 6% in the UFH group. The hemorrhagic risk was slightly greater in the UFH group (0.78%) than in the LMWH group (0%). Global mortality during the trial was 2.4%, but neither thrombotic nor hemorrhagic fatal events occurred. In this study coagulation parameters were measured. According to the authors, 2–4 hr after subcutaneous injection of LMWH, anti-Xa values were close to 0.16 ± 0.17 IU on day 1, on day 4–7, and on day 8–10. In the UFH-treated group, anti-Xa values were close to 0.04 ± 0.03 IU. In this study the values of AT III increased during administration of LMWH and decreased in the group treated with UFH.

Scala et al (1990) (27), in a randomized, double-blind clinical trial, included 25 patients with acute myocardial infarction. The authors compared the efficacy of LMWH treatment (dalteparin, 120 anti-Xa IU/kg, two subcutaneous injections daily) in a group of 13 patients. Another group of 12 patients was treated with UFH (continuous intravenous infusion in a dosage adapted to maintain APTT between 1.5 and 2.5 times the control value). The study lasted 7 days. ^{125}I-fibrinogen scanning and echocardiography were performed to diagnose DVT or left ventricular thrombosis. During the trial, neither DVT nor left ventricular thrombosis occurred. There was no mention of severe hemorrhagic complication.

Nesvold et al. (1991) (28), in an open dose-finding study, included 47 patients with acute myocardial infarction. The patients were treated with LMWH (dalteparin), 240–360 anti-Xa IU/kg/24 hr subcutaneously, divided in two or three injections per day [22 of the patients were treated also with aspirin (0.3 g) and streptokinase (1.5 million units intravenously)]. Echocardiography was performed. The treatment lasted 6–10 days. According to the authors, during the trial, left ventricular thrombosis (LVT) occurred in 6% of the patients and

2% had ischemic cerebral stroke. There was no mention of severe hemorrhagic complications, but minor bleedings occurred in patients receiving aspirin concomitantly. The authors suggest that 300 anti-Xa IU/kg/24 hr dalteparin, given in two or three subcutaneous injections per day, seems to be an effective and safe prophylactic treatment in patients with acute myocardial infarction.

V. DISCUSSION

The above 18 clinical trials included a total of 4619 patients receiving LMWH (2331 patients), placebo (1518 patients), UFH (749 patients), or oral anticoagulants (21 patients). Studies with LMWH are much more numerous in surgical than in medical patients. Moreover, some studies have been published in abstract form.

The evaluation of prophylactic antithrombotic treatment with LMWH in medical patients raises several questions. The available studies are dissimilar. The dose and the duration of treatment vary, as does the underlying pathology. Several studies, since they are double-blind, randomized, and include a rather large number of patients, allow statistical analysis. Furthermore, DVT and PE are well documented and the protocols well defined. However, the number of the patients included in some of the trials is small. In addition, not all studies followed their patients, and the clinical course after the cessation of the treatment was not always documented.

According to these studies, it is possible to point out that:

Preventive treatment with LMWH or LMW heparinoid seems effective. In all the studied categories of medical patients, the incidence of DVT and/or PE was lower in LMWH-treated groups than in placebo groups, and the difference was frequently significant. For instance, 3% versus 9.2% (p = 0.03) (11), 2.27% versus 30.4% (p = 0.002) (15), 20% versus 50% (p = 0.05) (16), 7.6% versus 15.7% (p = 0.02) (24) (see Tables 1–3).

In elderly patients, as well as in neurological and cardiological or other medical patients, the antithrombotic efficacy of the LMWH treatment was similar to that of the UFH. However, the incidence of thromboembolism ranged in different levels. Therefore, it is methodologically difficult to explain these variations, because the studied series are not comparable. Moreover, the protocols were not the same in each trial. It is remarkable that the higher incidence of DVT and/or PE appeared in patients with complete motor paralysis or acute thrombotic stroke treated with either UFH or LMWH.

All the studies demonstrate that tolerance of LMWH was at least as good as that of UFH, and in general, severe hemorrhagic accidents were rarely observed.

Table 1 Clinical Trials in Elderly Patients

First author, type of trial	Treatment	Dose	n	Duration	Diagnostic of DVT	DVT/PE	p	Severe hemor	Deaths thr-hem	Global mortality
Dahan, 1986 (11)	Enoxaparin	60 mg/0.5 ml 1 × 1 sc	132	10 days	Clinical exam.	3%	0.03	0	0.75%	4.5%
Randomized, double-blind trial	Placebo		131		^{125}I-Fg scan.	9.2%		0	2.29%	
Acquino, 1990 (12)	Nadroparin	3100 anti-Xa IU 1 × 1 sc	49	10 days	Clinical exam.	2%		0	0	
Prospective, comparative,					Phlebography		NS			2%
randomized open trial	UFH	5000 IU BW<60 kg 7500 IU BW>60 kg 1 × 1 sc	50		Lung scan, perfusion Doppler ultrasound	2%		4%	0	
Manciet, 1990 (13)	Nadroparin	3100 anti-Xa IU 1 × 1 sc	129	3 months	Clinical exam.	0		0.79%	1.55%	
Randomized, double-blind					Doppler ultrasound		NS			6.25%
clinical study	UFH	5000 IU 1 × 2 sc	127		Plethysmography Phlebography	0.78%		3.14%	1.57%	
Bergmann, 1992 (14)	Enoxaparin	20 mg 1 × 1 sc	216		Clinical exam.	5.6%		0.92%	0	
Randomized, double-blind				>7 days	^{125}I-Fg scan.		0.73			4%
trial	UFH	5000 IU 1 × 2 sc	226		Phlebography	4.9%		1.3%	0	

NS = not significant. Enoxaparin = Lovenox®; Nadroparin = Fraxiparine®.

Table 2 Clinical Trials in Neurological Patients

First author, type of trial	Treatment	Dose	*n*	Duration	Diagnostic of DVT	DVT/PE	*p*	Severe hemor	Deaths thr-hem	Global mortality
Turpie, 1987 (15) Randomized double-blind trial	Organon 10172	1000aXa IU loading dose iv 750 anti-Xa IU 2 × 1 sc	44	14 days	Clinical exam. ^{125}I-Fg scan. Impedance plethysmography	2.27%	0.002	2.27%	2.27%	4.4%
	Placebo		23		CT scan Phlebography Lung scan perfusion	30.4%		0%	4.3%	
Prins, 1990 (16) Randomized, double-blind trial	Dalteparin	2500 anti-Xa IU 2 × 1 sc	30	14 days	Clinical exam. CT scan	20%	0.05	13.3%[a]	?	
	Placebo		30		^{125}I-Fg scan Phlebography	50%		6.6%[a]	?	21.6%
Green, 1990 (17) Randomized, double-blind trial	Logiparin®	3500 anti-Xa IU 1 × 1 sc	20	8 weeks	Clinical exam. Impedance plethysmography	0	0.02	0	0	
	UFH	5000 IU 1 × 3 sc	21		Doppler ultrasound Phlebography	23.8%		9.5%	9.5%	4.8%
Sandset, 1990 (18) Randomized, double-blind trial	Dalteparin	3000–5500 anti-Xa IU 1 × 1 sc	52	14 days	Clinical exam. CT scan.	36%	NS	8%	7.6%	5.8%
	Placebo		51		Phlebography B-mode ultrasound Plethysmography	34%		6%	2%	
Yelnik, 1991 (19) Randomized, double-blind trial	Nadroparin	3100 anti-Xa IU 1 × 1 sc	17	45 days	Phlebography	41%	0.05	?	?	
	UFH	5000 IU 1 × 3 sc	89			29%		?	?	?
	AVK	?	21			24%		?	?	
	No treatment		20			55%				
Turpie, 1992 (20) Randomized, double-blind trial	Organon 10172	750 anti-Xa IU 2 × 1 sc	45	14 days	Clinical exam. ^{125}I-Fg scan.	13%	0.014	2% sev.hemor. 9%[2]	0	
	UFH	5000 IU 1 × 2 sc	42		CT scan. Impedance plethysmography	43%		5.6%[2]	0	?

[a] Hemorrhagic transformation of the infarction.

NS = not significant. Dalteparin = Fragmin®; Nadroparin = Fraxiparine®; Organon 10172 = Orgaran.

Table 3 Clinical Trials in Medical and Cardiological Patients

First author, type of trial	Treatment	Dose	n	Duration	Diagnostic of THR	DVT/PE	p	Severe hemor	Deaths thr-hem	Global mortality
Caulin, 1987 (21) Randomized, double-blind trial	Nadroparin	3100 anti-Xa IU 1 × 1 sc	1230	21 days	Clinical exam. Necropsy	2.93%	0.18	?	15.87%	10.80%
									$p = 0.12$	
	Placebo		1244			3.94%		?	28.33%	10.29%
Poniewierski, 1988 (22) Randomized, double-blind trial	Dalteparin	2500 anti-Xa IU 1 × 1 sc	100	7–10 days	Thermography Phlebography	0	?	0	0	0
	UFH	5000 IU 1 × 1 sc	100			0		0	0	0
Harenberg, 1989 (23) Open trial	Dalteparin after AVK	2500–15000 anti-Xa IU 1 × 1 sc adjusted dose	66	18 weeks	Clinical exam.	6%	?	0	0	0
Harenberg, 1989 (24) Randomized, double-blind trial	Nadroparin	3100 anti-Xa IU 1 × 1 sc	13	6 months		7.6%[a]	0.02	0	0	0
	Placebo		19			15.7%		0	0	0
Haas, 1990 (25) Open multicenter trial	Nadroparin after AVK	3100 anti-Xa IU 1 × 1 sc	44	164 days	Clinical exam.	4.5%		0	0	
Harenberg, 1990 (26) Randomized, double-blind trial	Sandoz	1500 aPTT U 1 × 1 sc	84	10 days	Clinical exam. Doppler ultrasound	3.4%		0	0	
	UFH	5000 IU 3 × 1 sc	82		Impedance plesthys-mography Phlebography	6%		0.78%	0	2.4%
Scala, 1990 (27) Randomized, double-blind trial	Dalteparin	120 aXaIU/kg/24 h 1 × 2 sc	13	7 days	^{125}I-Fg scan Echocardiography	0	—	0	0	0
	UFH	iv dose adjusted	12			0		0	0	0
Nesvold, 1991 (28) Open dose-finding trial	Dalteparin	240–360 anti-Xa IU/kg/24 h 1 × 2 or 1 × 3 sc	47	6–10 days	Echocardiography	6% LVT[b] 2% stroke		0	0	0

[a] Cerebral embolism [b] Left ventricular

Nadroparin = Fraxiparine®; Dalteparin = Fragmin®; THR = thrombosis

In elderly, neurological, and medical patients few deaths occurred due to thrombosis or bleeding during the treatment. The available results do not show a statistically significant difference in mortality rate among the studied series of patients. However, trials including large number of patients are required to demonstrate a possible reduction in mortality with prophylactic treatment.

It is remarkable that one study of neurological patients (18) demonstrated that prophylactic treatment with LMWH was not significantly effective in comparison with the placebo. The discrepancy between the results of heparin prophylaxis may reflect either unrecognized effects of paresis on the reliability of diagnostic screening tests or a false-negative result of this study. In addition, the prognosis index was significantly worse in the LMWH-treated group.

In all the studies, except one, the doses of LMWH were either fixed or adjusted according to body weight. LMWH was administered without any biological monitoring except in the Harenberg clinical trial (23).

At present, clinical and laboratory evidence shows that laboratory control is not required in patients receiving prophylactic treatment with LMWH. A recent study has shown that there is no strong correlation between plasma anti-Xa activity and hemorrhagic or thrombotic events in patients treated with LMWH (29). In addition, the correlation between anti-Xa activity and body weight in patients receiving a fixed dose of LMWH is highly significant. However, body weight is not the only parameter involved in the patient's response (29–31). Furthermore, since severe heparin-induced thrombocytopenia may occur in patients treated with LMWH, monitoring of platelet count before treatment and then every 2–3 days after its initiation is important (32). According to a retrospective medical record review (33), prophylaxis for venous thromboembolism is underused in hospitals. Since LMWH is an effective, safe, and easy administrated prophylactic treatment, its more frequent use could reduce the incidence of thromboembolism in medical patients.

VI. CONCLUSION

The results of clinical trials in medical patients suggest that prophylactic treatment with LMWH, administered subcutaneously once a day, is effective (even in high-risk patients), without frequent severe bleeding complications even in relatively long-term treatment. In addition, the benefit/risk ratio of this treatment is favorable. Administration of the treatment is simple and easy (usually one subcutaneous injection daily). It is striking that during the treatment, even fatal thrombotic or hemorrhagic events occurred only in high-risk groups such as neurological and elderly patients. Close clinical control is necessary for selected categories of treated patients (such as the elderly or paraplegics). Laboratory control regarding the measurement of anti-Xa plasma levels is not recommended except for high-risk patients, such as elderly or neurological patients or those with renal insufficiency. Moreover, in the absence of a reliable biological monitoring test, it is possible that dosage according to risk factors and the clinical situation of the patient may improve the effect of treatment, mainly in high-risk patients. Frequent control of platelets count is mandatory for all treated groups of patients. It is obvious that treatment with LMWH is of interest in the prevention of thromboembolism in medical patients, but further clinical and laboratory studies are required to demonstrate more clearly the effectiveness and the safety of the prophylactic antithrombotic approach.

REFERENCES

1. Odegard OR, Abildgaard UA. Antithrombin III: critical review of assay methods. Significance of variations in health and disease. Haemostasis 1978; 7 (2–3):127–134.
2. Conard J, Horellou MH, Samama MM. Screening for inherited disorders. Res Clin Lab 1989; 19:391–402.
3. Gallus AS, Hirsh J, Tuttle RJ, Trebilcock R, O'Brien SE, Carroll JJ, Minden JH, Hudecki SM. Small subcutaneous doses of heparin in prevention of venous thrombosis. N Engl J Med 1973; 288 (11):545–551.
4. Warlow C, Terry G, Kenmure ACF, Beattie AG, Ogston D, Douglas AS. A double-blind trial of low doses of subcutaneous heparin in the prevention of deep-vein thrombosis after myocardial infarction. Lancet 1973; 934–936.
5. Brown M, Glassenberg M. Mortality factors in patients with acute stroke. JAMA 1973; 224 (11):1493–1495.
6. Myllynen P, Kammonen M, Rokkanen P, Böstman O, Lalla M, Laasonen E. Deep venous thrombosis and pulmonary embolism in patients with acute spinal cord injury: a comparison with nonparalyzed patients immobilized due to spinal fractures. J Trauma 1985; 25(6):541–543.
7. Samama M, Michaut-Paterno F. La prophylaxie des accidents thromboemboliques veineux par les héparines de bas poids moléculaire. In: JEPU La maladie thromboembolique périoperatoire. Paris: Arnette, 1992:105–118.
8. Samama M, Babinet-Berthier A. Mise au point. Les nouvelles héparines. J Mal Vas 1992; 17:91–106.
9. Nurmohamed MT, Rosendaal FR, Büller HR, Dekker E, Hommes DW, Vandenbrouke JP, Briet E. Low-molecular-weight heparin versus standard heparin in general and orthopaedic surgery a meta-analysis. Lancet 1992; 340:152–156.
10. Leizorovicz A, Haugh MC, Chapuis F-R, Samama MM, Boissel J-P. Low molecular weight heparin in prevention of perioperative thrombosis. Br Med J 1992; 305:913–920.
11. Dahan R, Houlbert D, Caulin C, Cuzin E, Viltart C, Woler M, Segrestaa JM. Prevention of deep vein thrombosis in elderly medical inpatients by a low molecular weight heparin: a randomized double-blind trial. Haemostasis 1986; 16:159–164.

12. Aquino JP, Gambier A, Ducros JJ. Prevention of thromboembolic accidents in elderly subjects with Fraxiparine®. In: Bounameaux H, Samama M, Ten Cate JW, eds. Fraxiparin Second International Symposium. Recent Pharmacological and Clinical Data. Schattauer, 1990:51–54.
13. Manciet G, Vergnes C, Vaissié JH, Boisseau MR. A study on the efficacy and tolerance of Fraxiparine® during long-term therapy of the elderly. A randomized double-blind clinical trial. In: Bounameaux H, Samama M, Ten Cate JW, eds. Fraxiparine Second International Symposium. Recent Pharmacological and Clinical Data. Schattauer, 1990; 55–59.
14. Bergmann JF. Prophylaxis in medical geriatric patients. In: Symposium Clexane. RPR 16th World Congress of the International Union of Angiology, Paris, Sept 13–18, 1992.
15. Turpie AGG, Hirsh J, Jay RM, Andrew M, Hull RD, Levine MN, Carter CJ, Powers PJ, Magnani HN, Gent M. Double-blind randomised trial of ORG 10172 low-molecular-weight heparinoid in prevention of deep-vein thrombosis in thrombotic stroke. Lancet 1987; 523–526.
16. Prins MH, Den Ottolander GJH, Gelsema R, van Woerkom TCM, Sing AK, Heller I. Deep venous thrombosis prophylaxis with a LMW heparin (KABI 2165) in stroke patients. Abstract of XIth International Congress on Thromb. and Haemostasis. Brussels. Thromb. Haemost 1987; 58:117 (abstract 418).
17. Green D, Lee MY, Lim AC, Chmiel JS, Vetter M, Pang T, Chen D, Fenton L, Yarkony GM, Meyer PR. Prevention of thromboembolism after spinal cord injury using low-molecular-weight heparin. Ann Intern Med 1990; 113:571–574.
18. Sandset PM, Dahl T, Stiris M, Rostad B, Scheel B, Abildgaard U. A double-blind and randomized placebo controlled trial of low molecular weight heparin once daily to prevent deep vein thrombosis in acute ischemic stroke. Semin Thromb Hemost 1990; 16(Suppl):25–33.
19. Yelnik A, Dizien O, Bussel B, Schouman-Claeys E, Frija G, Pannier S, Held JP. Systematic lower limb phlebography in acute spinal cord injury in 147 patients. Paraplegia 1991; 29:253–260.
20. Turpie AGG, Gent M, Côte R, Levine MN, Ginsberg JS, Powers PJ, Leclerc J, Geerts W, Jay R, Neemeh J, Klimek M, Hirsh J. A low-molecular-weight heparinoid compared with unfractionated heparin in the prevention of deep vein thrombosis in patients with acute ischemic stroke. A randomized, double-blind study. Ann. Intern Med. 1992; 117:353–357.
21. Caulin C. Coordinator. Influence de l'administration de CY 216 sur la mortalité hospitalière des patients alités en médecine interne. Etude coopérative internationale en double—insu méthode et résultats préliminaires. In: Breddin K, Fareed J, Samama M, eds. Fraxiparine Premier Symposium International. Données Analytiques Structurales Pharmacologiques et Cliniques. Schattauer 1989:149–154.
22. Poniewierski M, Barthels M, Kuhn M, Poliwoda H. Über die wirksamkeit niedermolekularen Heparins (Fragmin®) in der thromboemboliepropyhlaxe bei internistischen patienten. Eine randomisierte doppelblindstudie. Med Klin 1988; 83:241–245.
23. Harenberg J, Leber G, Dempfle CE, Heene DL, Zimmermann R, Kübler W. Long term anticoagulation with low molecular weight heparin in outpatients with side effects on oral anticoagulants. Nouv Rev Fr Hematol 1989; 31:363–369.

24. Harenberg J, Weuster B, Pfitzer J, Oster P, Schlierf G. Efficacité et tolérance du CY 216 dans la prévention des accidents thrombo-emboliques chez les patients en fibrillation auriculaire. Résultats préliminaires. In: Breddin K, Fareed J, Samama M, eds. Fraxiparine Premier Symposium International. Données Analytiques Structurales Pharmacologiques et Cliniques. Schattauer 1987:16.
25. Haas S, Biegholdt M. Prevention of thromboembolism in out-patients with low molecular weight heparin. In: Bounameaux H, Samama M, Ten Cate JW, eds. Fraxiparine Second International Symposium. Recent Pharmacological and Clinical Data. Schattauer, 1990:41–50.
26. Harenberg J, Kallenbach B, Martin U, Dempfle CE, Zimmermann R, Kübler W, Heene DL. Randomized controlled study of heparin and low molecular weight heparin for prevention of deep-vein thrombosis in medical patients. Thromb Res 1990; 59:639–650.
27. Scala P-J, Thiollet M, Midavaine M, Kher A, Funck-Brentano C, Jaillon P, Robert A, Valty J. Deep venous thrombosis and left ventricular thrombosis prophylaxis by low molecular weight heparin in acute myocardial infarction. Haemostasis 1990; 20:368–369.
28. Nesvold A, Kontny F, Abildgaard U, Dale J. Safety of high doses of low molecular weight heparin (Fragmin) in acute myocardial infarction. A dose-finding study. Thromb Res 1991; 64:579–587.
29. Bara L, Leizorovicz A, Picolet H, Samama M. Correlation between anti-Xa and occurrence of thrombosis and haemorrhage in post-surgical patients treated with either Logiparin® (LMWH) or unfractionated heparin. Thromb Res 1992; 65:641–650.
30. Walenga JM, Hoppensteadt D, Fareed J. Laboratory monitoring of the clinical effects of low molecular weight heparins. Thromb Res 1991; (Suppl. XIV):49–62.
31. Samama MM, Combe S, Horellou MH, Augras D, Truc JB, Conard J, Girard P, Bara L, Poitout Ph. Anti Xa Activity and prothrombinase inhibition in patients treated with two different doses of enoxaparin in gynecologic surgery. Thromb Res 1991; (Suppl. XIV):29–37.
32. Lecompte T, Luo SK, Stieljes N, Lecrubier C, Burdin M, Samama M. Thrombocytopenia associated with low molecular weight heparin. Lancet 1991; 338:1271.
33. Anderson FA, Wheeler HB, Goldberg RJ, Hosmer DW, Forcier A, Patwardhan NA. Physician practices in the prevention of venous thromboembolism. Ann Intern Med 1991; 115:591–595.

12

Low-Molecular-Weight Heparins for Prevention of Venous Thromboembolism Following Lumbar Regional Anesthesia

Thomas Mätzsch
Lund University and Malmö General Hospital, Malmö, Sweden

David Bergqvist
University Hospital, Uppsala, Sweden

I. INTRODUCTION

Over the years there has been an impression among surgeons that the frequency of postoperative deep vein thrombosis (DVT) is lower if patients are operated on under regional anesthesia (spinal or epidural) than under general anesthesia. The Swedish surgeon Bohmansson suggested in 1943 (1) that patients at risk for developing postoperative thrombosis should be operated on under spinal anesthesia, and during the 1970s some uncontrolled studies indicated that epidural anesthesia could also have a prophylactic effect on postoperative thromboembolism (2–4). In prospective randomized studies during the 1980s this effect could be verified for patients undergoing total hip replacement (5–8), hip fracture surgery (9, 10) or open prostatectomy (11, 12). In a recent critical review of the literature, the type of anesthesia as a risk factor for DVT was analyzed (13). For hip surgery, the relative risk reduction for DVT in patients without prophylaxis was 46–55%. In patients receiving prophylaxis, no additional benefit was demonstrated with regard to a lower incidence of postoperative DVT if the operation was undertaken under regional anesthesia, but direct comparative studies for this group of patients are lacking. The frequency of postoperative DVT is, however, still high, and regional anesthesia should therefore not be regarded as a substitute for effective thromboprophylaxis. In other words, spinal/epidural anesthesia is better than nothing for preventing postoperative DVT, but cannot replace other means of thromboprophylaxis and is probably not additive in prophylactic effect.

The potential thromboprophylactic effect of spinal/epidural anesthesia has been ascribed to various mechanisms. In addition to hemodynamic effects with increased flow velocity in the femoral vein (12, 14, 15), a stimulation of fibrinolysis (6,12) and influence on coagulation (16, 17) have been cited. The reported influence on fibrinolysis is, however, controversial (18, 19). Furthermore, an influence on the red cell deformability and blood viscosity has been described (20). Thoracic epidural anesthesia including the segments T_4–S_5 has been demonstrated to block adrenalin secretion recorded during general anesthesia (21), but a thoracic epidural block is not associated with a decrease in incidence of postoperative DVT (22) and does not result in hyperkinetic blood flow in the lower limb, as described for lumbar epidural anesthesia (17).

II. LMWH IN ORTHOPEDIC AND NONORTHOPEDIC SURGERY

As of June 1992, the results of about 40 clinical trials on the thromboprophylactic effect of various low-molecular-weight heparins (LMWHs) in orthopedic and nonorthopedic surgery had been published (23). None of the studies were stratified on the basis of anesthesiological methods. From the 19 studies where the combination of LMWH with epidural/spinal anesthesia was stated, no influence of the type of anesthesia—either general, epidural, or spinal—on the frequency of postoperative DVT was reported. Only two published studies specifically addressed the issue of frequency of DVT after prophylaxis with LMWH or a low-molecular-weight heparinoid with regard to regional anesthesia (24,25). The question whether the effect of LMWH prophylaxis in preventing postoperative thromboembolism is influenced by the type of anesthesia given cannot therefore be answered owing to lack of available data. Future studies should address this point more specifically, both from safety aspects and in terms of efficacy.

Apart from the prophylactic effect of spinal/epidural anesthesia on postoperative DVT, although insufficient on its own, there are several other anesthesiological arguments for using this kind of anesthesia in preference to general anesthesia. Especially in vascular surgery patients, it has been reported that the rates of cardiovascular complications as well as the duration of intensive care unit stay were significantly reduced in patients receiving general anesthesia with postoperative epidural analgesia as compared with general anesthesia and on-demand narcotic analgesia (26). The question of risks in combining regional blocks with pharmacological methods of thromboprophylaxis thus arises. The safety aspects of combining a drug with potential bleeding-inducing effect with an invasive procedure form the theoretical basis for the concern and reluctance of many anesthetists to combine a regional anesthesia with pharmacological thromboprophylaxis in fear of causing an intraspinal hemorrhage with subsequent paraparesis. The issue has been debated for a long time and is still controversial.

III. COMBINATION LMWH AND EPIDURAL/SPINAL ANESTHESIA

As late as in 1981 Stanton-Hicks (15) stated ''that not only would [I] be reluctant to combine mini-dose heparin with major conduction anesthesia but that its concurrent use would indeed be contraindicated in the light of the foregoing risks.'' Whereas some anesthetists have followed this warning, others have shown no reluctance to use low-dose heparins in patients with spinal/epidural blocks, either before, during, or after. In 1989 it was reported from a German consensus conference that ''low-dose heparin prophylaxis is no contraindication to spinal or epidural anesthesia'' (27). The appropriateness of this standpoint could be confirmed in a survey among anesthetic departments in Denmark, which revealed that about 60% of the departments used the techniques of epidural/spinal lumbar analgesia in patients receiving prophylactic anticoagulant therapy with a low-dose heparin without any side effects (28).

From the cited consensus conference in Germany, an urgent warning was, however, issued not to use the combination of LMWH and epidural/spinal anesthesia and to remove an epidural catheter if thromboprophylaxis with LMWH was used (27). This combination ''should be performed in controlled studies only'' (27).

That this standpoint has already been superseded could be demonstrated in a questionnaire study in 1992 among all Swedish anesthetic departments where the attitude toward use of the combination was investigated (29). It was found that LMWH was the most common type of prophylaxis given in general, orthopedic, urological and gynecological surgery and that more than 140,000 epidural/spinal blocks had been performed without any reported cases of intraspinal hemorrhage; 84/89 and 85/89 departments found no contraindication in combining LMWH with epidural or spinal anesthesia, respectively. The same figures for low-dose heparin were 78/89 and 82/89, respectively. The attitude was expressed as ''the combination is practically risk-free and is no obstacle for the regional anesthesia and can be accepted if no anamnestic data speak against it'' by 79/89 of the departments for LMWH and 74/89 for low-dose heparin. The attitude and hence the use of the combination were thus even more liberal than in the cited Danish survey without any registered side effects regarding intraspinal hemorrhage.

When the problem of intraspinal hemorrhage is discussed in conjunction with the combination of epidural/spinal anesthesia and thromboprophylaxis, several factors must be taken into account. The frequency is extremely low and limited to case reports (30). Considering the seriousness and rareness of an intraspinal hematoma following regional blocks, readiness to report these cases can be assumed high and, thus, the number of unreported cases low. The most common cause of intraspinal hematomas is spontaneous bleeding of obscure etiology (31). Other causes include trauma, spinal canal tumors, or vascular anomalies and bleeding disorders. All these factors can hamper the judging of causality regarding anesthesiological technique and the complication and make it almost impossible to show a causal relationship. The rarity of this specific complication also makes it impossible to perform a prospective, randomized study on safety in this respect of various thromboprophylactic methods—with the low reported frequency of intraspinal hematomas after regional anesthesia, the number of patients to randomize would have to be at least 150,000 in each group! As a matter of fact, the rarity suggests that in the absence of bleeding disorders, epidural or spinal anesthesia virtually never causes symptomatic spinal hematoma, and the possibility of coincidental hematoma must be considered when evaluating case reports (32).

Heparinization with unfragmented heparin after diagnostic lumbar puncture has been reported to cause intraspinal hemorrhages in as much as 2% of the patients if a 20-gauge lumbar puncture needle was used (33, 34). Difficulty during puncture or a bloody tap appears in itself to be a risk factor for subsequent hematoma, at least in patients on anticoagulation (32).

Heparinization following spinal/epidural anesthesia appears to be a safe technique provided proper safety measurements are ensured, such as excluding bleeding diathesis, careful monitoring of the extent of heparinization, and removing the epidural catheter when heparin levels are low (32).

There are only two case reports of intraspinal hematomas in connection with low-dose conventional heparin and epidural blocks (35, 36).

Only one case of an intraspinal hematoma occurring during prophylaxis with LMWH has been reported after a procedure of combined lumbar spinal and epidural anesthesia and where a minimal amount of blood was seen at insertion of the catheter (27). Another case has been reported of a spontaneous intraspinal hemorrhage in a thrombocytopenic ($90{,}000 \times 10^9$/L) patient on LMWH prophylaxis, but where no attempt had been made for a lumbar puncture. No intraspinal hematomas were reported in those 19 studies comprising over 9000 patients where the combination of LMWH prophylaxis with a regional block was stated (30). Wolf and Welzel (37) analyzed in detail all patients with regional lumbar anesthesia from a large safety study comprising over 6000 patients receiving a fixed combination of LMWH and dihydroergotamine for thromboprophylaxis and observed no complication due to regional anesthesia.

Schwander and Bachmann (38) made a similar analysis and found no complications related to intraspinal bleedings after spinal/epidural anesthesia in almost 14,000 patients who received LMWH for thromboprophylaxis.

Thus, in view of the large number of patients treated with a combination of LMWH prophylaxis and spinal/epidural anesthesia, within and outside clinical studies, this combination must be considered safe. The initially proposed caution appears unjustified in the light of experience gained today. Nevertheless, some reluctance can be anticipated to prevail from some anesthetists from the theoretical reasoning of combining an invasive procedure with a hemostasis-interfering drug with potential, however minute, to cause bleeding. To some extent this is probably based on medicolegal considerations and understandable reluctance to experience even possible reproaches. This minimal theoretical risk must be balanced against the well-known risk of experiencing a fatal pulmonary embolism (about 0.8%) after general surgery if thromboprophylaxis is omitted.

Intensified and extensive observation routines with proposed daily neurological investigation during temporary cessation of administration of the analgetic agent (27) in order to exclude hemorrhage-related spinal paresis would almost certainly not be cost-effective in view of the extreme rareness of the complication.

Summing up the reported data in the literature, the experience gained with LMWH for prophylaxis, and the attitudes of many anesthetists, the combination of prophylaxis with LMWH with epidural/spinal anesthesia should not pose a problem provided normal safety precautions, also applying to the procedure on its own, are taken. It is not known whether the type of anesthesia has any influence on the efficacy of thromboprophylaxis with LMWH.

REFERENCES

1. Bohmansson G. Nord Med 1943; 17:182.
2. Lahnborg G, Bergström K, Friman L, Lagergren H. Lancet 1974; 1:329.
3. Lahnborg G, Bergström K. Acta Chir Scand 1975; 141:590.
4. Thorburn J, Loudon JR, Vallance R. Br J Anaesth 1980; 52:1117.
5. Modig J, Hjelmstedt ÅA, Sahlstedt B, Maripuu E. Acta Chir Scand 1981; 147:125.
6. Modig J, Borg T, Bagge L, Saldeen T. Br J Anaesth 1983; 55:625.
7. Modig J, Maripuu E, Sahlstedt B. Reg Anaesth 1986; 11:72.
8. David FM, Laurensen VG, Gillespie WJ, Wells JE, Foate J, Newman E. J Bone Joint Surg 1989; 71-B:181.
9. Davis FM, Laurensen VG. Anaesth Intens Care 1981; 9:352.
10. McKenzie PJ, Wishart HY, Gray I, Smith G. Br J Anaesth 1985; 57:853.
11. Hendolin H, Mattila MAK, Poikalainen E. Acta Chir Scand 1981; 147:425.
12. Poikalainen E, Hendolin H. Acta Chir Scand 1983; 149:361.
13. Prins M, Hirsh J. Thromb Haemost 1990; 64:497.
14. Haljamäe H, Frid I, Holm J, Åkerström G. Eur J Vasc Surg 1988; 2:395.
15. Stanton-Hicks M. JAMA 1981; 246:886.
16. Lindblad B, Bergqvist D, Hallböök T, Lindhagen A, Hedner U. Acta Chir Scand 1984; 150:525.
17. Modig J. Acta Chir Scand 1985; 151:589.
18. Bredbacka S, Blombäck M, Hägnevik K, Iwestedt L, Raake N. Acta Anaesthesiol Scand 1986; 30:204.
19. Engquist A, Askgaard B, Funding J. Br J Anaesth 1976; 48:903.
20. Drummond AR, Drummond MM, MacKenzie PJ, Lowe GDO, Smith G, Forbes CD, Wishart HY. In: Stoltz JE, Drouin P, eds. Haemorrheology and Diseases. Paris, 1980:445–450.

21. Engquist A, Brandt MR, Fernandes A, Kehlet H. Acta Anaesth Scand 1977; 21:330.
22. Mellbring G, Dahlgren S, Reiz S, Sunnergård O. Acta Chir Scand 1983; 149:263.
23. Bergqvist D. Eur J Surg 1992; 158:67.
24. Hoek JA, Henny CP, Knipscheer HC, ten Cate H, Nurmohamed MT, ten Cate JW. Thromb Haemost 1991; 65:122.
25. Planès A, Vochelle N, Fagola M, Feret J, Bellaud M. J Bone Joint Surg 1991; 73:418.
26. Tuman KJ, McCarthy RJ, March RJ, Dedania GA, Patel RV, Ivankovitch AD. Anesth Analg 1991; 73:696.
27. Tryba M, und die Teilnehmer des Workshops über hämostaseologische Probleme bei Regionalanaesthesien. Reg Anaesth 1989; 12:127.
28. Wille-Jørgensen P, Jørgensen LN, Rasmussen LS. Anaesthesia 1991; 46:623.
29. Mätzsch T, Bergqvist D, Johansson A. 1992 (submitted).
30. Bergqvist D, Lindblad B, Mätzsch T. Acta Anaesthesiol Scand 1992; 36:605.
31. Bruyn GW, Bosma NJ. In: Vinken PJ, Bruyn GW, eds. Handbook of Clinical Neurology, Vol 26. Amsterdam: North Holland, 1976:1–30.
32. Sage DJ. Anaesth Intens Care 1990; 18:319.
33. Ruff RL, Dougherty JH. Stroke 1981; 12:879.
34. Brem SS, Hafler DA, Van Uitert RL, Ruff RL, Rechert WH. N Engl J Med 1981; 304:1020.
35. Darnat S, Guzziari M, Grob R, Guillaume A, Viars P. Ann Fr Anesth Reanim 1986; 5:550.
36. Metzger G, Singbartl G. Acta Anaesthesiol Scand 1991; 36:105.
37. Wolf H, Welzel D. Perfusion 1991; 7:228.
38. Schwander D, Bachmann F. Ann Fr Anesth Reanim 1991; 10:284.

13

Low-Molecular-Weight Heparins in Extracorporeal Circuits

M. T. Nurmohamed, H. R. Büller, and J. W. ten Cate

Centre for Haemostasis, Thrombosis, Atherosclerosis and Inflammation Research, Academic Medical Centre, Amsterdam, The Netherlands

I. INTRODUCTION

Extracorporeal circulation requires anticoagulation to prevent activation of the coagulation system by the tubing system and membranes, which, without anticoagulants, will lead to deposition of fibrin clots and eventually to thrombotic obstruction. Hence, anticoagulation is required to maintain the filtration efficiency and to prevent the loss of red cells and platelets within the extracorporeal circuit. Standard (unfractionated) heparin, the routinely used anticoagulant, is a glycosaminoglycan with polysaccharide chains of different sizes and an average molecular weight of 12,000–15,000 Da. The administration of heparin is associated with a risk of bleeding and it may induce thrombocytopenia. This hemorrhagic potential is particularly cumbersome in patients requiring extracorporeal circulation, who are at high risk for bleeding, or who are actively bleeding.

Convincing evidence has been provided by various studies that low-molecular-weight heparins (LMWHs), which are fractions of standard heparin obtained by depolymerization, are at least as effective antithrombotics as standard heparin (1, 2). These fractions of heparin, with an average molecular weight of 2500–6000 Da, have a biological half-life that is approximately 2–3 times that of standard heparin and, in addition, they have, in contrast to standard heparin, minimal effects on coagulation parameters and platelet functions (1). These properties of LMWHs could eventually result in an increased benefit/risk ratio, i.e., less bleeding with an equal antithrombotic effect, also in patients undergoing extracorporeal circulatory procedures, which is the focus of this chapter. In addition, LMWHs may simplify the administration protocol since, owing to their prolonged half-life, a single bolus injection is expected to be adequate in hemodialysis patients, which is in contrast to the continuous infusion required for standard heparin therapy. Furthermore, standard heparin may play a role in the development of cardiovascular complications on long-term hemodialysis, by release of lipoprotein lipase from the capillary endothelium, thereby increasing the plasma lipolytic activity and causing increased plasma levels of free fatty acids and monoglycerides (3). Increased plasma levels of free fatty acids have, for example, been associated with cardiac arrhythmias (4). The activation of lipoprotein lipase caused by heparin seems to occur to a lesser extent with some LMWHs (1).

Before any compound can be applied as an anticoagulant in extracorporeal circuits, it needs to go through various phases of clinical investigation. In the dose-finding phase, the aim is to establish the effective dose in the target patient population. In the next phase, the efficacy and safety of this dose have to be confirmed in a larger patient sample, preferably in randomized comparison to the standard treatment with blinded end-point assessment. The final phase, in particular in chronic hemodialysis, is to investigate if drug accumulation and other adverse events occur during long-term use.

The anticoagulant doses required for extracorporeal circulatory procedures in children cannot simply be extrapolated from studies performed in adults, since the metabolism of standard heparin may differ and is unknown for LMWHs (5). Hence, it follows that LMWHs will have to go through the same phases of investigation in children.

Finally, a new drug will only replace the standard therapy if it is more efficacious or safer. In case of equal efficacy and safety, it will have to be more convenient or cost-effective.

A. Hemodialysis, Hemofiltration, and Related Techniques

In hemodialysis, blood is separated from the dialysate by the artificial semipermeable membrane of the dialyzer. Exchange between blood and dialysate of small molecules and water takes place across the membrane by diffusion. This process allows removal of metabolic waste products with concurrent correction of the patient's electrolyte disbalance. Hemofiltration (HF), continuous arteriovenous hemofiltration (CAVH), and continuous arteriovenous hemodialysis (CAVHD) are related techniques and are also applied in patients with severe renal failure.

In HF, metabolic toxins are removed by convective transport. Small filters with low resistance are used in CAVH without external blood pumps because the filtration pressure is maintained by the patient's own arterial blood pressure. CAVHD utilizes a dialyzer with a high flux membrane and combines both convective and diffusion transport. As for CAVH, no blood pumps are needed, which adds to the simplicity of the procedure. Both techniques can also be performed venovenous, but this requires blood pumps. HF, CAVH, and CAVHD are associated with less hemodynamic instability than hemodialysis. For this reason, they are preferred to hemodialysis in the unstable acute renal failure patient.

As for hemodialysis, each of these techniques requires adequate anticoagulation to prevent clotting within the extracorporeal circuit. With adequate anticoagulation it is possible to use the filters of CAVH and CAVHD continuously for several days. The available study reports in the literature reveal that there exists a limited experience with LMWHs in hemofiltration and other related techniques. Nevertheless, the few and small patient series or case reports indicated that no or minimal clot formation occurred in the course of hemofiltration and that the filter life was at least as long as during standard heparin therapy (6–14).

Because of the lack of adequate safety and efficacy studies, we will not further discuss the use of LMWH in these techniques. In studies investigating the anticoagulant effects of LMWH in hemodialysis as well as in hemofiltration procedures, the results of the hemofiltration sessions will be briefly summarized.

B. Low-Molecular-Weight Heparins

The great majority of studies in hemodialysis patients have been performed with the following LMWHs:

CY 222 (Choay, France)
CY 216 (Fraxiparine, Choay, France)
PK 10169 (Enoxaparin, Rhône-Poulenc-Rorer, France)
K 2165 (Fragmin, Kabi Pharmacia, Sweden)
ORG 10172 (Orgaran, Organon, the Netherlands)

Orgaran differs from the other LMWHs in that it is a mixture of the glycosaminoglycans heparan sulfate, dermatan sulfate, and chondroitin sulfate, though it has the same potential advantages as LMWH over standard heparin. For this reason, studies with ORG 10172 are also included in this chapter (15).

Only single dose-finding studies were published with two other LMWHs, i.e., LMW 21–23 (Braun, Germany) and Innohep (Leo, Denmark), and are therefore not taken into account in this review (16, 17).

The various LMWH preparations should be considered as different agents, because of their variations in molecular weights, half-lives, anti-factor IIa (aIIa) and anti-factor Xa (aXa) activity (18), and they will therefore be discussed separately. Dose-finding studies, heparin-controlled studies, long-term studies, and studies in pediatric patients are presented for each compound.

C. Efficacy and Safety Study End-Points

Different criteria were used for the assessment of efficacy in the various studies discussed in this chapter (Table 1). Monitoring of macroscopic clot formation in the bubble catcher, lines, and artificial kidney was the most frequently used

Table 1 Efficacy Assessments in Hemodialysis

Author	Ref.	Year	Macroscopic clot formation[a]	Creatinine washout	FPA[b]	β-TG[c]	Other efficacy assessments
CY 222							
Renaud et al.	6	1984	Yes	No	Yes	No	No
Dieval et al.	26	1987	Yes	No	Yes	No	No
Hory et al.	23	1987	Yes	Yes	No	No	Ultrafiltration rate; hemoglobin content of the dialyzer
Ireland et al.	27	1988	Yes	No	Yes	Yes	No
Morinière et al.	28	1990	Yes	No	No	No	No
CY 216							
Dieval et al.	24	1989	Yes	Yes	Yes	No	No
Schlegel et al.	30	1989	Yes	No	No	No	D-dimer
Steinbach et al.	7	1990	Yes	No	No	No	No
Nurmohamed et al.	29	1991	Yes	No	No	No	No
Grau et al.	25	1992	Yes	No	No	No	D-dimer, thrombin–antithrombin III complexes
PK 10169							
Pouzol et al.	31	1987	Yes	Yes	No	No	No
Briquel et al.	32	1987	Yes	Yes	Yes	No	No
Dechelette et al.	33	1987	Yes	No	No	No	No
Gamberoni et al.	34	1989	Yes	No	No	No	No
Bianchetti et al.	35	1990	Yes	No	No	No	No
K 2165							
Schrader et al.	36	1985	Yes	Yes	No	No	Fibrin monomers
Schrader et al.	44	1985	Yes	Yes	No	No	Fibrin monomers
Lane et al.	37	1986	Yes	Yes	Yes	Yes	No

Borm et al.	47	1986	Yes	No	No	Yes	No
Ljungberg et al.	39	1987	Yes	No	Yes	No	Fibrin monomers
Deuber et al.	52	1988	No	No	No	No	No
Schrader et al.	8	1988	Yes	No	No	No	Fibrin monomers
Anastassiades et al.	38	1988	Yes	No	Yes	No	No
Maurin et al.	45	1988	Yes	No	Yes	No	No
Laubenthal et al.	43	1989	Yes	No	No	No	No
Anastassiades et al.	38	1990	Yes	Yes	Yes	No	No
Suzuki et al.	46	1990	Yes	Yes	No	No	No
Bambauer et al.	50	1990	No	No	No	No	No
Baumann et al.	41	1991	Yes	No	No	No	No
Schneider et al.	48	1991	Yes	No	No	No	No
Deuber et al.	49	1991	Yes	No	No	No	No
Ljungberg et al.	40	1992	Yes	No	Yes	No	No
ORG 10172							
Henny et al.	19	1983	No	No	No	No	^{125}I-fibrinogen deposition within the dialyzer
ten Cate et al.	20	1985	Yes	No	Yes	Yes	pf4,[d] assessment of fibrin clots within the dialyzer[e]
Henny et al.	22	1985	Yes	No	No	No	Weight of clotted fibers within the dialyzer
Ireland et al.	54	1986	Yes	No	Yes	Yes	No
Frei et al.	21	1988	No	No	No	No	Radiolabeled erythrocytes deposition within the dialyzer
Bonsdorf et al.	55	1990	Yes	No	No	Yes	pf4

[a] In bubble catcher and/or dialyzer and/or tubing system.
[b] FPA = fibrinopeptide A.
[c] β-TG = β-thromboglobulin.
[d] pf4 = platelet factor 4.
[e] Detected by light microscopy.

Table 2 Safety Assessments in Hemodialysis Studies

Author	Ref.	Year	Measurement of compression time	Other assessments
CY 222				
Renaud et al.	6	1984	Yes	No
Dieval et al.	26	1987	Yes	No
Hory et al.	23	1987	Yes	No
Ireland et al.	27	1988	No	No
Morinière et al.	28	1990	No	No
CY 216				
Dieval et al.	24	1989	Yes	No
Schlegel et al.	30	1989	Yes	No
Steinbach et al.	7	1990	Yes	No
Nurmohamed et al.	29	1991	No	No
Grau et al.	25	1992	Yes	No
PK 10169				
Pouzol et al.	31	1987	Yes	No
Briquel et al.	32	1987	No	No
Dechelette et al.	33	1987	No	No
Gamberoni et al.	34	1989	No	No
Biachetti et al.	35	1990	No	No

K 2165				
Schrader et al.	36	1985	No	No
Schrader et al.	44	1985	No	No
Lane et al.	37	1986	No	No
Borm et al.	47	1986	No	Collagen-induced platelet adhesion
Ljungberg et al.	39	1987	Yes	No
Deuber et al.	52	1988	Yes	No
Schrader et al.	8	1988	No	Transfusion requirements
Anastassiades et al.	38	1988	No	No
Maurin et al.	45	1988	No	No
Laubenthal et al.	43	1989	Yes	No
Anastassiades et al.	38	1990	Yes	No
Suzuki et al.	46	1990	Yes	Collagen-induced platelet adhesion
Bambauer et al.	50	1990	No	Transfusion requirements
Baumann et al.	41	1991	Yes	No
Schneider et al.	48	1991	Yes	Collagen-induced platelet adhesion
Deuber et al.	49	1991	No	No
Ljungberg et al.	40	1992	No	No
ORG 10172				
Henny et al.	19	1983	No	No
ten Cate et al.	20	1985	No	Inhibition of platelet aggregation by factor Xa
Henny et al.	22	1985	No	No
Ireland et al.	54	1986	No	No
Frei et al.	21	1988	No	Occult blood loss measured by whole body counting (^{59}Fe)
Bonsdorf et al.	55	1990	No	No

efficacy end-point. Alternatively, fibrin formation within the dialyzer was assessed in several studies either by determining the deposition of radiolabeled fibrinogen or of radiolabeled erythrocytes (19–21) or by assessing the weight of clotted hollow fibers (22) or by determining the residual hemoglobin content within the dialyzer (23).

Another approach for determining the efficacy included measurement of biochemical markers for coagulation activation or the subsequent fibrinolysis.

Coagulation activation in the extracorporeal circuit leads to thrombin formation, which cleaves fibrinopetide A (FPA) from fibrinogen, thereby generating fibrin monomers that polymerize to a fibrin clot. Ultimately, the fibrin clots will be degraded by plasmin leading to D-dimer generation. In the presence of heparin, most of the thrombin will be inactivated by its main physiological inhibitor, antithrombin III, leading to thrombin–antithrombin III (TAT) complexes. In the last decade, several immunoassays have been developed for the quantitative assessment of all these intermediate activation products. In some hemodialysis studies, fibrin monomers, TAT complexes, and D-dimer plasma levels were assessed as substitution efficacy end-point. Increased levels of these activation products during dialysis are potentially more sensitive, albeit substitution for the more clinically relevant fibrin formation.

Also, platelets will be activated by direct contact with artificial surfaces and by thrombin generated in the course of extracorporeal circulation. This leads to release of β-thromboglobulin (β-TG) and platelet factor 4 (pf4) from the platelet granula with a subsequent rise in their plasma levels.

Some investigators have used these platelet parameters as an efficacy substitute end-point. Finally, efficacy has been assessed by measurement of creatinine and urea washout. For clarity, only clot formation in the extracorporeal circuit and FPA generation will be discussed as being the most appropriate and most frequently studied efficacy end-points.

Safety was assessed by monitoring clinical bleeding and determining hemoglobin levels and transfusion requirements. As a substitute measure for safety, the compression time to arrest bleeding from catheter puncture sites was used in many studies (Table 2). The safety end-points are of particular interest for studies performed in patients assumed to be at a higher risk for hemorrhage. In general, these patients may have one or more of the following: postoperative bleeding, uremic pericarditis, diffuse intravascular coagulation, gastrointestinal bleeding, coagulation disorders, recent major surgery, insertion of a deep vein catheter, liver or kidney biopsy, or recent arterial puncture.

D. Dosage Regimens

In the literature reviewed, K 2165 and ORG 10172 were expressed in anti-factor Xa (aXa) units and PK 10169 in milligrams. The compounds manufactured by

Choay have their own standard: the anti-Xa Institute Choay (aXa IC) unit. One aXa unit, as defined according to the First International Standard for LMWH, approximates 2.5 aXa IC units (18). It is important to note that a dose used for a particular compound cannot be extrapolated to another LMWH on a gravimetric or aXa or aIIa activity basis (1).

Since LMWHs give only a minimal prolongation of the conventional clotting times, such as the activated partial thromboplastin time (APTT), they require another type of monitoring to establish dose-response relationships with regard to efficacy and safety. The biological activity of LMWHs has usually been monitored by a chromogenic aXa assay and occasionally by a clot-based aXa assay.

With the exception of two of the considered studies, the routinely used anticoagulation regimen with standard heparin consisted of a predialysis bolus injection in a dose ranging from 1200 to 6400 IU, followed by a continuous infusion ranging from 375 to 2500 IU/hr. In two studies, standard heparin was given in two bolus injections of 4000–8000 IU, one at the start of dialysis and the other 2 hr later (24,25). Hence, a noteworthy variation in the dose regimens for standard heparin emerges, which may be related to differences in the execution of the dialysis procedures or in the body weights of the patients. Moreover, variation in criteria for efficacy used may explain the differences in heparin dosages. Some investigators focus on suppression of coagulation activation peptides such as FPA, whereas others focus on visible clot formation within the extracorporeal circuit. This latter criterion may obviously lead to a lower-dose regimen; i.e., a slight coagulation activation with elevated plasma levels of FPA may occur without visible clot formation within the extracorporeal circuit. Clearly, this wide range in dose regimens does not easily allow comparison of the results of different studies regarding efficacy and safety of LMWHs versus standard heparin. Therefore, we have not detailed the applied dose regimens of standard heparin throughout this chapter and use the term "standard heparin treatment" instead.

II. LMWH AND HEPARINOID STUDIES IN HEMODIALYSIS

A. CY 222

1. *Dose-Finding Studies*

A dose range of 75–300 aXa IC units/kg CY 222 given as a bolus injection with or without a continuous infusion of 1000 aXa IC units/hour was investigated and compared to standard heparin treatment in 21 chronic stable hemodialysis patients undergoing dialyses up to 4 hr (6, 26). Qualitative assessment of fibrin clots within the extracorporeal circuit revealed an approximately equal efficacy of 300 aXa IC units/kg with or without infusion of 1000 aXa IC units/hr versus standard heparin treatment.

Plasma FPA levels at the end of dialysis were almost normal with 300 aXa IC units/kg CY 222 single bolus injection, which was different from the standard heparin treatment, which was associated with significantly higher FPA levels at the end of the procedure.

Compression times to arrest bleeding from catheter puncture sites were comparable to those obtained in patients treated with standard heparin.

Further studies were undertaken in patients with acute or chronic renal failure and at high risk for bleeding: A considerably lower dose range was used, i.e., 33–150 aXa IC units/kg bolus injection with or without a continuous infusion of 1000 aXa IC units/hr in 214 patients undergoing 485 dialysis sessions and 53 hemofiltration sessions (26). The efficacy was considered satisfactory; extensive clot formation was observed in only 3.3 % of the sessions. A dose relationship was not found and no bleeding complications were encountered in these 214 patients.

In addition, a heparin-controlled study was performed in eight chronic dialysis patients undergoing a prolonged dialysis procedure lasting 5 hr or more (27). To be able to continue the dialyses for up to 6 hr, a dose of 20,000 aXa IC units as a bolus injection with a continuous infusion of 1500 aXa IC units/hr was required to inhibit (but not completely suppress) visible clot formation and FPA generation.

2. *Efficacy Studies in Patients Without an Enhanced Risk for Bleeding*

In a heparin-controlled crossover study in eight chronic hemodialysis patients, two dose regimens were investigated: 90 aXa IC units/kg as a bolus injection followed by continuous infusion of 1000 aXa IC units/hour versus 300 aXa IC units/kg as a single bolus injection. The clot formation within the extracorporeal circuit for the 300 aXa IC units/kg single predialysis bolus injection was comparable to that with standard heparin (23).

3. *Efficacy Study in Patients with a High Risk for Bleeding*

A large noncomparative study was performed in 343 patients with a high risk for hemorrhage, including six children (13). A single predialysis dose of 150 aXa IC units/kg was investigated in a total of 613 hemodialysis and in 66 hemofiltration procedures, lasting up to 4 hr. In this study, clotting within the extracorporeal circuit occurred in 23 sessions (3.4%), though without the necessity to replace the extracorporeal circuit. It is not indicated if a difference existed between hemodialysis and hemofiltration procedures for this end-point. No bleeding complications were observed in this study. However, without a comparison group the results remain difficult to interpret.

4. *Conclusion*

The available data suggest that CY 222 was effective and safe in chronic hemodialysis patients without a hemorrhagic tendency and in hemodialysis patients with a high risk for bleeding, though a properly designed heparin controlled study is still lacking in this last category of patients.

At present, the data regarding an optimal dose for hemodialysis procedures lasting 5 hr or more are not conclusive.

The optimal dose for hemodialysis procedures up to 4 hr appeared to be a single bolus injection of 300 aXa IC units/kg for patients without a bleeding tendency and 150 aXa IC units/kg for patients with a hemorrhagic risk. Appropriate long-term studies to investigate the eventual accumulation of CY 222, following repeated dialysis sessions, are needed. A preliminary study, in 10 patients, suggested a slight accumulation of aXa activity in the course of four consecutive dialysis procedures, though without clinical consequences (28).

This LMWH is at present not available for clinical use.

B. Fraxiparine, CY 216

The differences between CY 216 and CY 222 are: a molecular weight of 4500 Da for CY 216 versus 2500 Da for CY 222 and an aXa-aIIa ratio for CY 216 of 4 versus between 6 and 10 for CY 222 (1).

1. *Dose-Finding Studies*

A heparin controlled study was performed in eight patients, undergoing a total of 56 hemodialysis procedures, who received bolus injections ranging from 5000 to 15,000 aXa IC units (24). The efficacy of 10,000 aXa IC units (approximately 150 aXa IC units/kg) was comparable to that of standard heparin treatment for dialyses up to 4 hr. No visible clot formation occurred within the extracorporeal circuit in the majority of the sessions with either 10,000 aXa IC units, 15,000 aXa IC units, or standard heparin.

The compression times at the puncture sites were comparable to those under the standard heparin regimen.

2. *Efficacy Studies*

In a noncomparative study, 24 chronic and nine acute renal failure patients received CY 216 as a single predialysis bolus injection and underwent a total of 364 hemodialysis sessions, lasting up to 7 hr, and 39 hemofiltration procedures, lasting up to 5 hr. Approximately one-third of these 403 sessions were performed in patients with a high risk for hemorrhage (7). Initial doses were based on body weight, and subsequent doses were adjusted individually to prevent visible clot formation within the extracorporeal circuit. At a median dose of 250 aXa IC units/kg (range 100–330), a satisfactory response was obtained in 85% of the sessions, while in the remaining sessions minor clot formation occurred. No bleeding complications were observed.

In a recent heparin controlled, nonrandomized crossover study, 14 chronic dialysis patients were treated with heparin for 4 weeks, followed by a period of 6 weeks with CY 216. A dose of 250 aXa IC units/kg showed efficacy and safety results comparable to those with standard heparin treatment (25).

3. *Long-Term Randomized Heparin Controlled Efficacy Study*

A randomized heparin controlled, 6-month open follow-up study was performed in 70 chronic hemodialysis patients undergoing dialysis procedures up to 6 hr, with CY 216 as a single predialysis injection or standard heparin treatment (29). The optimal anticoagulant dose was 250 aXa IC units/kg for patients with a hematocrit $\geqslant 0.3$ or with a dialysis session lasting more than 4 hr whereas patients with a hematocrit below 0.3 received 200 aXa IC units/kg. The reason to use the hematocrit as an additional criterion for dose adaptation was derived from a single study in pediatric hemodialysis patients. Clotting of the extracorporeal circuit was observed in this study after the hematocrit was raised by transfusion of packed red cells (30).

During a total of approximately 4000 dialysis procedures (2000 with CY 216), a minimal, clinically not significant, clot formation was observed in 4% of the LMWH-treated patients and in 1% of the patients receiving standard heparin ($p > 0.05$). No major bleeding complications were observed in this long-term study. However, three patients (approximately 9%) in the CY 216 group had sustained minor bleeding from the puncture site after being in the study for several weeks. The LMWH dose could not be lowered in two of these patients without (minor) clotting within the extracorporeal circuit. These patients therefore received standard heparin for their further treatment.

Accumulation of CY 216 during consecutive dialysis procedures, measured by the predialysis aXa activity, was not observed.

4. *Pediatric Patients*

CY 216 was the first LMWH to be applied in a dose-finding study in pediatric chronic hemodialysis (30). A single predialysis dose of 300 aXa IC units/kg was used in 229 hemodialysis sessions, with a duration of 4 hr, in 16 children (mean age 10 years; range: 4–16) and revealed to be effective and safe; i.e., neither visible clot formation within the extracorporeal circuit nor hemorrhagic complications occurred.

5. *Conclusion*

The available studies demonstrate that a single predialysis bolus injection of CY 216 of 200–250 aXa IC units/kg, adapted according to the hematocrit, provides an adequate and safe anticoagulation during (chronic) hemodialysis for adult patients.

Only occasionally, the optimal dose in terms of efficacy and safety could not be established. The initial data obtained in pediatric patients are suggestive of adequate efficacy and safety for CY 216 in this category of patients, but final evidence will have to come from long-term heparin controlled investigations since comparative data are not available.

C. Enoxaparin, PK 10169

1. Dose-Finding Studies

In an open study, three randomly given bolus doses of 0.75 mg/kg, 1.0 mg/kg, and 1.25 mg/kg, respectively, were administered to 42 chronic hemodialysis patients dialyzing up to 4 hr. The optimal dose for PK 10169 appeared to be 1 mg/kg body weight (31).

2. Efficacy Studies in Patients Without an Enhanced Risk for Bleeding

A dose of 1 mg/kg was given in a study of 10 chronic renal failure patients, and three dialysis procedures per patient were investigated (32). Visible clot formation within the extracorporeal circuit was observed in 7 of 30 procedures (23%). Although this clot formation had no effect on the creatinine washout, markedly elevated FPA levels were observed in these cases. Higher or additional doses of PK 10169 during dialysis were not investigated.

3. Efficacy Studies in Patients with a High Risk for Bleeding

In an open noncomparative study, 46 chronic hemodialysis patients, undergoing 493 dialysis sessions, received a predialysis injection in a dose of 0.5 mg/kg in case of dual vascular access and in a dose of 0.75 mg/kg in case of single vascular access (33). Additional doses, which were half the bolus dose, were administered if visible clots appeared in the bubble catcher and were required in 98 dialysis sessions (i.e., in 20% of the procedures). Moreover, complete thrombotic obstruction of the extracorporeal circuit occurred in three dialysis sessions (0.6%), two of those during the 102 hemodialyses performed with a single access and one in 391 hemodialyses performed with a dual access. One patient had a PK 10169–related bleeding complication, i.e., excessive menstrual bleeding requiring transfusion.

The efficacy of the two PK 10169 doses was subsequently confirmed in a similar study in which a dose of 0.25 mg/kg was also investigated. However, the efficacy of this latter dose appeared less satisfactory; i.e., more visible clot formation within the extracorporeal circuit was noted (34).

4. Pediatric Patients

A noncomparative pilot study was performed in seven chronic hemodialysis children (mean age 13 years; range: 7–18), and 12 consecutive dialysis sessions with a duration of 4 hr were investigated per patient (35). In two children, the dose had to be increased from 24 to 36 mg/m^2 body surface area because of the appearance of visible clots within the bubble catcher. Bleeding complications were not observed, and the investigators therefore concluded that a single predialysis bolus injection of 24–36 mg/m^2 was efficacious and also safe.

5. *Conclusion*

Hitherto the results of hemodialysis studies with PK 10169 are promising, but the results of (long-term) heparin controlled studies have to be awaited to determine the eventual role of PK 10169 in hemodialysis. At present, no dose recommendations can be provided.

D. Fragmin, K 2165

1. *Dose-Finding Studies*

The largest experience with LMWH in hemodialysis comes from investigations with K 2165. Heparin-controlled studies were performed in Germany and England (36, 37). The German investigators determined the efficacy of K 2165 by suppression of visible clot formation within the extracorporeal circuit for dialysis procedures of up to 5 hr. They investigated 49 patients of whom 31 were treated by hemodialysis and 18 by hemofiltration. Of these patients, 14 had an enhanced risk for bleeding and 35 were without such a risk. The patients received, on aXa basis, a dose of 33–67% of their normal standard heparin dose, and no clinical relevant clotting in the extracorporeal circuit occurred in any of these patients. For patients without a bleeding risk the optimal dose regimen appeared to be 15–25 aXa units/kg bolus injection, followed by a continuous infusion of 8–12 aXa units/hr; for patients with a bleeding risk, a dose regime of 5–10 aXa units/kg bolus injection with a continuous infusion of 4–5 aXa units/hour appeared to be safe (36).

In the British studies, the efficacy criterion was based on inhibition of FPA generation (37, 38). A single bolus injection of 5000 aXa units inhibited FPA generation, to the same extent as standard heparin treatment, in dialysis procedures of 4-hr duration. The clinical efficacy of this dose was confirmed in one noncomparative study and one heparin controlled study (39, 40). However, this single dose appeared to be inadequate in a crossover study, and higher bolus injections of 85–90 aXa units/kg (approximately 7400–7900 aXa units) were required for dialyses of 4–5 hr, to effectively suppress visible clot formation (41).

Finally, a single bolus injection of 4000 aXa units with a continuous infusion of 750 aXa units/hr for dialyses lasting longer than 4 hr has been recommended by the British investigators (37).

2. *Efficacy Studies in Patients Without an Enhanced Risk for Bleeding*

The efficacy of the British dose regimen for dialysis of longer duration of 4000 aXa units bolus injection with 750 aXa units/hr continuous infusion was confirmed in a heparin controlled study in patients without an increased risk for bleeding (42).

In a heparin controlled efficacy study, the German dose regimen was also confirmed (43). However, some investigators had to use higher dose regimens (44, 45) whereas other investigators found a lower dose regimen to be adequate (46). This range of doses may be explained by interpatient variation, practical differences in the execution of the dialysis procedure, and differences in terms of efficacy end-points.

A dose regimen of 18 aXa units/kg bolus injection with 9 aXa units/kg/hr continuous infusion was evaluated in a crossover study versus standard heparin (47). With both treatments, minor clot formation in the extracorporeal circuit was observed in 40% of the hemodialysis procedures. Therefore, the dose regimens used in this study, both heparin and K 2165, seemed to be inadequate. Compression times at the puncture sites, as a substitute measure for safety, have been reported in seven of all reported K 2165 studies. The findings in these studies are contradictory; i.e., three studies reported a reduction of the compression time under K 2165 treatment, one study reported a prolongation, and finally, no significant difference versus standard heparin was observed in the remaining three studies. (39, 41–43, 46, 48, 49)

3. *Long-Term Heparin Controlled Studies*

K 2165 is the only LMWH for which long-term comparative studies of at least 1 year have been reported. In a randomized open study, 70 patients, who were new to hemodialysis or hemofiltration, were randomized to either K 2165 or standard heparin treatment for 1 year (8). Twenty-nine patients per group were treated by hemodialysis and six patients per group underwent hemofiltration. Dialyses lasted up to 5 hr and packed cell transfusions were given when the hemoglobin levels fell below 65 g/L. The anticoagulant doses were increased upon visible clot formation within the extracorporeal circuit. The optimal dose regimen appeared to be a bolus injection of 34 aXa units/kg and a continuous infusion of 12 aXa units/kg/hr. Clotting within the extracorporeal circuit occurred in 1.59% (80 of 5045 procedures) in the K 2165 group and in 1.33% (69 of 5187 procedures) in the standard heparin group. No accumulation of K 2165, as measured by consecutive predialysis aXa levels, was observed.

No major bleeding complications were encountered. However, 19 K 2165–treated patients and 16 heparin-treated patients needed packed cell transfusions. The number of transfusions was 76 in the K 2165 group and 88 in the standard heparin group ($p < 0.05$). This reduced transfusion requirement in the LMWH-treated patients was also observed in another heparin controlled study with K 2165 in chronic stable hemodialysis patients (50).

4. *The Effect of K 2165 on Lipid Metabolism*

In the long-term studies, significant differences in plasma lipid levels were found between the standard heparin and the K 2165–treated groups, i.e., an increase in plasma triglyceride levels and plasma lipolytic activity in heparin-treated patients (8, 50, 51), and a decrease of total cholesterol and LDL cholesterol and an increase in HDL cholesterol in K 2165–treated patients (48, 49, 51, 53).

However, most of these studies were small and had an open study design; therefore, these data are not conclusive.

5. *Conclusion*

K 2165 appeared to be an effective and safe anticoagulant for chronic hemodialysis patients. The following doses were most commonly applied: for chronic hemodialysis patients without a bleeding risk, a dose regimen of approximately 30–40 aXa units/kg bolus injection and 10–20 aXa units/hr continuous infusion; for patients with a bleeding risk, the dose regimen was adapted to approximately 5–10 aXa units/kg bolus injection and 4–5 aXa units continuous infusion; and for short dialysis procedures (up to 4 hr), a single bolus injection of 5000–7000 aXa units appeared to be sufficient.

The possible beneficial effects of K 2165 on the lipid profile are intriguing, but the results to date must be interpreted cautiously. Larger prospective studies with a crossover design are required to adequately investigate this issue.

E. Orgaran, ORG 10172

1. *Dose-Finding Studies*

The first clinical study with ORG 10172 was performed in acute hemodialysis patients and the heparinoid was administered as a single predialysis bolus injection of 300–600 mg in 12 patients with a high bleeding risk (19). The patients underwent 55 hemodialysis procedures, up to 4 hr, which were completed successfully without apparent enhancement of bleeding. The deposition of ^{125}-I-fibrinogen on the renal dialysis membrane was successfully inhibited in the four patients investigated.

In subsequent heparin controlled crossover studies ORG 10172 was administered as a single predialysis injection in a dose range of 22–70 aXa unit/kg. In a total of 49 chronic hemodialysis patients, 100 hemodialysis procedures, lasting up to 6 hr, were investigated and the antithrombotic efficacy of ORG 10172 was confirmed (22, 54).

2. *Efficacy Studies*

In two heparin controlled efficacy studies, both with a crossover design, ORG 10172 was administered as a single bolus injection of 34–40 aXa units/kg. A total of 69 patients, undergoing 223 hemodialysis sessions of up to 6.5 hr, were investigated (21, 55). The studies showed a similar efficacy of ORG 10172 and standard heparin.

Compression time at the puncture site was not used as a measure for safety in any of these studies. In one study, however, 7 of 14 patients had unexplained secondary bleeding from the puncture sites 24–36 hr after termination of the dialysis procedure (21). This observation might be related to the enhanced aXa levels that were observed for prolonged periods after dialysis; these prolonged periods may be due to the prolonged half-life of ORG 10172, which may even be as long as 31 hr in hemodialysis patients (21,54).

3. *ORG 10172 in Heparin-Induced Thrombocytopenia*

Heparin-induced thrombocytopenia (HIT) as a complication in hemodialysis patients might be a possible indication for ORG 10172. In a report comprising 57 patients with HIT of whom 21 required hemodialysis or hemofiltration, ORG 10172 was shown to be a safe, well-tolerated, effective anticoagulant. The hemodialysis patients were treated with an intravenous bolus injection of 3750 aXa units whereas the hemofiltration patients received an intravenous bolus of 2500 aXa units with an infusion of 200–600 aXa units/hr (56).

In 19 of these 21 patients the platelet counts normalized. One patient died suddenly of unknown cause 1 day after hemodialysis. Of the 19 patients in whom the thrombocytopenia resolved, eight died eventually of other causes than HIT. Compared to other LMWHs, Org 10172 has a much lower cross-reactivity rate with the HIT antibody (56, 57) and might therefore be preferred to other LMWHs in patients with HIT.

4. *Conclusion*

Because of its long half-life, exceeding 30 hr, in hemodialysis patients, ORG 10172 appeared to be less suitable for repeated use in chronic intermittent hemodialysis. However, in single dialysis procedures, it may be the anticoagulant of choice in HIT. An effective dose regimen was found to be a single bolus injection of 3750 aXa units.

III. CARDIOPULMONARY BYPASS SURGERY

Cardiopulmonary bypass surgery is a highly thrombogenic procedure in comparison to hemodialysis or hemofiltration, and therefore substantially higher doses of standard heparin are required. Serious postoperative hemorrhage remains a significant complication, despite technical improvements, the use of better surgical techniques, and the use of protamine sulfate for heparin neutralization. This postoperative complication is at least partly caused by the use of high doses of heparin. For this reason there is a continuous interest in development of alternative anticoagulants with a better safety profile.

Table 3 Dose and aXa Levels of Efficacy Studies in Hemodialysis

Author	Ref.	Year	Patient category	No. of patients[a]	No. of sessions[b,c]	Dose: Bolus	Dose: Infusion	aXa levels (units at the end of dialysis)
CY 222								
Morinière et al.	28	1990	With hemorrhagic risk	343	613	150 aXa IC/kg	—	1.3[d]
CY 216								
Steinbach et al.	7	1990	With/without hemorrhagic risk	32	364	250 aXa IC/kg	—	Not reported
Nurmohamed et al.	29	1991	Without hemorrhaghic risk	35	6 months	200–250 aXa IC/kg	—	Not reported
Grau et al.	25	1992	Without hemorrhaghic risk	14	231	235 aXa IC/kg	—	0.6
PK 10169								
Briquel et al.	32	1987	Without hemorrhagic risk	10	30	1 mg/kg	—	0.6
Dechelette et al.	33	1987	With hemorrhagic risk	46	493	0.5–0.75 mg/kg	—	Not reported
Gamberoni et al.	34	1989	With hemorrhagic risk	66	380	0.25–0.75 mg/kg	—	Not reported
K 2165								
Schrader et al.	36	1985	Without hemorrhagic risk	20	6 months	30–40 aXa/kg	8–15 aXa/kg/hr	0.5–0.6[g]
Borm et al.	47	1986	Without hemorrhagic risk	10	10	18 aXa/kg	9 aXa/kg/hr	0.4
Ljungberg et al.	39	1987	Without hemorrhagic risk	11	11	5000 aXa	—	0.8
Deuber et al.	52	1988	With/without hemorrhagic risk	20	18 months	20–80 aXa/kg[e]	10–20 aXa/kg/hr[e]	0.4–0.9
						1500–3000 aXa[f]	200–600 aXa/hr[f]	0.2–0.5

Schrader et al.	8	1988	With/without hemorrhagic risk	58	12 months	34 aXa/kg	12 aXa/kg/hr	0.6–0.7[g]
Maurin et al.	45	1988	Without hemorrhagic risk	6	72	23 aXa/kg	16 aXa/kg/hr	0.7
Laubenthal et al.	43	1989	Without hemorrhagic risk	8	56	22 aXa/kg	11 aXa/kg/hr	0.4
Anastassiades et al.	38	1990	Without hemorrhagic risk	21	1 month	3000–4000 aXa	750 aXa/hr	0.9
Suzuki et al.	46	1990	Without hemorrhagic risk	61	419	15–20 aXa/kg	7.5–10 aXa/kg/hr	0.4
Bambauer et al.	50	1990	Without hemorrhagic risk	21	6 months	Not reported	Not reported	0.2–0.3
Baumann et al.	41	1991	Without hemorrhagic risk	60	360	85–90 aXa/kg	—	0.9
Schneider et al.	48	1991	Without hemorrhagic risk	21	6 months	1500 aXa	675 aXa/hr	Not reported
Deuber et al.	49	1991	Without hemorrhagic risk	5	4 years	17–95 aXa/kg	7–20 aXa/kg/hr	0.4–1.0
Ljungberg et al.	40	1992	Without hemorrhagic risk	11	22	5000 aXa	—	0.6
ORG 10172								
Henny et al.	22	1985	Without hemorrhagic risk	55	55	34 aXa/kg	—	0.5
Frei et al.	21	1988	Without hemorrhagic risk	14	168	35–40 aXa/kg	—	Not reported

[a] Number of LMWH-treated patients.
[b] Number of sessions investigated with LMWH.
[c] For studies of 1 month or longer, the time on LMWH is reported.
[d] Institut Choay aXa unit.
[e] For patients with no hemorrhagic risk.
[f] For patients with a hemorrhagic risk.
[g] Two hours after start of the dialysis.

Thus far, limited experience is available with the use of LMWHs in cardiopulmonary bypass surgery. One open noncomparative study with LMWH and a few case reports have been published (58–63).

A. PK 10169

In an open study 15 patients received a total dose of 80–267 mg PK 10169 (58). This wide dose range was due to great differences in body surface area, duration of cardiopulmonary bypass, and hypothermia. These high doses were administered mainly to prevent clotting in the extracorporeal circuit, which was not observed in any patient. However, three patients experienced excessive postoperative blood loss, despite the administration of protamine sulfate. Although the APTT activity of LMWHs is completely neutralized by protamine sulfate, the aXa activity is only partly neutralized. This persisting aXa activity might be the cause for the observed abnormal postoperative bleeding, but this still remains to be established.

B. CY 216, ORG 10172

A few case reports have been published regarding the successful application of CY 216 (59) and ORG 10172 (60–63) in patients with HIT undergoing cardiopulmonary bypass surgery.

C. Conclusion

From the available data, LMWHs can only be considered experimental in patients with HIT undergoing cardiopulmonary bypass surgery. Obviously, further studies are needed to investigate whether there is indeed a place for LMWHs in cardiopulmonary bypass surgery.

IV. GENERAL CONCLUSIONS

At present convincing evidence exists that in hemodialysis patients LMWHs have at least similar efficacy and safety as standard heparin. No LMWH-induced thrombocytopenia or other adverse events were reported in the studies discussed in this chapter.

For long-term use, however, CY 222 and ORG 10172 seem less suitable because of their gradually accumulating anticoagulant activity in the course of consecutive dialysis procedures, and PK 10169 needs further investigation because a long-term study is still lacking.

In chronic stable hemodialysis patients, some open studies may indicate that LMWHs are associated with a lower bleeding tendency; however, these data are not conclusive. In addition, the recent introduction of recombinant

Table 4 Methodological Criteria of the Efficacy Studies in Hemodialysis

						Blind assessment of end-points	
Author	Ref.	Year	Comparative	Randomized	Crossover	Efficacy	Safety
CY 222							
Morinière et al.	28	1990	No	—	—	No	No
CY 216							
Steinbach et al.	7	1990	No	—	—	No	No
Nurmohamed et al.	29	1991	Yes	Yes	No	No	No
Grau et al.	25	1992	Yes	No	Yes	No	No
PK 10169							
Briquel et al.	32	1987	No	—	—	No	No
Dechelette et al.	33	1987	No	—	—	No	No
Gamberoni et al.	34	1989	No	—	—	No	No
K 2165							
Schrader et al.	36	1985	No	No	No	No	No
Borm et al.	47	1986	Yes	Yes	Yes	Yes	No
Ljungberg et al.	39	1987	Yes	No	Yes	No	No
Deuber et al.	52	1988	No	—	—	No	No
Schrader et al.	8	1988	Yes	Yes	No	No	No
Maurin et al.	45	1988	Yes	No	Yes	No	No
Laubenthal et al.	43	1989	Yes	No	Yes	No	No
Anastassiades et al.	38	1990	Yes	Yes	Yes	No	No
Suzuki et al.	46	1990	Yes	No	Yes	No	No
Bambauer et al.	50	1990	Yes	No	Yes	No	No
Baumann et al.	41	1991	Yes	Yes	Yes	No	No
Schneider et al.	48	1991	Yes	No	Yes	No	No
Deuber et al.	49	1991	No	No	No	No	No
Ljungberg et al.	40	1992	No	—	—	No	No
ORG 10172							
Henny et al.	22	1985	Yes	Yes	Yes	Yes	No
Frei et al.	21	1988	Yes	Yes	Yes	No	No

erythropoietin markedly improved hemostasis and has significantly reduced the transfusion requirements for chronic stable hemodialysis patients (64). This reduces the bleeding risk in this category of patients, thereby limiting the significance of an eventual lower bleeding tendency in LMWH-treated patients.

Hence, the main advantage of LMWHs, so far, is the further simplification of the anticoagulant regimen in chronic hemodialysis patients, because of the efficacy of a single predialysis bolus injection. Moreover, there is no need for laboratory monitoring.

Whether the safety of LMWHs is better in hemodialysis patients with a high bleeding risk needs to be further confirmed in properly designed comparative studies.

A noteworthy variation in the optimal dose regimen emerges from the available studies (Table 3), which may be due to practical differences in the execution of the dialysis and to the different criteria for efficacy, such as inhibition of FPA generation or of visible clotting within the extracorporeal circuit. This latter criterion may obviously result in a lower dose regimen.

Furthermore, most of the studies had methodological imperfections and were therefore subject to bias (Table 4). Only 7 of 23 studies had a randomized comparative design, and only two of these studies had a blind assessment of the efficacy end-point. Therefore, the reported advantages of LMWHs over standard heparin treatment must be interpreted with caution.

There are some indications that K 2165 had beneficial effects on the lipid profile. However, larger prospective long-term, heparin controlled studies are mandatory before any conclusion can be reached.

In pediatric patients, at present, the available experience is too limited to allow meaningful conclusions concerning potential benefits of LMWH.

For hemofiltration and related techniques, preliminary data suggest equal efficacy and safety for LMWHs compared to heparin.

For cardiopulmonary bypass surgery even less information is available. Clearly, this potential indication needs further investigation.

Finally, none of the reported studies addressed the cost-effectiveness of LMWH versus standard heparin.

REFERENCES

1. Verstraete M. Drugs 1990; 40:498.
2. Nurmohamed MT, Rosendaal FR, Büller HR, Dekker E, Hommes DW, Vandenbroucke JP, Briët E. Lancet 1992; 340:152.
3. Persson E, Norderström J, Nilsson-Ehle P, Hagenfeldt L. Eur J Clin Invest 1985; 15:215.
4. Tansey MJB, Opie LH. Lancet 1983; 2:419.
5. McDonald MM, Hathaway WE. J Pediatr 1982; 101:451.

6. Renaud H, Moriniere P, Dieval J, Abdull-Massih Z, Dkhissi H, Toulemonde F, Delobel J, Fournier A. Proc EDTA-ERA 1984; 21:276.
7. Steinbach G, Bosc C, Caraman PL, Azoulay E, Olry L, d'Azamar P, Chopin J. Néphrologie 1990; 11:17.
8. Schrader J, Stibbe W, Armstrong VW, Kandt M, Muche R, Köstering H, Siedel D, Scheler F. Kidney Int 1988; 33:890.
9. Ryzlewich T, Saupe J, Fuchs G, Eichhorn HM. Dial Transplant 1991; 20:124.
10. Journois D, Safran D, Castelain MH, Chanu D, Drévillon C, Barrier G. Ann Fr Anesth Réanim 1990; 9:331.
11. Lorenzini JL, Freysz M, Honnart D, Zeller V, Dutrillaux F. Int J Clin Pharmacol Ther Toxicol 1991; 29:89.
12. John G, Shehabi Y, Mudaliar Y. Anaesth Intens Care 1991; 19:588.
13. Morinière PH, Dieval J, Renaud H, Westeel PF, Tondriaux A, Boudailliez B, Schmit JL, Hocine Ch, Nahle M, Bayrou B, Delobel J, Fournier A. Réan Soins Intens Méd Urg 1990; 6:135.
14. Hory B, Cachoux A, Toulemonde F. Nephron 1985; 41:125.
15. Nurmohamed MT, Fareed J, Hoppensteadt B, Walenga JM, ten Cate JW. Semin Thromb Hemost 1991; 17(Suppl 2):214.
16. Ryan KE, Lane DA, Flynn A, Shepperd J, Ireland HA, Curtis JR. Thromb Haemostas 1991; 66:277.
17. Schrader J, Stibbe W, Kandt M, Warneke G, Armstrong V, Müller HJ, Scheler F. Trans Am Soc Artif Intern Organs 1990; 36:28.
18. Thomas DP. Thromb Haemostas 1989; 61:648.
19. Henny CP, ten Cate H, ten Cate JW, Surachno S, van Bronswijk H, Wilmink JM, Ockelford PA. Lancet 1983; 1:890.
20. ten Cate H, Henny Ch.P, ten Cate JW, Büller HR, Mooy MC, Surachno S, Wilmink JM. Thromb Res 1985; 38:211.
21. Frei U, Wilks MF, Boehmer S, Crisp-Lindgren N, Schwarzrock R, Stiekema JCJ, Koch KM. Nephrol Dial Transplant 1988; 3:435.
22. Henny CP, ten Cate H, Surachno A, Stevens P, Büller HR, den Hartog M, ten Cate JW. Thromb Haemost 1985; 54:460.
23. Hory B, Cachoux A, Saunier F, Kieffer Y, Laroze M, Henriet MT, Toulemonde F, Bayrou B, Perol C. Presse Méd 1987; 16:955.
24. Dieval J, Morinière P, Bayrou B, Roussel B, Fournier A, Delobel J. In: Breddin K, Fareed J, Samama M, eds. Fraxiparine, First International Symposium. Stuttgart: Schattauer, 1989:169.
25. Grau E, Sigüenza F, Maduell F, Linares M, Angels Olaso M, Martinez R, Caridad A. Nephron 1992; 62:13.
26. Dieval J, Morinière P, Roussel B, Bayrou B, Fournier A, Delobel J. J Mal Vasc 1987; 12:114.
27. Ireland H, Lane DA, Flynn A, Pegrum AC, Curtis JR. Thromb Haemost 1988; 59:240.
28. Morinière P, Dieval J, Bayrou B, Renaud H, Roussel B, Gross S, Hocine C, Nahle M, Delobel J, Fournier A. Réan Soins Intens Méd Urg 1990; 6:129.
29. Nurmohamed MT, ten Cate J, Stevens P, Hoek JA, Lins RL, ten Cate JW. Trans Am Soc Artif Intern Organs 1991; 37:M459.

30. Schlegel N, Macher MA, Hurtaud MF, Maisin A, Bara L, Loirat C. In: Breddin K, Fareed J, Samama M, eds. Fraxiparine, First International Symposium. Stuttgart: Schattauer, 1989:177.
31. Pouzol P, Polack B, Dechelette E, Jurkovitz C, Cusin E. J Mal Vasc 1987; 12:108.
32. Briquel ME, Kessler M, André E, Cao Huu T, Alexandre P, Renoult E, Jonon B. J Mal Vasc 1987; 12:111.
33. Dechelette E, Pouzol P, Jurkovitz C, Kuentz F, Polack B, Cuzin E, Woler M. J Mal Vasc 1987; 12:105.
34. Gamberoni J, Jonon B, Cao Huu T, Kessler M. Ann Med Nancy 1989; 28:187.
35. Bianchetti MG, Peck S, Müller R, Oetliker OH. Schweiz Rundschau Med 1990; 23:730.
36. Schrader J, Valentin R, Tönnis HJ, Hildebrand U, Stibbe W, Armstrong VW, Kandt M, Köstering H, Quellhorst E. Kidney Int 1985; 28:823.
37. Lane DA, Ireland H, Flynn A, Anastassiades E, Curtis JR. Neprol Dial Transplant 1986; 1:179.
38. Anastassiades E, Lane DA, Ireland H, Flynn A, Curtis JR. Clin Nephrol 1989; 32:290.
39. Ljungberg B, Blombäck M, Johnsson H, Lins LE. Clin Nephrol 1987; 27:31.
40. Ljungberg B, Jacobson SH, Lins LE, Pejler G. Clin Nephrol 1992; 38:97.
41. Baumann D, Frühsorger A, Glass W, Zielke E. Nieren-Hochdruckkrankheit 1991; 1:36.
42. Anastassiades E, Ireland H, Flynn A, Lane DA, Curtis JR. Nephrol Dial Transplant 1990; 5:135.
43. Laubenthal E, Plum J, Spreger KBG, Grabensee B. Nieren-Hochdruckkrankheit 1989; 11:488.
44. Schrader J, Rieger J, Müschen H, Stibbe W, Köstering H, Kramer P, Scheler F. Klin Wochenschr 1985; 63:49.
45. Maurin N, Kierdorf H. Klin Wochenschr 1988; 66:246.
46. Suzuki T, Ota K, Naganuma S, Koshikawa S, Hirasawa Y, Nakagawa S, Otsubu O, Akizawa T. Semin Thromb Hemost 1990; 16(Suppl):46.
47. Borm JJJ, Krediet R, Sturk A, ten Cate JW. Haemostasis 1986; 16(Suppl 2):59.
48. Schneider H, Schmitt Y. Klin Wochenschr 1991; 69:749.
49. Deuber HJ, Schulz W. Kidney Int 1991; 40:496.
50. Bambauer R, Rücker S, Weber U, Köhler M. Trans Am Soc Artif Intern Organs 1990; 36:M646.
51. Stibbe W, Schrader J, Armstrong VW, Kandt M, Walli A, Seidel D, Scheler F. Nieren-Hochdruckkrankheit 1990; 2:81.
52. Deuber HJ, Schulz W. Nieren-Hochdruckkrankheit 1988; 7:262.
53. Nikolay J, Schulz E, Traut G, Nieth N, Biesel E, Zielke E. Nieren-Hochdruckkrankheit 1990; 12:519.
54. Ireland H, Lane DA, Flynn A, Anastassiades E, Curtis JR. Thromb Haemost 1986; 55:271.
55. von Bonsdorff M, Stiekema J, Harjanne A, Alapiessa U. Int J Artif Organs 1990; 13:103.
56. Chong BH, Magnani HN. Haemostasis 1992; 22:85.
57. Chong BH, Aust NZ. J Med 1992; 22:145.

58. Massonnet-Castel S, Pelissier E, Bara L, Terrier E, Abry B, Guibourt P, Swanson J, Jaulmes B, Carpentier A, Samama M. Haemostasis 1986; 16:139.
59. Gouault-Heilmann M, Huet Y, Contant G, Payen D, Bloch G, Rapin M. Lancet 1983; 1:1374.
60. Deryck YLJ-M, van Krugten RJ, Schepp RM, Movhtar B. Acta Anaesthesiol Belg 1990; 41:54.
61. Doherty DC, Ortel TL, de Bruijn N, Greenberg CS, van Trigt P, III. Anesthesiology 1990; 73:562.
62. Rowlings PA, Evans S, Mansberg R, Murray B, Rozenberg MC, Aust NZ. J Med 1991; 21:52.
63. Marshall LR, Cannell PK, Herrmann RP. Thromb Haemost 1992; 67:587.
64. Moia M, Manucci PM, Vizzotto L, Casati S, Cattaneo M, Ponticelli C. Lancet 1987; 2:1127.

14

Low-Molecular-Weight Heparins for Prevention of Restenosis Following Coronary Angioplasty

F. W. Amann, B. J. Meyer, C. Neuenschwander, and H. Drexel
University Hospital, Zurich, Switzerland

I. PERCUTANEOUS TRANSLUMINAL CORONARY ANGIOPLASTY

Percutaneous transluminal coronary angioplasty (PTCA) was first applied clinically in 1977 by Andreas Grüntzig at our institution (1). The principle of PTCA is to place a catheter-guided balloon in the lumen adjacent to a coronary stenosis and to dilate the lesion. The procedure provides an efficient means for nonoperative dilation of atherosclerotic coronary narrowings. Due to advances in operator experience and technical equipment, the primary success rate now approaches 95% in most centers. However, the initial gain in lumen size is jeopardized by acute reocclusions and late restenosis (2).

A. Complications of PTCA

Acute reocclusions occur with about 5% of lesions and are caused by thrombosis, intimal dissection, medial and subintimal hemorrhage, vascular recoil, and vasoconstriction (2). The pathogenesis of these complications has been partly elucidated by intravascular ultrasound imaging. It was observed (3) that angioplasty achieves luminal enlargement primarily by overstretching the arterial wall with the lesion volume remaining practically unchanged. Overstretching explains intimal dissections whose surfaces initiate thrombus formation. Unfractionated heparin limits, but does not completely prevent, this early thrombotic response (2).

Late restenosis is different from reocclusion in many respects, such as clinical time course, pathophysiology, and treatment.

II. RESTENOSIS

A. Magnitude of the Clinical Problem

The first follow-up studies indicated a rate of 33% of restenosis within 6 months after the procedure (4, 5). Although intercenter differences in restenosis rates persist (6), there is now a consensus that restenosis occurs in about 30–40% of patients (2, 7). Apparently, all recurrences have developed by 3 months after PTCA (8). Data from multivessel angioplasty clearly indicate that restenosis is a lesion-related problem and not a patient-related problem; i.e., every individual lesion faces the same risk of restenosis (9). However, a remarkable and significant ($p < 0.01$) difference in restenosis rate between men (36%) and women (22%) has been reported (8). In addition to male sex, further risk factors for restenosis have been identified, including diabetes mellitus, stenosis in the left anterior descending coronary artery or in a venous bypass graft, and absence of an intimal dissection after PTCA (6). Somewhat surprisingly, indeed, dissection after PTCA confers an advantage in prognosis (10). There is no sound evidence that procedural factors (balloon size, number, duration, or pressure of inflation) are capable of reducing restenosis rates (6).

B. Symptoms and Diagnosis

Restenosis is often, but not always, symptomatic; exertional angina is the most frequent symptom. In a follow-up study of 229 patients, 71% of those with symptoms developed restenosis but only 14% of those without did (11). Although restenosis correlates well with the recurrence of symptoms, the two factors are not identical (6). Studies using quantitative angiography established the definition for restenosis of a loss of >1 mm^2 corresponding to a 70% narrowing of the cross-sectional lumen. On the basis of this morphological definition, a restenosis rate of 33% was described (12, 13).

C. Pathophysiology

The pathophysiology of restenosis is incompletely understood. First clues pointing to a proliferative process came from autopsy studies. In the previously dilated segments of two patients who died 17 and 62 days, respectively, after angioplasty, focal proliferation of vascular smooth muscle cells was prominent on neointimal surfaces (14). In another patient who died 5 months after PTCA, the restenosis was caused by fibrocellular tissue (15). With an increase of information on restenosis a picture emerges (Fig. 1) involving not only platelet activation and thrombin generation (2), but also release of mitogens (2) with subsequent fibrocellular intimal hyperplasia (2, 16). The latter is caused by proliferation of endothelial and vascular smooth muscle cells (17) and alterations of intimal extracellular matrix (18). It was shown in rat experiments that platelet-

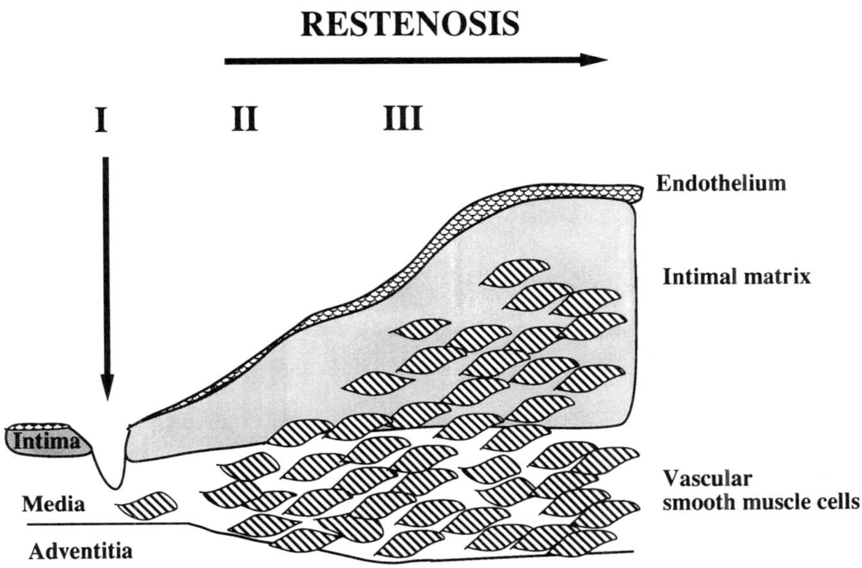

Figure 1 Schematic view of the restenosis process. (I) Intimal lesion; (II) proliferation of vascular smooth muscle cells (VSMC); (III) migration of VSMC from media into the intima. Restenosis involves increased matrix formation, proliferation of VSMC, and migration of VSMC from the media into the intima.

derived growth factor induces migration of smooth muscle cells into the intima where basic fibroblast growth factor initiates their proliferation (19). Recently, a model for restenosis was proposed attributing the main role to leukocytes and smooth muscle cells producing a cascade of cytokines and growth factors (20). According to this model, restenosis is an exaggerated, but otherwise natural, reaction to vascular injury. Whether there is a role for dyslipoproteinemia in the development of restenosis is still a matter of debate (21).

D. Prognosis and Treatment

Restenosis is rarely life-threatening provided it is diagnosed and treated promptly. The incidence of myocardial infarction during the first 2 years after PTCA is 4% and the incidence of death is 1–2% (4, 22). Moreover, myocardial infarction and death are rarely the first manifestations of restenosis. Restenosis in most instances is treated by repetition of PTCA. The second PTCA is more often successful than the first one, which explains why continued success rates increase from 63% after the first to 78% after the second dilation (4). Alternative treatment modalities for restenosis include coronary artery venous bypass grafting and transluminal atherectomy. In a large series reported from Grüntzig's group,

Table 1 Compounds Used for Restenosis Prevention

Compound	Model	Effect	Ref.
Warfarin	Human	No	23
Aspirin	Human	No	23
Omega-3 fatty acids	Human	No	26,27
Cilazapril	Animal	Yes	30
Cilazapril	Human	No	31
Unfractionated heparin	Human	No	32
Low-molecular-weight heparin	Animal	Yes	35,36,37
Low-molecular-weight heparin	Human	No	39,41

bypass grafting was necessary in only 5% of patients after a first PTCA (4). Although restenosis is not life-threatening, its high incidence and treatment costs make its prevention desirable.

E. Pharmacological Prevention

Many attempts have been made to reduce the incidence of restenosis after PTCA. An ideal strategy would inhibit smooth muscle cell migration and proliferation without affecting reendothelialization of the injured vessel site. Significant improvement of post-PTCA outcome is to be expected from a feasible pharmacological prevention of restenosis. Warfarin (23), aspirin, and other antiplatelet agents (23, 24) have been tested and were apparently no better than placebo. Alternatively, omega-3 fatty acids are good candidates for prevention of reocclusion because of their platelet inhibitory, anti-inflammatory (2), and antiproliferative properties (25). However, these compounds were not effective when given after PTCA (26, 27). A beneficial effect was only demonstrated when treatment was begun 1 week before PTCA (28, 29). Because proliferation and migration of vascular smooth muscle cells are mediated in part by angiotensin II, it has been suggested that angiotensin-converting-enzyme inhibitors may prevent restenosis (30). In rats, cilazapril and captopril were indeed shown to reduce the degree of restenosis after vascular injury by 80% (30). In humans, however, cilazapril failed to reduce restenosis after PTCA and offered no clinical benefit over placebo (31). Table 1 lists some of the compounds that have been used in an attempt to prevent restenosis.

Heparin appears particularly promising because, in addition to its antithrombotic effect, it inhibits both smooth muscle cell proliferation and migration and produces an alteration in matrix composition (18). However, studies using unfractionated heparin reportedly failed to prevent restenosis after angioplasty. Gimple et al. (32) administered heparin both subcutaneously and intramurally after balloon angioplasty of rabbit femoral arteries. Both treatment modalities failed to reduce restenosis after angioplasty. One explanation for this failure may be that the animals were extremely hypercholesterolemic at the time of angioplasty, a state that alters composition of the injury-induced lesion with an increase of foam cells and a decrease in smooth muscle cells (18). Such a lesion would be relatively resistant to heparin treatment. In humans, however, prolonged treatment (> 48 hr) with unfractionated heparin has not been tested for prevention of restenosis. In conclusion, thus, none of the above-mentioned approaches considerably reduced rates of restenosis.

III. LOW-MOLECULAR-WEIGHT HEPARIN

Low-molecular-weight heparin (LMWH) appears a good candidate to reduce late restenosis after PTCA for three important reasons: First, the benefit-to-risk ratio is higher than with unfractionated heparin, especially with respect to bleeding complications (33). Second, because of its long action, LMWH can be administered once daily. Third, the low-molecular-weight fraction retains the full antiproliferative potential of heparin (34).

Because of these features, LMWH has been used in animal models to prevent reocclusions. Indeed, a reduction in the proliferative response to vascular injury has been reported in rabbits (35) and minipigs (36), the animal model with the closest resemblance to the human situation (7). Hanke et al. (35) administered 164 IU/kg/day of logiparin to 20 male New Zealand White rabbits for 7 days after balloon dilatation and compared the intimal wall thickness after 28 days to that of 20 controls not receiving LMWH. Treated animals had a mean increase in intimal wall thickness to 20 ± 6 cell layers after 28 days, whereas control animals had an increase to 35 ± 15 cell layers ($p < 0.01$). In a similar study, Buchwald et al. (36) administered 82–123 IU/kg/day of dalteparin to minipigs after coronary stent implantation. Maximal neointimal thickness was 0.44 ± 0.18 mm with dalteparin compared to 0.80 ± 0.14 mm in control animals ($p < 0.01$). Similarly, Guyton et al. (37) demonstrated a 77% decrease in myointimal proliferation by a heparin preparation similar to LMWH in rat carotid arteries injured by air drying. Finally, in similar studies Dryjski et al. (38) showed that all the antiproliferative potential of heparin was recovered in the low-molecular-weight fraction.

These promising results prompted the use of LMWH in humans. So far two studies have been reported. Faxon et al. (39) conducted a multicenter placebo-controlled trial of 3417 IU/day over 28 days in 459 patients undergoing PTCA. Preliminary results (40), with a restenosis rate of 52% after nadroparin versus 51% under placebo, are discouraging. In our own open pilot study (41), 20 patients with chronic stable coronary artery disease undergoing a first elective

PTCA were included. Nadroparin, 6150 IU/day, was started 1 day before PTCA, and additional 3075 IU was given 2 hr prior to dilation. During angioplasty, unfractionated heparin was given at a dose adjusted to achieve an activated clotting time of at least 300 sec. After PTCA, nadroparin was continued for 28 days at a daily dose of 6150 IU. All patients had an uneventful hospital course and were free of angina or relevant silent ischemia on a bicycle stress test before discharge. Three months after PTCA, all patients underwent reangiography. Six of our 20 patients (30%) had angiographic evidence for restenosis (defined as >50% stenosis). Four of these six patients with restenosis had developed stable angina between 4 and 12 weeks after angioplasty. Thus, when compared to the spontaneous restenosis rate after PTCA of 30–40% (2, 7), our patients probably did not experience much benefit from LMWH. However, because of our small study population and the open study design, no firm conclusion can be drawn. One important aspect of our study was that LMWH was well tolerated over a period of 4 weeks and there were no bleeding complications or other adverse effects. This favorable experience compares well with the high safety reported by Faxon et al. (39) and makes a larger controlled trial of LMWH worthwhile in patients after PTCA.

For such a trial, three strategies appear promising: modification of dosage, alternative application regimens, and combined treatment. Dosage in the human studies, where LMWH failed to prevent restenosis, was 50–80 IU/kg (39, 41) whereas the successful animal studies used LMWH at a dose of 120–160 IU/kg (18, 19). Thus, on a body weight basis, humans received only about one-half of the dose operative in animals. Such low doses can hardly be effective since it has been demonstrated that vascular smooth muscle cells of patients with restenosis exhibit decreased sensitivity to heparin (42). Therefore, and because a high level of safety has been demonstrated for LMWH, higher doses are worth being tested as a first-line strategy. Second, so far no consensus exists on start and duration of LMWH treatment, and various approaches appear justified. Third, use of LMWH in combination with other agents such as omega-3 fatty acids appears promising. Such trials are underway (7). Thus, different doses of LMWH, different protocols of delivery, and combination regimens will, it is hoped, significantly decrease the rate of restenosis after PTCA (18).

REFERENCES

1. Grüntzig AR, Senning A, Siegenthaler WE. Nonoperative dilation of coronary artery stenosis: percutaneous transluminal coronary angioplasty. N Engl J Med 1979; 301:61–68.
2. Ip JH, Fuster V, Israel D, Badimon L, Badimon J, Chesebro JH. The role of platelets, thrombin and hyperplasia in restenosis after coronary angioplasty. J Am Coll Cardiol 1991; 17:77B–88B.

3. The SHK, Gussenhoven EJ, Zhong Y, et al. Effect of balloon angioplasty on femoral artery evaluated with intravascular ultrasound imaging. Circulation 1992; 86:483–493.
4. Meier B, King III SB, Grüntzig AR, et al. Repeat coronary angioplasty. J Am Coll Cardiol 1984; 4:463–466.
5. Holmes DR, Vliestra RE, Smith HC, et al. Restenosis after percutaneous transluminal coronary angioplasty (PTCA): a report from the PTCA Registry of the National Heart, Lung, and Blood Institute. Am J Cardiol 1984; 53:77C–81C.
6. Meier B. Restenosis after coronary angioplasty: review of the literature. Eur Heart J 1988; 9(Suppl C):1–6.
7. Popma JJ, Califf RM, Topol EJ. Clinical restenosis after coronary angioplasty. Circulation 1991; 84:1426–1436.
8. Cowley MJ, Mullin SM, Kelsey SF, et al. Sex differences in early and long-term results of coronary angioplasty in the NHLBI PTCA Registry. Circulation 1985; 71:90–97.
9. Hollmann J, Galan K, Franco I, Simpfendorfer C, Fatica K, Beck G. Recurrent stenosis after coronary angioplasty. J Am Coll Cardiol 1986; 7:20A (abstract).
10. Leimgruber PP, Roubin GF, Anderson HV, et al. Influence of intimal dissection on restenosis after successful coronary angioplasty. Circulation 1985; 72:530–535.
11. Mabin TA, Holmes Dr, Smith HC, et al. Follow-up clinical results in patients undergoing percutaneous transluminal coronary angioplasty. Circulation 1985; 71:754–760.
12. Fleck E, Dirschinger J, Rudolph W. Quantitative Koronarangiographie vor und nach PTCA. Restenosierungsrate. Analyse beeinflussender Faktoren. Herz 1985; 10:313–320.
13. Johnson MR, Brayden GP, Ericksen EE, et al. Changes in cross-sectional area of the coronary lumen in the six months after angioplasty: a quantitative analysis of the variable response to percutaneous transluminal angioplasty. Circulation 1986; 73:467–475.
14. Austin GE, Ratliff NB, Hollman J, Tabei S, Phillips DF. Intimal proliferation of smooth muscle cells as an explanation for recurrent coronary artery stenosis after percutaneous transluminal coronary angioplasty. J Am Coll Cardiol 1985; 6:369–375.
15. Essed CD, Van den Brand M, Becker AE. Transluminal coronary angioplasty an early restenosis. Fibrocellular occlusion after wall laceration. Br Heart J 1983; 49:393–396.
16. Liu MW, Roubin GS, King SB. Restenosis after coronary angioplasty: potential biologic determinants and role of intimal hyperplasia. Circulation 1989; 79:1374–1387.
17. Ueda M, Becker AE, Tsukada T, Numano F, Fujimoto T. Fibrocellular tissue response after percutaneous transluminal coronary angioplasty. Circulation 1991; 83:1327–1332.
18. Clowes AW. Heparin. Will it control intimal thickening after angioplasty? Circulation 1992; 86:1657–1658.
19. Reidy MA, Fingerle J, Lindner V. Factors controlling the development of arterial lesions after injury. Circulation 1992; 86(Suppl III):III-43–III-46.

20. Libbey P, Schwartz D, Brogi E, Tanaka H, Clinton SK. A cascade model for restenosis. A special case of atherosclerosis progression. Circulation 1992; 86(Suppl III):III-47–III-52.
21. Austin GE. Lipids and vascular restenosis. Circulation 1992; 85:1613–1615.
22. Kent KM, Bentivoglio LG, Block PC, et al. Long-term efficacy of percutaneous transluminal coronary angioplasty (PTCA): report from the National Heart, Lung, and Blood Institute PTCA Registry. Am J Cardiol 1984; 53:27C–31C.
23. Thornton MA, Gruentzig AR, Hollmann J, et al. Coumadin and aspirin in prevention of recurrence after transluminal coronary angioplasty: a randomized study. Circulation 1984; 69:721–727.
24. Schwartz L, Lesperance J, Burassa MG, et al. The role of antiplatelet agents in modifying the extent of restenosis following percutaneous transluminal angioplasty. Am Heart J 1990; 119 232–236.
25. Winer BH, Ockene IS, Levine PH, et al. Inhibition of atherosclerosis by cod-liver oil in a hyperlipidemic swine model. N Engl J Med 1986; 315:841–846.
26. Grig LE, Kay TWH, Valentine PA, et al. Determinants of restenosis and lack of effect of dietary supplementation with eicosapentaenoic acid on the incidence of coronary artery restenosis after angioplasty. J Am Coll Cardiol 1989; 13:665–672.
27. Reis GS, Sipperly ME, Boucher TM, et al. Results of a randomized double-blind placebo-controlled trial of fish oil for prevention of restenosis after PTCA. Circulation 1988; 78(Suppl II):II-291 (abstract).
28. Dehmer GJ, Popma JJ, van der Berg EK, et al. Reduction in the rate of early restenosis after coronary angioplasty by a diet supplemented with n-3 fatty acids. N Engl J Med 1988; 319:734–740.
29. Milner MR, Cillino RA, Leffingwell A, Pichard AD, Rosenberg J, Lindsay J. High dose omega-3-fatty acid supplement reduces clinical restenosis after coronary angioplasty. Circulation 1988; 78(Suppl I):I-634 (abstract).
30. Powell JS, Clozel J-P, Müller RKM, et al. Inhibitors of angiotensin-converting enzyme prevent myointimal proliferation after vascular injury. Science 1989; 245:186–188.
31. MERCATOR Study Group. Does the new angiotensin converting enzyme inhibitor cilazapril prevent restenosis after percutaneous transluminal coronary angioplasty? Circulation 1992; 86:100–110.
32. Gimple LW, Gertz SD, Haber HL, et al. Effect of chronic subcutaneous or intramural administration of heparin on femoral artery restenosis after balloon angioplasty in hypercholesterolemic rabbits. Circulation 1992; 86:1536–1546.
33. Leizorovicz A, Haugh MC, Chapuis F-R, Samama M M, Boissel J-P. Low molecular weight heparin in prevention of perioperative thrombosis. Br Med J 1992; 305:913–920.
34. Karnovsky MJ, Wright TO Jr, Castellot JJ, Choay J, Lormeau JC, Petitou M. Heparin, heparin sulfate, smooth muscle cells, and atherosclerosis. Ann NY Acad Sci 1989; 556:268–281.
35. Hanke H, Oberhoff M, Hanke S, et al. Inhibition of cellular proliferation after experimental balloon angioplasty by low-molecular-weight heparin. Circulation 1992; 85:1548–1556.

36. Buchwald AB, Unterberg CH, Nebendahl K, Gröne HJ, Wiegand V. Low-molecular-weight heparin reduces neointimal proliferation after coronary stent implantation in hypercholesterolemic minipigs. Circulation 1992; 86:531–537.
37. Guyton JR, Rosenberg RD, Clowes AW, Karnowsky MJ. Inhibition of rat arterial smooth muscle cell proliferation by heparin: in vivo studies with anticoagulation and nonanticoagulant heparin. Circ Res 1980; 46:625–634.
38. Dryjski M, Mikat E, Bjornsson TD. Inhibition of intimal hyperplasia after arterial injury by heparins and heparinoid. J Vasc Surg 1988; 8:623–633.
39. Faxon J, Spiro T, Minor S, et al. Enoxaparin, a low molecular weight heparin, in the prevention of restenosis after angioplasty: results of a double blind randomized trial. Am Coll Cardiol 1991; 19:258A (abstract).
40. Talley JD. Progress in interventional cardiology. J Interven Cardiol 1992; 5:245–251.
41. Amann FW, Neuenschwander Ch, Meyer BJ. Fraxiparin for prevention of restenosis after percutaneous transluminal coronary angioplasty. Semin Thromb Hemost 1993; 160–163.
42. Chan P, Patel M, Betteridge L. Abnormal growth regulation of vascular smooth muscle cells by heparin in patients with restenosis. Lancet 1993; 341:341–342.

15

Low-Molecular-Weight Heparins for Treatment of Established Venous Thromboembolism

Dieter Lockner
University Hospital, Huddinge, Sweden

I. INTRODUCTION

The most frequently used and established treatment of deep venous thrombosis (DVT) of the leg is continuous intravenous (i.v.) infusion of unfractionated heparin (UFH) with roughly 30,000 IU/24 hr, with an initial bolus dose of 5000 IU. The dose is adjusted during infusion with repeated determinations of the APT time, keeping it between 1.5 and 2.5 times greater than the initial (normal) value (1).

With the development of the low-molecular-weight heparins (LMWH) the most immediate important question was the merit of LMWHs compared with the established UFH in the treatment of DVT.

The treatment of DVT with LMWH was preceded by several years by its use as a prophylactic agent against thromboembolism. In 1982, Kakkar et al. (2) published the first paper on the prophylactic use of LMWH to prevent postoperative thromboembolism. Results of the first study on the treatment of established DVT did not appear until 1985 (3).

The LMWHs were first developed in Europe; therefore, early studies were performed there. It was not until 1992 that the first study from the United States was published (4). In many European countries LMWHs are already registered for use as either a prophylactic or a treatment. In the United States it will take some years until a sufficient number of American studies have been performed to allow registration.

The randomized studies hitherto published and registered on Medline will be reviewed here. A short description of the studies will be given in the text, and the most important results will be presented in tables grouped according to the different treatment forms. The level of evidence of the studies will be classified according to Cook et al (5).

Weighted means for the results collected in the tables will be calculated where the number of studied patients influences the weight of the mean value. The results will be evaluated in the discussion and their common merits will be compared. Uncontrolled studies will not be included as they allow no comparison.

II. CONTINUOUS INTRAVENOUS INFUSION OF LMWH COMPARED WITH INTRAVENOUS INFUSION OF UFH

The first study on the use of the new LMWHs in the treatment of established DVT was published by Bratt et al. in 1985 (3). The DVTs were venographically verified, and the patients were randomized between the LMWH from Kabi, Sweden (Kabi 2165) and UFH. Both drugs were infused intravenously in identical doses, 240 anti-FXa/IU/kg/12 hr. Warfarin treatment was started when the patient had been randomized. It was known that the LMWH inhibited thrombin less than factor Xa and that the APT time was therefore an inaccurate measurement of the anticoagulant activity of LMWH. There was, however, at this time no sufficiently rapid method available to measure the LMWH activity, thus enabling dose adjustment. The authors therefore allowed only a slight elevation of the APT time in the LMWH group.

Two recently operated patients, however, had major bleedings, and the study was discontinued when 33 patients had been randomized. Later 30 more patients were randomized but with the LMWH-treated patients receiving only half the dose, that is, 120 anti-FXa IU/kg/12 hr. UFH or LMWH treatment was continued for at least 5 days or until the prothrombin value had been therapeutic for 2 days. This duration of the UFH treatment had been shown to be sufficient in an earlier study (6). Venography was immediately repeated after heparin treatment was finished, and its change was analyzed according to Marder et al. (7) and used as the end-point. The UFH-treated patients are considered as one group. The patients studied were too few to allow statistical calculations. The results are summarized in Table 1.

Vogel and Machulik reported on the congress of the International Society for Thrombosis and Haemostasis (ISTH) in 1987 (8) about 28 randomized DVT patients who were intravenously treated with 3000 IU/day of the LMWH from Sandoz compared with 30,000 IU UFH/day for 10 days. Venography was checked before and after treatment.

The groups did not differ in phlebographic outcome. Five patients in the UFH group had large hematomas; none occurred in the LMWH group. The results are not included in the table as no details are reported.

In 1989, Albada et al. (9) reported the results of a study of 194 patients, randomized in a double-blind mode, who received the LMWH from Kabi (Sweden), now called Fragmin, or UFH. Not only patients with DVT were treated, but even those with axillary vein thrombosis and pulmonary embolism (PE). The authors determined anti-FXa activity 4 hr after every change of dose. Patients with risk for bleeding complications were placed into a high-risk group in regard to bleeding, the rest in a low-risk group. An anti-FXa value of 0.4–0.9 IU/ml was allowed for the high-risk group and 0.3–0.6 IU/ml for the low-risk group. Diagnosis was usually established by impedance plethysmography (IPG), but in some cases by venography or ultrasound. In cases of suspected pulmonary embolism, the diagnosis was made with pulmonary scintigraphy or angiography. Oral anticoagulants were started immediately after diagnosis at the discretion of the patient's physician. When sufficient anticoagulation was achieved, LMWH or UFH was stopped, but treatment was given for a minimum of 5 days. After treatment was finished, IPG and/or a lung scan was repeated.

Of the 194 patients analyzed, 115 had a DVT, 70 a PE, and nine an axillary thrombosis. The planned anti-FXa values were reached with 31,000 IU/24 hr of UFH and 15,000 IU/24 hr of Fragmin. The groups did not differ in anticoagulation intensity. No figures for progress of DVT after treatment are reported.

UFH and Fragmin did not differ statistically in therapeutic efficacy with respect to DVT or lung scan. There was a 21% reduction in bleeding, but this reduction was not significant. The results are summarized in Table 1.

Conclusion: Taken together, the studies show that with intravenous LMWH doses of approximately 200–240 IU/kg/24 hr similar improvements of the Marder score after treatment of DVT can be achieved as with i.v. UFH. Progress is less often found in the LMWH group, and the number of major bleeds is similar (Table 1).

III. TWICE-DAILY SUBCUTANEOUS ADMINISTRATION OF LMWH COMPARED WITH CONTINUOUS INTRAVENOUS INFUSION OF UFH

The longer half-life and higher bioavailability of LMWH compared with UFH made its subcutaneous use very attractive (10). In the following randomized studies, LMWH was injected twice daily s.c. and compared with conventional continuous i.v. infusion of UFH.

In 1989 Aiach et al. (11) reported on 66 patients with DVT, who were randomized between Fragmin, s.c. twice daily, and UFH, continuously i.v. Fragmin, at a dose of 100 anti-FXa IU/kg/12 hr, was injected s.c. and adjusted to result in anti-FXa values of 0.5–0.8 IU/ml plasma 3 hr after injection; 240 IU/kg/12 hr UFH was infused i.v. and the dose adjusted by APT-time determinations. The use of oral anticoagulants is not discussed. The efficacy of the treatment was studied by performing venography before and 10 days after treatment.

Table 1 DVT Patients Randomized Between Continuous UFH and LMWH Intravenously

Ref.	LMWH used	Mean dose LMWH/day	AC start	Patients analyzed	UFH score (%)		LMWH score (%)		Level of evidence	Major bleeds (%)	
					I	W	I	W		UFH	LMWH
Bratt et al. (3)	Fragmin	480	1	27	48	11	50	0	II	0	17
		240		27			77	0		7	15
Albada et al. (9)	Fragmin	204	1	93	51		56		II	13	10
			Weighted mean:		**50**	**11**	**59**	**0**		**10**	**12**
			Total number of patients analyzed: 147								

A standard dose of UFH was infused and adjusted with APTT determinations. The LMWH dose is in anti-FXa IU/kg/24 hr. AC start = day oral anticoagulants were started. Comparison of the venographic score according to Marder or of the impedance plethysmogram before and after treatment = score. I = improved; W = worse. The level of evidence of the venographic scores of the studies is estimated according to Cook et al. (5).

The treatments did not differ significantly from each other. The results are summarized in Table 2.

In 1990 Bratt et al. published a study (12) in which 119 patients with DVT were randomized between Fragmin, 120 anti-FXa IU/kg s.c. twice daily, and UFH, 480 anti-FXa IU/kg/24 hr i.v. The doses were adjusted to keep the anti-FXa value in plasma between 0.2 and 0.4 IU/ml immediately before the next Fragmin injection. In the UFH-treated patients APT time guided dose adjustments. Oral anticoagulants were given from the first day. Phlebography was performed to diagnose the DVT and repeated 5–7 days later. The Marder scores were determined and compared. The treatment results did not differ significantly for the two groups. The results are given in Table 2.

The same year Harenberg et al. (13) reported a study in which 50 patients were randomized between an i.v. infusion of 450 anti-FXa U/kg intravenously and 150 anti-FX U/kg LMWH from Sandoz twice daily for 10 days. Doses where adjusted to maintain peak levels of 0.5–1.0 anti-FXa U/ml plasma. The use of an anticoagulant is not indicated. Phlebographies and sonographies were performed before and after treatment. The treatments did not differ statistically. The results are presented in Table 2.

In 1991 Simonneau reported for the TYPENOX group on the ISTH congress (14) about a multicenter study including 134 patients with venographically verified proximal DVT. The patients were randomized between Enoxaparin, 1 mg/kg = 105 anti-FXa IU twice daily, and i.v. UFH. The Enoxaparin dose was fixed; UFH was adjusted by APT-time determinations. The outcome was measured by phlebography 10 days later. Enoxaparin treatment resulted in a significantly better phlebographic outcome than UFH. The results are summarized in Table 2.

The results of a collaborative European multicenter study were reported by Duroux in 1991 (15). A total of 166 patients with a DVT of less than 5 days' duration went through bilateral venography for diagnosis. Eighty-one patients received UFH as continuous i.v. infusion adjusted by APT-time determinations; 85 patients received about 100 anti-FXa IU/kg CY 216 (Fraxiparine) twice daily s.c. The CY 216 doses were kept constant and the treatment was not monitored. Oral anticoagulants were not started before the 10th day. On the same day phlebography was performed again. Seventy-one patients could be analyzed according to Marder in the UFH group and 77 in the CY 216 group. Fraxiparine was significantly more effective than UFH on the basis of the venographies and the lung scans. The results are presented in Table 2.

In 1992 Prandoni et al. published a study on 170 patients with proximal DVT (16). Eighty-five patients were treated with UFH continuously i.v. and 85 with Fraxiparine s.c. In each group there are 15 patients previously included in the above-mentioned study (15). Diagnosis was made by venography. Perfusion lung scans were performed. The UFH dose was adjusted according to APT-time

Table 2 DVT Patients Randomized Between Continuous UFH i.v. and LMWH s.c. Twice Daily

Ref.	LMWH used	Mean dose LMWH/day	AC start	Patients analyzed	UFH score (%)		LMWH score (%)		Level of evidence	Major bleeds (%)	
					I	W	I	W		UFH	LMWH
Aiach et al. (11)	Fragmin	183	?	60	79	3	71	6	II	4	0
Bratt et al. (12)	Fragmin	232	1	94	61	4	76	6	II	4	2
Harenberg et al. (13)	Sandoz	300	0	28	77	0	87	7	II	7	15
Simonneau (14)	Enoxaparin	210	?	134	37	—	57	—	II	0	0
Duroux (15)	Fraxiparine	212	10	148	62	7	70	7	I	5	2
Prandoni et al. (16)	Fraxiparine	208	7	170	43	16	60	5	II	4	1
			Weighted mean:		**54**	**9**	**66**	**6**		**4**	**2**
			Total number of patients analyzed: 634								

A standard dose of UFH was infused and adjusted by means of APTT determinations. The LMWH dose is in anti-FXa IU/kg/24 hr. AC start = day oral anticoagulants were started. Comparison of the venographic score (= score) according to Marder before and after treatment. The level of evidence of the venographic scores of the studies is estimated according to Cook et al. (5).

determinations, and Fraxiparine was given in a fixed s.c. dose related to body weight, 110 anti-FXa IU/kg twice daily. Oral anticoagulants were started on day 7. Heparin treatment was discontinued on day 10. Venography and a perfusion lung scan were repeated the same day and up to 6 months after treatment whenever an extension of the thrombosis or a new pulmonary embolus was suspected. After initial treatment oral anticoagulants were adjusted by the patient's general physician and given between 3 and 6 months.

Fraxiparine was significantly more effective than UFH on the basis of repeat venographies and lung scans after initial treatment. The frequency of bleeding or late recurrence of thromboembolism did not differ significantly between the heparins. Significantly less patients died of cancer after Fraxiparine than after UFH. The results are shown in Table 2.

Conclusion: In the above-mentioned studies UFH i.v. was compared with LMWH s.c. twice daily. Improvement of the venograms after treatment with LMWH was better than after UFH. The percentage of progress and the frequency of major bleeds was about the same in the two groups.

IV. TWICE-DAILY SUBCUTANEOUS ADMINISTRATION OF LMWH VERSUS UFH

In a number of early studies, treatment with two s.c. injections of UFH daily was effective in comparison with continuous i.v. UFH (17). For this reason, s.c. administration of UFH twice daily has been compared with the same mode of administration of LMWH.

As early as 1986 Holm et al. (18) published a multicenter study on 56 patients with venographically diagnosed DVT. They were randomized between UFH and Fragmin s.c. twice daily for 7 days, after an i.v. course of UFH up to 24 hr. The doses were selected according to the sex and age of the patient, with doses between 8000 and 15,000 IU UFH and 4000 and 7500 IU Fragmin (about 500 IU/kg/24 hr UFH and 200 IU/kg/24 hr Fragmin) adjusted according to anti-FXa determinations. Venography was repeated after 7 days of treatment. Warfarin treatment was started on day 1. The venographic outcome of the two treatments did not differ statistically. The results are shown in Table 3.

In 1988 Faivre et al. (19) reported on 68 patients with phlebographically diagnosed DVT, who were randomized between s.c. treatment with UFH or CY 222 twice daily. The dose was 500 anti-FXa IU/kg/24 hr of UFH and 750 Choay IU of CY 222 (about 300 anti-FXA IU/kg/24 hr). Treatment was given for 10 days without oral anticoagulants. At the end of the treatment, venography was repeated. There was no statistical difference between the two treatments. The results are shown in Table 3.

In 1992 Lopaciuk et al. reported a Polish multicenter trial in which 134 patients with venographically diagnosed DVT were treated s.c. for 10 days with

Table 3 DVT Patients Randomized Between s.c. UFH and s.c. LMWH Twice Daily

Ref.	LMWH used	Mean dose LMWH/day	AC start	Patients analyzed	UFH score (%)		LMWH score (%)		Level of evidence	Major bleeds (%)	
					I	W	I	W		UFH	LMWH
Holm et al. (18)	Fragmin	200	1	50	48	8	40	4	II	0	0
Faivre et al. (19)	CY 222	300	?	59	65	7	64	0	II	5	0
Lopaciuk et al. (20)	Fraxiparine	184	7	134	49	18	66	15	II	1	0
				Weighted mean:		**53**	**13**	**60**	**9**	**2**	**0**
				Total number of patients analyzed:				**243**			

LMWH dose is in anti-FXa IU/kg/24 hr. The day oral anticoagulants were started = AC start. Comparison of the venographic score according to Marder before and after treatment = score. The level of evidence of the venographic scores of the studies is estimated according to Cook et al. (5).

either UFH or Fraxiparine twice a day. The daily dose was 500 IU/kg UFH or 184 IU/kg Fraxiparine (20). The UFH was monitored using the APT time, Fraxiparine was not monitored. The UFH-treated patients received a bolus injection of 5000 IU when the UFH treatment was initiated. Oral anticoagulation was started on the 7th day and continued for at least 3 months. Patients were ambulating on the 3rd day wearing elastic support stockings. A new venography was performed 1–2 days after heparin treatment was finished. There was no statistical difference between the two treatments. The results are shown in Table 3.

Conclusion: In the studies cited above, s.c. UFH was compared with s.c. LMWH, both injected twice daily. The venography improved somewhat more with LMWH. Progress of the DVTs and major bleedings was seen less often in this group.

V. SUBCUTANEOUS ADMINISTRATION OF LMWH: ONCE VERSUS TWICE DAILY

In 1989 Lockner et al. presented the first 60 patients with DVT randomized between Fragmin s.c. once or twice daily, with similar outcomes in both groups (21). The results are included in the complete study referred to below (23).

The same year Siegbahn et al. published a study including 20 patients with venographically diagnosed DVT (22). The patients were randomized between Logiparin 75 anti-FXa IU/kg s.c. twice daily or 150 anti-FXa IU/kg once daily for 5 days. An oral anticoagulant was given from the first day. A new phlebogram was performed on day 7. Nineteen of 20 patients were reinvestigated according to Marder score. There was no statistical difference between the two treatments. The results are shown in Table 4.

In 1992 Holmström et al. published the complete study referred to above (23). A total of 101 patients with venographically diagnosed first-time DVTs not extending into more than two-thirds of the femoral vein were included. The patients were randomized to treatment for a minimum of 5 days: 200 anti-FXa IU/kg Fragmin was injected s.c. once or 100 anti-FXa IU/kg Fragmin twice daily. Before randomization, a continuous infusion of UFH was given intravenously for up to 24 hr. The plasma anti-FXa concentrations immediately before the next injection were maintained between 0.1 and 0.3 anti-FXa IU/ml plasma by dose adjustments. Oral anticoagulants were started together with Fragmin. The patients were mobilized on the second day of the study. Venography was repeated immediately after the end of Fragmin treatment and the Marder score determined. There was no statistical difference between the two treatments. The results are summarized in Table 4.

Conclusion: The patients treated with LMWH s.c. once daily more often showed an improved venogram and somewhat less progress and major bleeding then those injected with LMWH s.c. twice a day. The patients studied are, however, few.

Table 4 DVT Patients Randomized Between LMWH s.c. Once or Twice Daily

Ref.	LMWH used	Patients analyzed	AC start	Mean dose LMWH		Improved (%)		Progress (%)		Level of evidence	Major bleeds (%)	
				12 hr	24 hr	12 hr	24 hr	12 hr	24 hr		12 hr	24 hr
Siegbahn et al. (22)	Logiparin	19	1	75	150	30	60	0	0	II	0	0
Holmström et al. (23)	Fragmin	87	1	100	200	51	55	4	0	II	2	0
				Weighted mean:		**47**	**56**	**3**	**0**		**2**	**0**
				Total number of patients analyzed: 106								

AC start = day when oral anticoagulants were started. LMWH doses given are in anti-FXa U/kg. Comparison of the venographic score according to Marder before and after treatment. Percentage of patients improved or showing progress of DVT. The level of evidence of the venographic scores of the studies is estimated according to Cook et al. (5).

VI. SUBCUTANEOUS ADMINISTRATION OF LMWH AS COMPARED WITH CONTINUOUS INTRAVENOUS INFUSION OF UFH LATE RECURRENCES

In 1992 Hull et al. published a double-blind multicenter trial (4) in which 432 patients with venographically diagnosed proximal DVT were randomized between adjusted continuous i.v. UFH infusion and a fixed dose of 175 anti-FXa IU/kg Logiparin once a day. Adjustment of the UFH was by APT-time determinations. The LMWH was not monitored. All patients had a lung scan within 48 hr after admission. The treatment was finished earliest on the 6th day, later if effective oral anticoagulation was not achieved. Warfarin was started on the second day and administered for at least 3 months. After the 6th day adjustment of the warfarin dose was made by the primary physician. The patients were followed for 3 months with respect to recurrent DVT and embolism. If symptoms developed, lung scan or angiography, or IPG or venogram was repeated. The number of patients not included is not reported. The patients in the LMWH group had statistically fewer late recurrences and early major hemorrhages. The death rate was lower in the LMWH group. The results are presented in Table 5.

Prandoni et al. (16) not only studied changes in the phlebographic score and lung scan during the initial heparin treatment, as presented above, but even recorded thromboembolic recurrences for 6 months afterward. Coumarin was administered under control of the primary physician for at least 3 months. UFH and LMWH did not differ statistically in the rate of thromboembolic recurrences; the death rate was statistically lower after LMWH than after UFH treatment, mainly by a reduction in cancer deaths. This later part of the study is combined with the results of Hull et al. (4) in Table 5.

Conclusion: The two studies show that fewer recurrences of thromboembolic events occur if LMWH is given, irrespective of whether it is injected once or twice daily subcutaneously. The recurrence of DVT and PE together was significantly reduced in one study (4) but not in the other (16), as were the major bleeds. The difference in death rate reached significance in the Prandoni study. There were fewer deaths in cancer patients in both studies. In a meta-analysis of the two studies, Lensing et al. (24) found significantly lower odds ratios for thromboembolic recurrences, severe bleeding, and death after LMWH compared to UFH. Green et al. (25) analyzed the same two studies and found a lower odds ratio for cancer deaths after LMWH.

VII. THE EFFECT OF LMWH ON PULMONARY EMBOLISM

Only one randomized study had the direct intention of comparing the use of UFH with LMWH in pulmonary embolism (PE) (26). In the other few studies reported, the main intention was to treat DVT, and the effect on PE was reported as a side

Table 5 Patients with DVT Treated with i.v. UFH or s.c. LMWH Once (4) or Twice Daily (16)

Ref.	LMWH used	Mean dose LMWH	AC start	Patients analyzed	Recurrent DVT (%)		Recurrent PE (%)		Level of evidence	Major bleeds (%)		Death from cancer (%)	
					UFH	LMWH	UFH	LMWH		UFH	LMWH	UFH	LMWH
Hull et al. (4)	Logiparin	175/24 hr	2	432	4	1	3	1	II	5	0.5	29	15
Prandoni et al. (16)	Fraxiparine	104/12 hr	7	170	6	2	8	5	II	4	1	44	7
			Weighted mean:		**5**	**1**	**4**	**2**		**5**	**0.6**	**33**	**13**
			Total number of patients analyzed: 602										

The LMWH doses given are in anti-FXa IU/kg. AC start = day oral anticoagulants were started. Comparison of the recurrence rates of DVT and PE as well as death from cancer, after finishing initial treatment. The level of evidence of the recurrence rate is estimated according to Cook et al. (5). The study of Prandoni et al. (16) is summarized in Table 2.

result. The last-mentioned studies are described below and summarized in Table 6. The study by Théry et al. (26) is summarized in Table 7.

In the study of Bratt et al. (3), all patients with DVT had a lung scan, and the influence of continuous i.v. UFH or LMWH treatment on the positive scans and the appearance of new positive scans was studied. The patients studied were too few to allow statistical calculations.

Albada et al. (9) did a repeated lung scan on most of their patients, who were treated as above. The treatments did not differ statistically.

Duroux (15) treated his patients with either UFH continuously i.v. or LMWH s.c. twice daily. The author performed lung scans in 148 patients before and 10 days after treatment. The scans improved significantly after both treatments, but there was no significant difference between the treatments. No detailed results are presented; for this reason, the results are not included in Table 6.

Prandoni et al. (16) treated their patients in the same way as above. All patients were screened with lung scans before and after treatment. There were significantly more new segmental defects in the UFH group than in the LMWH group.

In the study by Théry et al. (26), where only pulmonary embolism was treated, the diagnosis was made by pulmonary angiography and the effect of therapy was determined on day 8 with a new angiography. LMWH was injected s.c., with 160, 240, and 360 anti-FXa IU/kg/day, in three divided doses. The treatment with the two higher doses was stopped because of major bleedings. There was no statistical difference in the angiographic outcome between the treatments. The results are summarized in Table 7.

Conclusion: The only study with the direct plan to treat PE and to compare the effects of LMWH and UFH found no statistical difference between the treatments. One study in which the effects of PE were evaluated as a side result found a statistical favor for LMWH. The effect of LMWH on PE thus has not been sufficiently studied.

VIII. DISCUSSION

To validate the role of LMWHs in the treatment of established DVT of the leg, the LMWHs have to be compared with the established treatment in use, that is, intravenous or subcutaneous UFH. There are four conditions that alone or in combination should be considered when comparing the two heparins studied: efficacy, safety, usability, and economic considerations. I would like to discuss these different items in relation to the studies presented.

A. Efficacy

The two complications of DVT are PE and disabling venous insufficiency. PE is uncommon with the intravenous heparin treatment of today. For example,

Table 6 Comparison of Lung Scans Before and After Treatment of Patients with DVT

Ref.	LMWH used	LMWH dose	LMWH applied	UFH applied	Patients analyzed	Scintigram UFH I	Scintigram UFH W	Scintigram LMWH I	Scintigram LMWH W	Level of evidence
Bratt et al. (3)	Fragmin	240	i.v.	i.v.	15	73	9	50	0	II
		120	i.v.	i.v.	15			50	25	
Albada et al. (9)	Fragmin	204	i.v.	i.v.	80	74	15	77	9	II
Prandoni et al. (16)	Fraxiparine	104	s.c. × 2	i.v.	160		19		5	II
				Weighted mean:		**74%**	**17%**	**70%**	**7%**	
				Total number of patients analyzed: 270						

The patients were randomized between UFH and LMWH. The LMWH doses are given in anti-FXa U/kg. The mode of administration of LMWH and UFH is indicated. The scintigrams are classified as percent I = improved and W = worsened. The level of evidence of the studies is estimated according to Cook et al. (5).

Table 7 Comparison of Pulmonary Angiograms Before and After Treatment of Patients with Pulmonary Embolism

Ref.	LMWH used	Dose (anti-FXa U/kg)	LMWH application	UFH application	Patients analyzed	Angiogram (UFH)			Angiogram (LMWH)			Angiogram (LMWH—all)			Level of evidence
						I	U	W	I	U	W	I	U	W	
Théry et al. (26)	Fraxiparine	80	s.c. × 2	i.v.	57	100	0	0	94	0	6	94	0	6	II

The patients were randomized between UFH and LMWH. The LMWH dose is given in anti-FXa IU/kg. The frequency and type of application of LMWH and UFH is noted, as is the method of administration of UFH. The angiograms are classified as percent I = improved, U = unchanged, and W = worsened. The level of evidence of the study with respect to the difference between angiograms after UFH or LMWH treatment is classified according to Cook et al. (5).

Holmström et al. (27) found, in a recently performed investigation, that of 1393 patients treated from 1973 to 1986 at our hospital, only 0.36% died of PE. This means that large numbers of patients must be treated to determine if a difference between treatments exists. No studies reported are large enough to answer this question.

The second complication, venous insufficiency, takes 10–15 years to develop. Such studies require much patience and large patient numbers as well. LMWHs have not been in use long enough to allow results of such studies.

An indirect way to demonstrate the efficacy of the treatment of DVT is to study the diseased veins before and after the treatment. One tries to show that the thrombus becomes smaller, or at least does not become larger, after treatment, and then the two treatment results are compared. This suggests, but does not prove, that a larger visible or measurable thrombus means a greater risk of developing venous insufficiency later. Venography is considered the standard for measurement of the extension of a thrombus, and most of the studies cited have used this technique. But even IPG is considered an adequate measure of the extension of at least a proximal thrombus (28). In only two of the cited studies was this technique used (4, 9). Different methods have been used to quantitate the venographic findings. The method most often applied is that of Marder et al. (7), but even the method of Arnesen et al. (29) was used in one of the studies reviewed here.

Fifteen randomized studies have been published in which LMWHs were compared with UFH to study the efficacy of these heparins. It must, however, be kept in mind that the different LMWH preparations are not identical, and one must be careful not to extend the comparisons too far. The first two studies tried to find out if LMWH had an effect comparable to that of UFH when both were infused intravenously in 147 patients. LMWH was slightly, but not significantly, more effective. Even progress of the thrombus was less often seen when LMWH was used (3, 8, 9).

Pharmacokinetic studies taught us about the longer half-life and higher bioavailability of LMWH (10). This made the LMWHs especially well suited for subcutaneous application. LMWHs were injected s.c. twice daily and compared with UFH infused i.v. or injected s.c. In six studies where i.v. UFH was compared with LMWH s.c. twice daily, LMWH gave a statistically better phlebographic outcome in three of the studies with 452 of 634 patients (11–16). When UFH was injected s.c. twice daily as well as LMWH in 243 patients, the LMWHs induced a better phlebographic outcome, but the difference was not significant (18–20).

In 106 patients s.c. LMWH twice daily was compared with one s.c. LMWH injection a day. LMWH once a day gave somewhat better results and less progress of the thrombus, but significance was not found (22, 23).

In two studies (4, 16) the recurrence of thromboembolism was studied after the initial UFH or LMWH treatment. In the study of Hull et al. (4) with 423 patients, during the 3 months after initial treatment, significantly fewer recurrences occurred with LMWH (Logiparin) s.c. once daily than with UFH. In the study of Prandoni et al. (16), with subcutaneous LMWH (Fraxiparine) twice daily, during 6 months after initial treatment there were fewer thromboembolic recurrences; oral anticoagulants were given for at least 3 months. It is not stated how many of the recurrences occurred in patients after oral anticoagulants were stopped. The difference in number of recurrences was not significant in this study.

In a meta-analysis, Lensing et al. (24) pooled the results of these two studies and studies and found that the common relative odds were significantly lower for recurrent thromboembolism, initial major bleeding, and death (mainly caused by cancer) when LMWH was used instead of UFH. Green et al. (25) analyzed the same studies for the odds ratio of deaths from cancer and found significantly lower odds after initial LMWH treatment than after UFH treatment. The authors conclude that an increase of the death rate caused by UFH is not probable but well a reduction of cell growth by LMWH. There are observations that heparins inhibit angiogenesis leading to tumor regression (30). These findings are interesting and need further investigation.

In both studies oral anticoagulants were administered by the primary physician. It is of importance that oral anticoagulation after the initial treatment is of the same intensity if the initial treatment is made responsible for the differences between the groups. Prandoni et al. (16) state that 70% of the measurements in 70 respective 73% of the patients are therapeutic, that is about 50%. Hull et al. (4) state that before recurrence most of the patients had therapeutic prothrombin values, but no details are reported in any of the two studies. It has been shown that the efficacy of anticoagulant treatment increases with the number of patients treated and decreases with the number of physicians involved (31), an observation that is not in favor of patients treated by a primary physician, as illustrated by the low figure of Prandoni et al. (16). Another problem is standardization of the prothrombin determinations. It has been shown that only 21% of the laboratories in the United States have properly standardized prothrombin determinations (32). The prothrombin standardization that the primary physicians used in the above-mentioned studies has not been reported.

Summing up, it can be said that LMWH in all forms of application, even when injected once daily, presumably is moderately more efficacious than UFH, causes possibly fewer recurrences, causes moderately fewer bleedings, and reduces the death rate by reducing death from cancer within 3–6 months after treatment for unexplained reasons.

B. Safety

The measure of safety for all authors has been bleeding. The definition of the degree of bleeding is, however, quite different in each study and comparison of the studies published therefore uncertain. Many authors include, for example, the indication for transfusion. As the indication for transfusion differs between physicians, this is a bad definition. It would be much easier to compare different studies if, for example, only the decrease in hemoglobin concentration combined with signs of cerebral and retroperitoneal bleeding were taken as a sign of major bleeding. Because of the diffuse definitions of bleeding used, only major bleedings are considered here.

Generally, the major bleeding frequencies in the studies reviewed are below 5% and somewhat in favor of patients treated with LMWH. Most studies are too small to make statistical calculations meaningful. The few calculations presented show no difference in the frequency of major bleedings. Only the large study of Hull et al. (4) shows a statistical favor of LMWH during initial treatment. This statistical advantage of LMWH is even demonstrable in the meta-analysis (24) of the combined studies by Hull et al. (4) and Prandoni et al. (16).

Does the LMWH dose influence the bleeding frequency? It is interesting that intravenous LMWH shows higher bleeding frequencies than subcutaneous LMWH with similar doses (3,9), but generally the LMWH doses show no correlation with the frequency of major bleeding.

This raises the question of the optimal LMWH dose. UFH is routinely dosed by means of APTT determinations, which are insensitive to LMWHs because of their low anti-FII activity (10). Instead anti-FXa determinations for dosing LMWHs have been used, where an activity of 0.4–0.7 anti-FXa IU/ml plasma has produced effective inhibition of experimental thrombus growth (10). Similar anti-FXa concentrations in plasma have been used in the studies cited in this review. The LMWH doses that result in the above-mentioned anti-FXa values were somewhat lower than half the usual UFH dose in anti-FXa units, that is, about 200 anti-FXa IU/kg/24 hr. When UFH was administered, APTT values 1.5–2.5 times the normal value were aimed for. In only one study was the anti-FXa concentration in plasma used to dose LMWH as well as UFH treatment (9). Even in this study a LMWH dose somewhat lower than half the UFH dose in anti-FXa units was necessary to reach the same anti-FXa concentration in plasma. In all studies performed in recent years, LMWHs have been administered per kilogram of body weight. This was not the case with UFH. It is possible that this has played a roll in reducing the bleeding risk and may make it possible to administer LMWHs without monitoring.

With the above-mentioned doses somewhat better effects on the thrombus and somewhat fewer major bleedings result.

The lowest effective LMWH dose has not been determined. Three large studies, as well as studies that used higher doses, report good and comparable effects on phlebographic thrombus size: Aiach et al. (11) has used 183 anti-FXa IU/kg/day, Lopaciuk et al. (20) 184 IU, and Hull et al. (4) 175 IU. Siegbahn et al. (22) have used as little as 150 IU, but the study is too small to allow conclusions.

Another safety problem is thrombocytopenia. In all studies presented here, a total of 16 cases of thrombocytopenia have been reported after UFH and nine cases after LMWH. Only one case in each group was serious [in Simonneau's study. (14)] but no details are given. All other cases showed only reduced platelet values without complications. Eight other cases of thrombocytopenia after LMWH were found in the literature (33). The risk for thrombocytopenia seems to increase with the length of heparin treatment. Whether this is also the case with LMWH needs further observation.

As LMWHs are cleared principally by the renal route (10), reduction of the dose is necessary to protect renal function. This is best correlated with determinations of the anti-FXa concentration in plasma.

In summary, despite a somewhat higher efficacy of LMWHs, the risk for major bleeds tends not to be increased; it is moderately decreased instead. The lowest LMWH dose effective in the treatment of DVT has not yet been found. The lowest effective dose used in a larger study is 175 anti-FXa IU/kg/day in the study of Hull et al. (4). Thromocytopenia has been observed in a few cases after LMWH, but not in a higher frequency than when UFH is used. Serious complications of thrombocytopenia after LMWH have not been described.

C. Ease of Use

From the results presented above (Tables 2 and 3), it can be concluded that LMWHs can be injected s.c. twice daily with somewhat better effect and greater safety compared to UFH. Earlier the i.v. route was considered the best and safest for UFH, but recently it has been shown in a meta-analysis that UFH s.c. twice daily is more effective and as safe as UFH i.v. in the treatment of DVT (17). This makes intravenous administration of UFH unnecessary in uncomplicated cases. Two daily injections of LMWHs have a moderate advantage over s.c. UFH, but the question is whether it is worthwhile for this advantage to change to the more expensive LMWH. It has, however, been shown by Lockner et al. (21) and Siegbahn et al. (22), in 1989, and later by Holmström et al. (23) and Hull et al. (4), in 1992, that LMWHs can be injected subcutaneously only once a day to treat DVT with at least the same (21–23) or even better (4) efficacy than with UFH. Only a few dose changes were necessary in the study of Holmström et al.. Siegbahn et al. and especially Hull et al. in their large study used fix doses with good results.

In summary, this means that one injection per day with a fixed dose without monitoring may be possible in the future. This reduces the workload of the staff and the number of blood samples that must be analyzed.

D. Economic Considerations

As the production of LMWHs is more complicated, their price is generally 3–4 times that of UFH. The question is how the cost of continuous intravenous UFH treatment compares to that of LMWH treatment in a clinical setting. We have measured the time it takes the staff at two university hospitals (Karolinska and Huddinge hospitals in Stockholm, Sweden) to administer UFH intravenously or LMWH once daily subcutaneously. A number of nurses noted every minute it took to administer the two treatments and to take the necessary samples in a treatment lasting 6.5 days. The cost of UFH and LMWH was included, as was the cost of the X-ray investigations and the hospital cost. In 1993 we arrived at $2,860 for the UFH treatment and $2,790 for the LMWH treatment, practically the same cost. But if the patient can be treated as an outpatient after 3 days in the hospital, the cost for the whole initial treatment is $1,960 instead. This means that UFH i.v. and LMWH s.c. once daily generate practically the same total cost in the clinical setting despite a higher cost and easier use of LMWH. When the patient can be treated all or part of the time as an outpatient, substantial savings are possible, as the hospital cost is the only important factor. Whether outpatient treatment is possible, safe, and effective in a substantial number of patients has yet to be shown.

IX. SUMMARY

All hitherto published randomized studies in which LMWH was used to treat DVT have been reviewed, comprising about 1500 patients.

LMWH was found to be moderately more effective than UFH when comparing measurements before and after initial treatment; even thromboembolic recurrences occur less often after LMWH than after UFH. Major bleedings occur somewhat less often after LMWH than after UFH.

Thrombocytopenia is at least as uncommon after LMWH as after UFH.

LMWHs have at least the same positive effect on pulmonary embolism as UFH has, but this conclusion is based on very few patients.

Patients with cancer die less often after a DVT if it is treated with LMWH rather than with UFH.

These positive effects of LMWH can even be shown when LMWH is injected subcutaneously once daily without monitoring. Doses as low as 175 anti-FXa IU/kg/day seem sufficient, but effective and safe dosages must be established for each LMWH brand.

The superiority of LMWH over UFH is not so impressive that a change from the inexpensive UFH to the much more expensive LMWH would be warranted. The cost to treat a patient with UFH i.v. continuously or LMWH s.c. once daily in a hospital is the same. If the patient can be entirely or partly treated with LMWH once daily as an outpatient without monitoring, the cost is substantially reduced. That this is a real possibility has to be shown.

REFERENCES

1. Hirsh J Heparin. N Engl J Med 1991; 324:1565–1574.
2. Kakkar VV, Djazaeri B, Fok J, Fletcher M, Scully MF, Westwick J. Low-molecular-weight heparin and prevention of postoperative deep vein thrombosis. Br Med J 1982; 284:375–379.
3. Bratt G, Törnebohm E, Granquist S, Åberg W, Lockner D. A comparison between low molecular weight heparin (KABI 2165) and standard heparin in the intravenous treatment of deep venous thrombosis. Thromb Haemost 1985; 54:813–817.
4. Hull RD, Raskob GE, Pineo GF, Green D, Trowbridge AA, Elliott CG, Lerner RG, Hall J, Sparling T, Bretell HR, Norton J, Carter CJ, George R, Merli G, Ward J, Mayo W, Rosenblom D, Brant R. Subcutaneous low-molecular-weight heparin compared with continuous intravenous heparin in the treatment of proximal-vein thrombosis. N Engl J Med 1992; 236:975–982.
5. Cook DJ, Guyatt GH, Laupacis A, Sackett DL. Rules of evidence and clinical recommendations on the use of antithrombotic agents. Chest 1992; 102:305S–311S.
6. Schulman S, Lockner D, Bergström K, Blombäck M. Intensive initial oral anticoagulation and shorter heparin treatment in deep vein thrombosis. Thromb Haemost 1984; 52:276–280.
7. Marder VJ, Soulen RL, Atichartakarn V. Budzynski AZ, Parulekar S, Kim JR, Edvard N, Zahavi J, Algazy KM. Quantitative venographic assessment of deep venous thrombosis in the evaluation of streptokinase and heparin therapy. J Lab Clin Med 1977; 89:1018–1029.
8. Vogel G, Machulik M. Efficacy and safety of a low molecular weight heparin (LMW-heparin Sandoz) in patients with deep vein thrombosis. Thromb Haemost 1987; 59:120.
9. Albada J, Nieuwenhuis HK, Sixma JJ. Treatment of acute venous thromboembolism with low molecular weight heparin (Fragmin). Circulation 1989; 80:935–940.
10. Hirsh J, Levine MN. Low molecular weight heparin. Blood 1992; 79:1–17.
11. Aiach M, Fiessinger JN, Vitoux JF, Derlon A, Grollier G, Le Querrec A, Gouault-Heilmann M, Huet Y, Franco A, Polack B, Pouzol P, Dubios A, Schved JF, Boneu B, Guittard J, Sie P, Heilmann JJ, Kher A, Haye I. Traitement des thromboses veineuses profondes constituées. Étude comparative d'un fragment d'héparine de bas poids moléculaire (Fragmine®) administrée par voie sous-cutanée et de l'héparine standard administrée par voie intraveineuse continue. Étude multicentrique. Rev Med Int 1989; 10:375–381.
12. Bratt G, Åberg W, Johansson M, Törnebohm E, Granquist S, Lockner D. Two daily subcutaneous injections of Fragmin as compared with intravenous standard heparin in the treatment of deep venous thrombosis (DVT). Thromb Haemost 1990; 64:506–510.
13. Harenberg J, Huck K, Bratsch H, Stehle G, Dempfle CE, Mall K, Blauth M, Usadel K-H, Heene DL. Therapeutic application of subcutaneous low-molecular-weight heparin in acute venous thrombosis. Haemostasis 1990; 20:205–219.

14. Simonneau G. Subcutaneous fixed dose Enoxaparine (E) versus intravenous adjusted dose of unfractionated heparin (UH) in the treatment of deep venous thrombosis (DVT). Thromb Haemost 1991; 65:754.
15. Duroux P. A randomised trial of subcutaneous low molecular weight heparin(CY 216) compared with intravenous unfractionated heparin in the treatment of deep vein thrombosis. A collaborative European multicentre study. Thromb Haemost 1991; 65:251–256.
16. Prandoni P, Lensing AWA, Büller HR, Carta M, Cogo A, Vigo M, Casara D, Ruol A, Ten Cate JW. Comparison of subcutaneous low-molecular-weight heparin with intravenous standard heparin in proximal deep-vein thrombosis. Lancet 1992; 339:441–445.
17. Hommes DW, Bura A, Mazzolai L, Büller HR, Ten Cate JW. Subcutaneous heparin compared with continous intravenous heparin administration in the initial treatment of deep vein thrombosis. A meta analysis. Ann Intern Med 1992; 116:279–284.
18. Holm HA, Ly B, Handeland GF, Abildgaard U, Arnesen KE, Gottschalk P, Hoeg V, Aandahl M, Haugen K, Laerum F, Scheel B, Sortland O, Vinje B. Subcutaneous heparin treatment of deep venous thrombosis: a comparison of unfractionated and low molecular weight heparin. Haemostasis 1986; 16:30–37.
19. Faivre R, Neuhart Y, Kieffer Y, Apfel F, Magnin D, Didier D, Toulemonde F, Bassand JP, Maurat JP. Un nouveau traitement des thromboses veineuses profondes: les fractions d'héparine de bas poids moléculaire. Etude randomisée. Presse Méd 1988; 17:197–200.
20. Lopaciuk S, Meissner AJ, Filipecki S, Zawilska K, Sowier J, Ciesielski L, Bielawiec M, Glowinski S, Czestochowska E. Subcutaneous low molecular weight heparin versus subcutaneous unfractionated heparin in the treatment of deep vein thrombosis: a Polish multicenter trial. Thromb Haemost 1992; 68:14–18.
21. Lockner D, Johansson M, Åberg W, Bratt G, Granquist S, Fragmin (Kabi) subcutaneously once or twice daily in the treatment of deep venous thrombosis (DVT). Thromb Haemost 1989; 62:526.
22. Siegbahn A, Y-Hassan S, Boberg J, Bylund H, Neerstrand HS, Östergaard P, Hedner U. Subcutaneous treatment of deep venous thrombosis with low molecular weight heparin. A dose finding study with LMWH-Novo. Thromb Res 1989; 55:767–778.
23. Holmström M, Berglund M-C, Granquist S, Bratt G, Törnebohm E, Lockner D. Fragmin once or twice daily subcutaneously in the treatment of deep venous thrombosis of the leg. Thromb Res 1992; 67:49–55.
24. Lensing A, WA, Prins M, Koopman MMW, Büller H. Which heparin for proximal deep-vein thrombosis? Lancet 1992; 340:311–312.
25. Green D, Hull RD, Brant R, Pineo GF. Lower mortality in cancer patients treated with low-molecular-weight versus standard heparin. Lancet 1992; 339:1476.
26. Théry C, Simonneau G, Meyer G, Hélénon O, Bridey F, Armagnac C, d'Azemar P, Coquart JP. Randomized trial of subcutaneous low-molecular-weight heparin CY 216 (Fraxiparine) compared with intravenous unfractionated heparin in the curative treatment of submassive pulmonary embolism. A dose-ranging study. Circulation 1992; 85:1380–1389.
27. Holmström M, Bratt G, Törnebohm E, Rhedin A-S, Lockner D. Fatal pulmonary

embolism caused by streptokinase treatment of deep vein thrombosis of the leg? J Intern Med 1990; 228:647–649.

28. Hull RD, Taylor DW, Hirsh J. Impedance plethysmography: the relationship between venous filling and sensitivity and specificity for proximal vein thrombosis. Circulation 1978; 58:898–902.
29. Arnesen H, Heilo A, Jacobsen E, Ly B, Skaga E. A prospective study of streptokinase and heparin in the treatment of deep vein thrombosis. Acta Med Scand 1978; 203:457–463.
30. Folkman J, Langer R, Linhardt RJ. Angiogenesis inhibition and tumor regression caused by heparin or a heparin fragment in the presence of cortison. Science 1983; 221:719–725.
31. Carlsson A, Gustafsson C. Bleeding complications with anticoagulant treatment. Information from the Swedish Drug Agency 1992; 31:21–24.
32. Bussey HI, Force RW Bianco TM, Leonard AD. Reliance on prothrombin time ratios causes significant errors in anticoagulation therapy. Arch Intern Med 1992; 152:278–282.
33. Lecompte T, Luo SK, Stieltjes N, Lecrubier C, Samama MM, Tardy B, Zeni F, Reynaud J, Tardy-Poncet B, Comtet C, Bertrand JC. Thrombocytopenia associated with low-molecular-weight heparin. Lancet 1991; 338:1217.

16

Conclusion

Current Controversies About Low-Molecular-Weight Heparins in Prevention and Therapy of Venous Thromboembolism

Henri Bounameaux
Geneva University School of Medicine and University Hospital of Geneva, Geneva, Switzerland

I. INTRODUCTION

The aim of this volume was to present the current opinion of experts in the field of low-molecular-weight heparins (LMWH) and to cover both prophylaxis and therapy of thromboembolic diseases. Despite the great care taken by the editor and the publisher, collecting and processing the chapters took more time than anticipated. Because of this unavoidable delay, important data were sometimes omitted in some chapters because they were published during that processing period.

In this last chapter, we, therefore, present a latest update or summary on a few selected, controversial issues in the field that may have been only partly covered in the corresponding chapters.

II. EFFICACY AND SIDE EFFECTS OF LMWH IN PREVENTION OF VENOUS THROMBOEMBOLISM: RESULTS OF META-ANALYSES

Individual studies on prevention of venous thromboembolism following general surgery, orthopedic surgery, and neurosurgery, as well as in immobilized medical patients, were presented and discussed in the respective chapters of this book. Alternatively, meta-analyses allow the systematic, quantitative summary of data from individual studies, which may supply the answers that individual trials

Table 1 Results of Two Meta-analyses (1, 2) of the Use of LMWH for Prevention of Postoperative Venous Thromboembolism

Critical event	No. of patients evaluated		No. of patients with outcome		RR (95% CI)
	LMWH	UFH	LMWH	UFH	
General surgery					
DVT					
Nurmohamed (1)	3467	3411	184	230	0.79 (0.65–0.95)
Leizorovicz (2)	5103	4575	248	267	0.86 (0.72–1.04)
PE					
Nurmohamed	2888	2843	9	20	0.44 (0.21–0.95)
Leizorovicz	4841	4305	12	25	0.62 (0.33–1.15)
Major bleedings					
Nurmohamed	1977	1966	52	51	1.01 (0.70–1.48)
Leizorovicz	5108	4575	649	596	1.02 (0.90–1.16)
Orthopedic surgery					
DVT					
Nurmohamed	672	622	93	132	0.68 (0.54–0.86)
Leizorovicz	1369	1323	224	256	0.83 (0.68–1.02)
PE					
Nurmohamed	590	582	10	24	0.43 (0.22–0.82)
Leizorovicz	1239	1236	17	28	0.53 (0.27–1.03)
Major bleedings					
Nurmohamed	672	622	6	8	0.75 (0.26–2.14)
Leizorovicz	1236	1187	145	143	1.09 (0.76–1.58)

LMWH = low-molecular-weight heparin; UFH = unfractionated heparin; RR = relative risk; 95% CI = 95% confidence interval; DVT = deep venous thrombosis; PE = pulmonary embolism.

cannot because of the increased statistical power afforded by the larger sample size.

Recently two meta-analyses compared subcutaneous low-dose LMWH and unfractionated heparin (UFH) for prevention of postoperative venous thromboembolism (1, 2). The main results of these analyses are presented in Table 1.

Briefly, the data in patients undergoing general surgery show a marginally statistically significant (1) to nonsignificant (2) difference in efficacy of LMWH on the incidence of postoperative deep venous thrombosis (DVT) and pulmonary embolism (PE) as compared with UFH. Both pooled analyses are consistent with a clinically relevant reduction of postoperative thromboembolic risk following general surgery as compared with low-dose UFH. The risk reduction might be as high as 21% for DVT and 56% for PE. In patients who underwent total hip arthroplasty, both meta-analyses (1, 2) agreed on the superiority of LMWH with respect to the incidence of postoperative DVT (risk reduction 17–32%) and PE (risk reduction about 50%). Following both general and orthopedic surgery, the incidence of major bleeding was almost identical for LMWH and UFH (Table 1).

The results of any meta-analysis can be influenced or even flawed by many factors, including publication bias and heterogeneity of the studies pooled. There is one additional concern in the particular case of LMWH, that is, the heterogeneity of the drug. LMWH are distinct compounds that differ from one another in their molecular weight distribution, specific activities (anti-Xa to antithrombin ratio), and plasma clearance. Thus, as emphasized by Verstraete in the Foreword, a meta-analysis of clinical results conducted with different LMWH compounds might not be appropriate. However, it provides some kind of overview and may be very helpful if the pooled results are not immediately used to support one particular drug.

III. COMPARISON OF LMWH FRACTIONS

LMWH fractions have been compared in thromboprophylactic studies with UFH (1, 2), dextran (2), or even placebo (2), but very few data exist regarding the comparison of different dosages of the same LMWH fraction or between different LMWH fractions (Table 2). This issue is crucial because there is no biological marker that reliably correlates with the antithrombotic action of these compounds.

In the frame of a multicenter, double-blind trial, Leizorovicz et al. (3) compared the prophylactic effects of 2500 IU and 3500 IU (both once daily subcutaneously) of Logiparin in medium-to high-risk patients undergoing a general surgical procedure. Abnormal fibrinogen uptake test (FUT) was recorded before the 8th postoperative day in 34/431 (7.9%) (with venographic confirmation

Table 2 Results of Thromboprophylactic Studies Comparing Various Types and Dosages of LMWH Fractions

	LMWH/daily dosage (s.c.)	No. of DVT (%)	*p* level
Leizorovicz (3)			
Regimen I	Logiparin/2500 IU	34/431 (7.9)	
Regimen II	Logiparin/3500 IU	16/430 (3.7)	$p < 0.01$[a]
Bounameaux (4); Wicky (5)			
Regimen I	Dalteparin/2500 IU	30/93 (32.3)	
Regimen II	Nadroparin/3075 IU	15/92 (16.3)	$p = 0.012$[a]
Regimen III	Dalteparin/5000 IU	13/92 (14.1)	$p = 0.006$[a]

[a] Compared with regimen I. DVT diagnosis was based on an abnormal FUT (3) or on venographic findings (4, 5).

in 24/34) in the patients given 2500 IU/day compared with 16/430 (confirmed in 10/16) in those receiving 3500 IU daily. The difference was both statistically significant ($p < 0.01$) and clinically relevant.

In a monocenter, single-blind study with systematic venography on the 8th postoperative day (4), we recently reported an incidence of 30 DVT/93 patients [32.3%, 95% confidence interval (CI): 23–43%] in medium-to high-risk patients given prophylaxis with one daily s.c. injection of 2500 IU of Dalteparin compared with 15/92 (15.3%, 95% CI: 9–25%) in patients given 3075 IU of Nadroparin. Again, the difference was significant ($p = 0.012$) and of potential clinical relevance. A subsequent open trial (5) revealed that increasing the dosage of Dalteparin to 5000 IU daily was associated with a rate of phlebographically proven DVT of 13/92 patients (14.1%, 95% CI: 7–21%), which did not differ from the rate previously observed with 3075 IU of Nadroparin but was significantly ($p = 0.006$) lower than the frequency recorded with 2500 IU of Dalteparin in the previous trial.

The results of these studies point to the facts that (1) dosage (expressed in anti-Xa IU) might not be the sole determinant of the antithrombotic efficacy of LMWHs; (2) double-blind thromboprophylactic studies comparing different dosages and different LMWH fractions are needed; (3) the venographic DVT rate following general surgery may be 3–4 times higher than the rate based on a FUT. The latter issue will be discussed below.

IV. DIAGNOSIS OF POSTOPERATIVE DVT IN THROMBOPROPHYLACTIC TRIALS

Accurate diagnosis of postoperative, mainly asymptomatic, calf vein thrombosis is of great clinical relevance because this end-point is often used as a surrogate end-point for clinically more relevant critical events—clinically manifest DVT and nonfatal or fatal PE. The quantitative relation between asymptomatic DVT and fatal PE during the perioperative period is tentatively shown in Figure 1.

A. Critical Appraisal of the FUT

All thromboprophylactic studies with LMWH fractions that were considered for the meta-analyses (1, 2) of the efficacy and safety of these compounds following general (abdominal) surgery used the FUT for screening of postoperative DVT. Two trials (4, 5) that used systematic venography reported a 3–4 times higher DVT frequency than was anticipated from results of trials using the FUT (1,2). This discrepancy may result (1) from the relatively small sample size of these two studies (about 300 patients) as compared with many thousands in the pooled analyses; (2) from differences in the selection of patients, with more high-risk patients in the two trials using venography as end-point; (3) from a lower sensitiv-

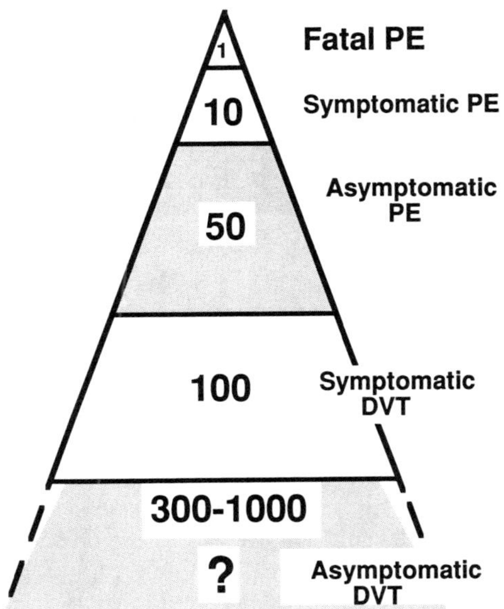

Figure 1 Tentative representation of the quantitative relationship between asymptomatic deep venous thrombosis (DVT), symptomatic DVT, asymptomatic pulmonary embolism (PE), symptomatic nonfatal PE, and fatal PE in the perioperative period.

ity of the FUT compared with venography. Although the first two hypotheses cannot be ruled out with certainty, the latter possibility deserves further comment.

Indeed, most of the postoperative DVTs are asymptomatic, essentially because stasis is less likely to occur in supine subjects, because postoperative DVT usually starts in the below-knee veins, and also because many of them are at least initially nonocclusive. Detection of asymptomatic DVT by screening with FUT (leg scanning) was introduced in the seventies and was subsequently largely used for the evaluation of prophylactic tools in the perioperative period (6). Initial studies reported a high accuracy of FUT to detect calf vein thrombosis. These studies had a poor methodology, and recent trials have challenged their results by demonstrating a rather low sensitivity of the FUT for the presence of calf vein thrombosis in patients who underwent total hip replacement, which might be extended to the situation in general abdominal surgery. A careful reassessment of the performances of the FUT from the available literature (6) revealed that this method is globally insensitive for screening of postoperative DVT following orthopedic surgery. The review article also pointed to the insufficiency of the existing data regarding its use in general surgical patients. In fact, only two studies with a total of 183 patients assessed the performances of the

FUT in this kind of patient. The reported 100% sensitivity of the method to the presence of calf vein thrombosis was based on a subgroup of eight (!) patients, whereas the overall sensitivity of 93% to all DVTs was derived from 40 accurately detected cases among 43 patients (6). Beside its poor accuracy, the FUT also carries a potential risk of transmission of viral particles via the blood-donor-derived fibrinogen. Thus, even ethical arguments strongly discourage its use as a screening tool in clinical trials.

B. Ultrasound Imaging of the Leg Veins

With an accuracy of over 95% for proximal vein thrombosis, B-mode real-time ultrasound (US) alone or in combination with pulsed doppler (Duplex), with or without color coding, is progressively replacing the other diagnostic tools in patients clinically suspected of having DVT (7). It was therefore tempting to use these techniques for the surveillance of asymptomatic postoperative high-risk patients. The results of venographically controlled studies (8–10), however, did not confirm the initial hopes (Table 3). The sensitivity of US to the presence of venographically diagnosed proximal vein thrombosis following high-risk orthopedic surgery ranged from 38% to 57%, which is disappointingly low and precludes the use of these methods for postoperative screening in thromboprophylactic trials.

C. Systematic Ascending Venography

There is thus a consensus as to the need to use bilateral ascending venography for screening of postoperative DVT in thromboprophylactic studies following hip surgery (11). After general abdominal surgery, looking for alternative tools like liquid crystal contact thermography or plasma measurement of D-dimer, a fibrin-specific derivative, was rather disappointing (12), although the negative predictive value of a D-dimer plasma concentration of less than 3000 μg/L on the 8th postoperative day was as high as 93%. Thus, venography—possibly only in patients with a D-dimer plasma level above the cutoff of 3000 μg/L—might be the sole diagnostic tool also after general surgery (4). Moreover, since this technique is likely to reveal higher frequencies of postoperative DVT than the FUT, the fear of using an invasive method as a screening tool might be obviated by the advantage of diagnosing asymptomatic DVT in a substantial proportion of postoperative patients, thereby allowing early treatment.

However, using venography as a screening method for postoperative DVT does not solve all problems. The interobserver variability of interpretation of 185 venograms that were obtained in such a thromboprophylactic study was recently assessed (13). Blinded films were submitted to three experts from different centers, and their diagnoses were compared with one another and with the initial evaluation during the study. Despite a prevalence of DVT of 24% in the

Table 3 Accuracy of Ultrasound With and Without Color Doppler in the Detection of DVT Following Hip or Knee Replacement as Compared with Venography

Ref.	No. limbs	No. DVT	No. prox	Method	Sv (%)	Sp (%)	PPV (%)	NPV (%)
Mattos (8)	190	44	3	Color	55	98	89	88
Agnelli (9)	187	49	21	US	25	99	92	79
					57[a]	99[a]	93[a]	95[a]
Davidson (10)	319	80	21	Color	20			
					38[a]	92[a]	26[a]	95[a]

[a] For proximal DVT

prox = proximal vein thrombosis; US = B-mode real-time ultrasound; color = color-coded duplex examination; Sv = sensitivity; Sp = specificity; PPV = positive predictive value; NPV = negative predictive value.

population studied, apparent pairwise agreement between the four readings ranged from 87 to 93% with corresponding "true" coefficients of agreement kappa of 0.63–0.74. This considerable degree of disagreement among experienced readers should be taken into account in calculating sample sizes in prospective thromboprophylactic studies. Indeed, one of the two prophylactic regimens proved to be significantly ($p = 0.012, p = 0.031, p = 0.043$) or nonsignificantly ($p = 0.073$) superior to the other one, depending on the reader (13), which, however, does not affect the clinical relevance of the data in the particular trial.

V. DURATION OF POSTOPERATIVE THROMBOEMBOLISM PROPHYLAXIS

Systematic perioperative prophylaxis with low-dose UFH reduced the incidence of DVT following surgery by about two-thirds (14, 15), a figure that is probably further improved when LMWH fractions are used instead of UFH (1, 2). These figures concern in-hospital incidences of postoperative thromboembolism. While prophylactic regimens are usually stopped at discharge, it has been suggested that the risk of developing thromboembolic events after surgery might extend beyond the hospital stay. Table 4 summarizes the data from five trials that addressed this important issue. The proportion of afterdischarge events to the total number of postoperative thromboembolic events ranges in these series from 3% to 68% (16–20). The extreme values both originate from small studies. The two largest trials, which studied 19,061 patients and 3809 patients, respectively, report figures of 23% (16) and 38% (20), respectively, which is far from negligible. Indeed, assuming a 25% proportion of afterdischarge events among all symptomatic postoperative PEs (not prevented by heparin prophylaxis) and a

Table 4 Frequency of Postoperative Venous Thromboembolism Occurring After Discharge from Hospital

Ref.	No. of patients	VTE ratio (in-hospital/ afterdischarge)	Afterdischarge events (%)	End-point
Huber (16)	19,161	80/24	23	Symptomatic PE
Scurr (17)	57	6/13	68	FUT-DVT
Clarke-Pearson (18)	281	12/10	45	FUT-DVT
Clarke-Pearson (19)	382	61/2	3	FUT-DVT
Kakkar (20)	3,809	41/25	38	Symptomatic VTE

FUT = fibrinogen uptake test; DVT = deep venous thrombosis; PE = pulmonary embolism; VTE = venous thromboembolism

66% efficacy of the prophylaxis, the overall proportion of afterdischarge PEs among all (prevented and unprevented) postoperative symptomatic PEs will be about 10%. Although Kakkar et al. (20) conclude that the risk is too low to justify prolonged prophylaxis following hospital discharge, we feel that a placebo-controlled, randomized trial during the 4 weeks following discharge from hospital, or at least a careful cost-benefit analysis, should be performed to assess the potential need of prolonged prophylaxis. Such an analysis seems appropriate at a time when postoperative hospital stay tends to be reduced and ambulatory surgery becomes more and more popular. This trend should not obscure the fact that "afterdischarge period" does not necessarily mean "ambulatory period": many convalescent patients, albeit early discharged, may remain confined to bed at home, thereby promoting delayed thromboembolism.

VI. EFFICACY AND SIDE EFFECTS OF LMWH IN THERAPY OF VENOUS THROMBOEMBOLISM

In Chapter 15, Lockner reviewed the present state of the use of LMWH fractions for treatment of established DVT and concluded that these compounds applied subcutaneously are at least as effective and safe as unfractionated heparin given as continuous i.v. infusion. In a pooled analysis of the two therapeutic trials with clinically relevant end-points (21, 22), Lensing et al. (23) suggested that LMWHs are associated with a statistically significant ($p = 0.015$) and clinically relevant reduction of the risk of thromboembolic recurrence (odds ratio 0.38, 95% CI: 0.20–0.85). The main additional advantages of the novel regimens are (1) the s.c. application, which allows a higher mobility of the patient, and (2) the absence of laboratory controls of the anticoagulant effect since the LMWHs are given according to body weight.

Unresolved issues include (1) the possibility of applying the daily dosage in one instead of two injections of the drug; (2) the possibility of treating proximal vein thrombosis in an ambulatory setting; (3) the possibility of treating patients with symptomatic pulmonary embolism. The two last issues deserve to be addressed in specific clinical trials. Outpatient treatment of proximal vein thrombosis with LMWH is presently being tested in large-scale studies in the Netherlands and in France. Preliminary data regarding the use of LMWH in patients with established nonmassive pulmonary embolism (24) are already available from a dose-ranging study that showed that daily doses of 240 IU/kg and 320 IU/kg of nadroparin are associated with an unacceptably high rate of major bleedings (5/26 and 4/7, respectively). At day 8, the improvement of the pulmonary vascular obstruction and the frequency of major bleedings were similar in the group of patients given 150 IU/kg/day ($n = 35$) (in two s.c. applications) of nadroparin and in the group of patients treated with continuous i.v. UFH ($n = 33$). These data need to be confirmed in larger trials.

With respect to the reduction of the number of s.c. applications of the LMWH compounds (two applications in most trials) to one single daily administration, one large-scale, double-blind trial (22) clearly showed that a single s.c. administration of logiparin (175 IU/kg/24hr) is superior to continuous i.v. UFH for treatment of proximal vein thrombosis. Six recurrent thromboembolic events were recorded among the 213 patients given the LMWH while 15 events occurred among the 219 patients given UFH ($p = 0.07$). Major bleedings occurred in 0.5% and 5%, respectively, in the two groups ($p = 0.006$). In a smaller trial, Holmström et al (25) concluded that a total daily dosage of 200 IU/kg of dalteparin had a similar efficacy and tolerance when it was given in one or two s.c. administrations. However, the trial included only 101 patients in total and the end-point, the improvement of the venographic Marder score after 5–7 days, is of limited clinical relevance. A large-scale, double-blind trial comparing one versus two injections (same daily dosage) of nadroparin was started in April 1993 in 50 European centers. It is planned to study 650 patients with proximal vein thrombosis over a period of 18 months. Establishing the efficacy of the once-daily regimens for treatment of proximal DVT is crucial if outpatient treatment of this condition is to be widespread in the future.

VII. LMWH, MORTALITY, AND CANCER

In the two largest studies of the use of LMWH fractions for treatment of established DVT (21, 22), mortality rates were lower in patients randomized to LMWH. It has been suggested that this could be due to a decreased cancer-related mortality in this group. Green et al. (26) calculated that cancer deaths from the two studies were 21/67 (31%) for UFH and 7/62 (11%) for LMWH ($p = 0.005$) with a 95% CI for odds ratio of 1.4–9.2. Since fatal thrombotic and hemorrhagic events occurred with a similar frequency in both groups, the difference in mortality cannot be ascribed to the hemostatic properties of the compounds. Although an unbalanced assignment of patients with more advanced tumors in the UFH group cannot be absolutely excluded, this hypothesis is unlikely, since the number of patients with tumor who were randomly allocated in the two treatment groups was substantial ($n = 129$). LMWH might exert an antitumor effect via different mechanisms, including inhibition of proliferation of smooth muscle cells and inhibition of angiogenesis (26). Although these data are preliminary, they certainly justify careful assessment as to whether LMWHs should be studied as potential antineoplastic agents.

VIII. WILL (SHOULD) LMWH REPLACE UFH?

UFH is used not only for prevention and treatment of venous thromboembolism, but also for treatment of established acute arterial thromboembolic events, such as acute myocardial infarction, alone or in conjunction with a thrombolytic agent, acute cerobravascular accident, and acute obstruction of a peripheral artery. At present, there are no convincing data about the use of LMWH fractions in these various indications. Thus, clinical studies are urgently needed to assess the potential place of LMWHs in these arterial indications before the ''old'' UFH can be generally replaced by the novel compounds.

IX. CONCLUDING REMARKS

In his remarkable Foreword, Marc Verstraete addressed a long series of questions he hoped to find answers for in this book. He may be only partly satisfied. This final chapter aimed at suggesting some clues to some of the issues he addressed. There is still some work to be done regarding both basic mechanisms and clinical problems. As usual in such situations an attempt to summarize the present state of knowledge also revealed a large field of ignorance. We hope that this recognition will stimulate further research in the field.

REFERENCES

1. Nurmohamed MT, Rosendaal FR, Büller HR, et al. Low-molecular-weight heparin versus standard heparin in general and orthopedic surgery: a meta-analysis. Lancet 1992; 340:152–156.
2. Leizorovicz A, Haugh MC, Chapuis FR, Samama MM, Boissel JP. Low molecular weight heparin in prevention of perioperative thrombosis. Br Med J 1992; 305:913–920.
3. Leizorovicz A, Picolet H, Peyrieux JC, Boissel JP, and the HBPM Research Group. Prevention of perioperative deep vein thrombosis in general surgery: a multicentre

double blind study comparing two doses of Logiparin and standard heparin. Br J Surg 1991; 78:412–416.

4. Bounameaux H, Huber O, Khabiri E, Schneider PA, Didier D, Rohner A. Unexpectedly high rate of phlebographic deep venous thrombosis following elective general abdominal surgery among patients given prophylaxis with low-molecular-weight heparin. Arch Surg 1993; 128:326–328.
5. Wicky J, Couson F, Ambrosetti P, Didier D, Rohner A, Bounameaux H. Postoperative deep venous thrombosis (DVT) and low-molecular-weight heparin (LMWH) type and dosage. Thromb Haemost 1993; 69:402–403.
6. Lensing AWA, Hirsh J. 125I-Fibrinogen leg scanning: reassessment of its role for the diagnosis of venous thrombosis in post-operative patients. Thromb Haemost 1993; 69:2–7.
7. Becker DM, Philbrick JT, Abbitt PL. Real-time ultrasonography for the diagnosis of lower extremity deep venous thrombosis. The wave of the future? Arch Intern Med 1989; 149:1731–1734.
8. Mattos MA, Londrey GL, Leutz DW, Hodgson KJ, Ramsey DE, Barkmeier LD, Stauffer ES, Spadone DP, Summer DS. Color-flow duplex scanning for the surveillance and diagnosis of acute deep venous thrombosis. J Vasc Surg 1992; 15:366–376.
9. Agnelli G, Volpato R, Radicchia S, Veschi F, Di Filippo P, Lupatelli L, Nenci GG. Detection of asymptomatic deep vein thrombosis by real-time B-mode ultrasonography in hip surgery patients. Thromb Haemost 1992; 68:257–260.
10. Davidson BL, Eliott CG, Lensing AWA, for the RD Heparin Arthroplasty Group. Low accuracy of colour doppler ultrasound in the detection of proximal leg vein thrombosis in asymptomatic high-risk patients. Ann Intern Med 1992; 117:735–738.
11. Büller HR, Lensing AWA, Hirsh J, ten Cate JW. Deep vein thrombosis: new non-invasive diagnostic tests. Thromb Haemost 1991; 66:133–137.
12. Bounameaux H, Khabiri E, Huber O, Schneider PA, Didier D, de Moerloose P, Reber G. Value of liquid crystal contact thermography and plasma level of D-dimer for screening of deep venous thrombosis following general abdominal surgery. Thromb Haemost 1992; 67:603–606.
13. Couson F, Bounameaux C, Didier D, Geiser D, Meyerovitz MF, Schmitt HE, Schneider PA, Bounameaux H. Influence of variability of interpretation of contrast venography for screening of postoperative deep venous thrombosis on the results of a thromboprophylactic study. Thromb Haemost 1993 (in press).
14. Clagett GP, Reisch JS. Prevention of venous thromboembolism in general surgical patients. Ann Surg 1988; 208:227–240.
15. Collins R, Scrimgeour A, Yusif S, Peto R. Reduction in fatal pulmonary embolism and venous thrombosis by perioperative administration of subcutaneous heparin: overview of results of randomized trials in general, orthopedic, and urologic surgery. N Engl J Med 1988; 318:1162–1173.
16. Huber O, Bounameaux H, Borst F, Rohner A. Postoperative pulmonary embolism after hospital discharge. An underestimated risk. Arch Surg 1992; 127:310–313.
17. Scurr JH, Coleridge-Smith PD, Hasty JH. Deep venous thrombosis: a continuing problem. Br Med J 1988; 297:28.
18. Clarke-Pearson DL, Jelovsek FR, Creasman WT. Thromboembolism complicating

surgery for cervical and uterine malignancy: incidence, risk factors, and prophylaxis. Obstet Gynecol 1983; 61:87–94.

19. Clarke-Pearson DL, Synan IS, Coleman RE, Hinshaw W, Creasman WT. The natural history of postoperative thromboemboli in gynecologic oncology: a prospective study of 382 patients. Am J Obstet Gynecol 1984; 148:1051–1054.
20. Kakkar VV, Cohen AT, Edmonson RA, Phillips MJ, Cooper DJ, Das SK, Maher KT, Sanderson RM, Ward VP, Kakkar S, on behalf of the thromboprophylaxis Collaborative Group. Low molecular weight versus standard heparin for prevention of venous thromboembolism after major abdominal surgery. Lancet 1993; 341:259–265.
21. Prandoni P, Lensing AW, Büller HR, Carta M, Cogo A, Vigo M, Casara D, Ruol A, ten Cate JW. Comparison of subcutaneous low-molecular weight heparin with intravenous standard heparin in proximal deep-vein thrombosis. Lancet 1992; 339:441–445.
22. Hull RD, Raskob GE, Pineo GF, Green D, Trowbridge AA, Elliott G, Lerner RG, Hall J, Sparling T, Brettell HR, Norton J, Carter CJ, George R, Merli G, Ward J, Mayo W, Rosenbloom D, Brant R. Subcutaneous low-molecular-weight heparin compared with continuous intravenous heparin in the treatment of proximal-vein thrombosis. N Engl J Med 1992; 326:975–982.
23. Lensing AWA, Prins M, Koopman MMW, Büller HR. Which heparin for proximal vein thrombosis? Lancet 1992; 340:311–312.
24. Théry C, Simonneau G, Meyer G, Hélénon O, Bridey F, Armagnac C, d'Azemar P, Coquart JP. Randomized trial of subcutaneous low-molecular-weight heparin CY 216 (Fraxiparine) compared with intravenous unfractionated heparin in the curative treatment of submassive pulmonary embolism. A dose-ranging study. Circulation 1992; 85:1380–1389.
25. Holmström, Berglund MC, Granqvist S, Bratt G, Törneböhm E, Lockner D. Fragmin once or twice daily subcutaneously in the treatment of deep venous thrombosis of the leg. Thromb Res 1992; 67:49–55.
26. Green D, Hull RD, Brant R, Pineo GF. Lower mortality in cancer patients treated with low-molecular-weight versus standard heparin. Lancet 1992; 339:1476.

Index

ACE-inhibitors, 276
α_2-antiplasmin, 147
Alteplase, 159
Ancrod, 100
Anesthesia, 242
Angioplasty (*see* PTCA)
Anti-factor Xa activity (*see also* Monitoring of LMWH), 11, 39, 300
  amidolytic assays, 46
  clotting assays, 45
Antithrombin activity, 49
Antithrombin III, 131
  concentrates, 101
Aprotinin, 156
APSAC, 147
APTT (*see also* Monitoring of LMWH), 11, 12, 35, 45, 300
Argatroban, 156
Aspirin, 101

Bernard-Soulier syndrome, 98
β-thromboglobuline (β-TG), 254
Bioavailability, 11
Bleeding under LMWH
  and anti-Xa level, 177
  in general surgery, 176, 307
  in hemodialysis, 254
  and lumbar anesthesia, 243
  in orthopedic surgery, 192, 307
  during treatment of DVT, 299
Bleeding time, 82

Calcium, 37
Cancer, 130, 299, 315
Calf vein thrombosis, asymptomatic, 64
Cardiopulmonary bypass surgery, 263
Chain length material (CLM), 23
Chondroitin sulfate, 91, 130
Chronic venous insufficiency, 69, 176
Clearance, 10, 13
Cost-effectiveness, 69, 302
CY 222 (*see* LMWH, brands)

DDAVP, 157
D-Dimer, 52

Deep venous thrombosis (DVT) (*see also* Prophylaxis of DVT and Treatment of DVT)
  asymptomatic, 59, 311
  diagnosis of, 55, 189, 310
  epidemiology of, 55, 187
  following orthopedic surgery, 189
  pathogenesis, 213, 225
  prophylaxis of, 3, 6, 69
  proximal, 205
  symptomatic, 59
  thrombolysis in, 62
Dermatan sulfate (*see also* Glycosaminoglycans), 28, 30, 75, 81
DIC (Disseminated intravascular coagulation), 94
Dihydroergotamine (DHE), 218
Dose-effect relationship, 21
Dose regimens, 179
  in general surgery, 179
  in hemodialysis, 254
  in orthopedic surgery, 190
  weight-adjusted, 43, 208
Duteplase, 160

Elderly, 226
Endothelial cells, 129
  and binding of heparins, 132
  and fibrinolysis, 150
  proliferation of, 138
  and t-PA/PAI secretion, 153
Enoxaparin (*see* LMWH, brands)
ϵ-aminocaproic acid, 156
Euglobulin lysis time, 157
Extracorporeal circulation, 6, 247

Factor VIII, 30
Factor V, 30
Factor Xa, 7, 27
Factor XIII, 147
Fibrin, 149
Fibrinolysis (*see also* Thrombolysis), 143
Fibrinopeptide A, 2, 6, 52, 188, 254
Fibroblast growth factors, 133
Fragmin (*see* LMWH, brands)
Fraxiparine (*see* LMWH, brands)
Free fatty acids, 248
FUT (fibrinogen uptake test), 170, 189, 213, 310

GAG (*see* Glycosaminoglycans)
GISSI-2, 160
Glycoproteins, 78, 79
Glycosaminoglycans (*see also* Dermatan sulfate), 129
  and antithrombin III, 130
Glycosyl-phosphatidyl-inositol, 139
GUSTO, 160

Hemiplegia, 225
Hemodialysis, 6, 248
  in children, 258
Hemofiltration, 248
Hemorrhage (*see* Bleeding time and Bleeding under LMWH)
Heparan sulfate (*see also* Glycosaminoglycans), 75, 81
Heparin
  anticoagulant effect of, 28
  antithrombotic effect of, 28, 50
  binding to endothelial cells, 132
  and bleeding time, 82
  and cell growth, 137
  and cell migration, 137
  chemistry, 23
  dosage of (*see also* Dose regimens), 65
  and fibrinolysis, 151

Heparin (*cont.*)
  low-dose, 70, 216
  monitoring, 35, 43, 50
  pharmacokinetics, 136
  and plasminogen activation, 151
  and platelets (*see also* HIT), 78
    immune activation, 84
    nonimmune activation, 81
  resistance to, 94
  and thrombolysis, 154, 157, 159
  units, 11, 22, 34, 37, 39, 51
Heparin cofactor II, 27, 153
Heptest, 45
High-affinity material (HAM), 23, 37
Hip fracture, 200
Histidin-rich glycoprotein (HRG), 25, 27, 78, 153
HIT (heparin-induced thrombocytopenia)
  antiplatelet therapy in, 101
  clinical features, 89
  definition, 85
  diagnosis, 98
  dose dependence of, 91
  epidemiology, 86, 177
  and Fc receptor, 96
  pathogenesis, 95
  and preparations of heparin, 87
  prevention of, 103, 105
  reexposition to heparin in, 103
  treatment, 99, 263

Iloprost, 101
Immunoglobulins, intravenous high-dose, 101
INR (international normalized ratio), 65
International standards for heparins, 48
ISIS-3, 160

Laboratory control (*see* Monitoring of LMWH)
Left ventricular thrombus, 232
Lipoprotein A, 149
Lipoproteinlipase, 29, 248
Liver enzymes, 179
Logiparin (*see* LMWH, brands)
LMWH (*see also* Prophylaxis of DVT and Treatment of DVT)
  and affinity for endothelial cells, 134
  and cancer, 315
  mechanism of action, 7, 27
  and mortality, 315
  and lumbar anesthesia, 243
  bioavailability of, 12
  brands
    comparison of, 309
    CY 222, 255
    Enoxaparin (PK 10169), 5, 50, 134, 193, 227, 259, 266
    Fragmin (K 2165, dalteparin), 50, 193, 231, 260, 277
    Fraxiparine (CY 216, nadroparin), 52, 134, 208, 227, 231, 257, 266
    Logiparin (tilziparin), 52, 193, 229
    Organ (ORG 10172, lomoparan), 5, 79, 101, 193, 219, 262
    Sandoparin, 232
  therapeutic range, 51
Low-affinity material (LAM), 23
Low-molecular-weight heparins (*see* LMWH)
Lumbar anesthesia, 241
Lumbar puncture, 244

Mast cells, 129
Molecular weight, 10, 23

Monitoring of LMWH, 43, 210, 237
 in treatment of DVT, 300
Multidisciplinary approach to DVT, 71
Myocardial infarction, 159

Neutralization of LMWH, 181

Oral anticoagulation
 and cancer, 67
 control, 65
 and lactation, 66
 and pregnancy, 66
 and prophylaxis of DVT, 71
Orgaran (*see* LMWH, brands)
Outpatients, prophylaxis in, 208

PAI (*see* Plasminogen activators inhibitors)
Paraplegia, 225
Pentasaccharide, 10, 28, 36
Pentosan polysulfate, 80, 83, 91
PF4 (platelet factor 4), 24, 27, 78, 140, 254
 and ACLM neutralization, 35
 and diagnosis of HIT, 97
Pharmacodynamics, 10, 38
Pharmacokinetics, 11, 38
Phlebography (*see* Venography)
Plasmapheresis, 101
Plasmin, 144, 146
Plasminogen, 143
Plasminogen activators, 143
 inhibitors, 143, 148
Prophylaxis of DVT
 duration of, 181, 313
 in general surgery, 169
 after hip fracture, 200
 in knee surgery, 201
 mechanical, 69, 214, 217
Prophylaxis of DVT (*cont.*)
 in medical patients, 225
 meta-analyses of studies on, 307
 in myocardial infarction, 232
 in neurosurgery, 213
 in orthopedic surgery, 187
 under plaster cast, 208
 by regional anesthesia, 242
 after spinal cord trauma, 216
 in stroke patients, 218
Prostacyclin, 82
Protamine (*see* Neutralization of LMWH)
Protein C, 31, 65
Proteoglycans, 130, 136
Prothrombin, 4
 activation of, 8, 13, 32
Prothrombinase, 2, 7, 13, 31
Prothrombin fragment 1 + 2 (F_{1+2}), 2, 4, 52
Proximal DVT, selective prophylaxis of, 205
Pseudothrombocytopenia, 80
PTCA
 reocclusion after, 273
 restenosis after, 277, 293
Pulmonary embolism, 55
 prevention of, 176
 treatment with LMWH, 293

Renal insufficiency, 10, 266
Reocclusion (*see* PTCA)
Restenosis (*see* PTCA)

ScuPA, 150
^{14}C-Serotonin release, 85, 98
Serpins, 148
Skin necrosis, 93
Spinal cord injury, 230
Streptokinase, 63, 147, 160

Thrombin, 2, 7, 35
generation, 30
potential, 35, 44, 51
Thrombin-antithrombin III complexes, 2, 6, 53, 188, 254
Thrombolysis, 62, 144, 154, 157
Thrombosis, pathogenesis in hip surgery, 188
Thrombocytopenia (*see* HIT)
Tissue factor pathway inhibitor (TFPI), 29, 45
Tissue-type plasminogen activator (t-PA), 62, 146
Transforming growth factor β, 140
Treatment of DVT
with LMWH, 282, 314
with UFH, 64

UFH (*see* Heparin)
Ultrasonography, 59, 312
Urokinase, 63, 146

Vena caval interruption, 67
Venography, 59, 189, 312
indication to, 59
and thrombolysis, 62
Venous occlusion test, 157
Vitronectin, 25, 27, 78
von Willebrand factor, 78

Warfarin, 65
White clot syndrome (*see also* HIT), 92

About the Editor

HENRI BOUNAMEAUX is Chief of the Division of Angiology and Hemostasis in the Department of Medicine at the University Hospital of Geneva and Privat-Docent at the University of Geneva School of Medicine, Switzerland. The author or coauthor of over 200 original journal articles, literature reviews, book chapters and abstracts, Dr. Bounameaux is a Fellow of the International Society on Thrombosis and Hemostasis, the International Society on Fibrinolysis and Thrombolysis, and the International Union of Angiology, among others, and a President of the Swiss Society of Angiology (1993–1994). The recipient of the Karl-Rohr Award of the Swiss Society of Hematology (1991) and the Swiss Angiology Award (1991), he received the M.D. degree (1978) from Basel University School of Medicine, Switzerland.